WITHDRAWN

Date Due

Anger and Hostility in Cardiovascular and Behavioral Disorders

The Series in Health Psychology and Behavioral Medicine

Charles D. Spielberger, *Editor-in-Chief*

Chesney, Rosenman Anger and Hostility in Cardiovascular and Behavioral Disorders
Lonetto, Templer Death Anxiety
Morgan, Goldston Exercise and Mental Health

IN PREPARATION

Elias, Marshall Cardiovascular Disease and Behavior
Hobfoll Ecology of Stress
Pancheri, Zichelli Biorhythms and Stress in the Physiopathology of Reproduction

Anger and Hostility in Cardiovascular and Behavioral Disorders

Edited by

Margaret A. Chesney, Ph.D.
Ray H. Rosenman, M.D.
SRI International
Menlo Park, California

● HEMISPHERE PUBLISHING CORPORATION, Washington
A subsidiary of Harper & Row, Publishers, Inc.

Cambridge   New York   Philadelphia   San Francisco
London   Mexico City São Paulo   Singapore   Sydney

ANGER AND HOSTILITY IN CARDIOVASCULAR AND BEHAVIORAL DISORDERS

Copyright © 1985 by Hemisphere Publishing Corporation. All rights reserved. Printed in the United States of America. Except as permitted under the United States Copyright Act of 1976, no part of this publication may be reproduced or distributed in any form or by any means, or stored in a data base or retrieval system, without the prior written permission of the publisher.

3 4 5 6 7 8 9 0   E B E B   8 9 8 7 6

This book was set in Press Roman by Hemisphere Publishing Corporation. The editors were Christine Flint and Susan Dittbrenner; the production supervisor was Miriam Gonzalez; and the typesetter was Shirley J. McNett. Edwards Brothers, Inc., was printer and binder.

Library of Congress Cataloging in Publication Data

Main entry under title:

Anger and hostility in cardiovascular and behavioral disorders.

  (The Series in health psychology and behavioral medicine)
  Based on the proceedings of a research planning workshop entitled: Prevention research on the assessment, health correlates, and treatment of disabling anger, held January 1983 in Menlo Park, Calif.
  Includes bibliographies and index.
  1. Cardiovascular system—Diseases—Psychosomatic aspects—Congresses. 2. Cardiovascular system—Diseases—Psychological aspects—Congresses. 3. Hostility (Psychology)—Congresses.
4. Anger—Congresses. I. Chesney, Margaret A. II. Rosenman, Ray H. date. III. Title: Prevention research on the assessment, health correlates, and treatment of disabling anger. [DNLM:
1. Anger—congresses. 2. Behavioral Medicine—congresses.
3. Cardiovascular Diseases—etiology—congresses. 4. Cardiovascular Diseases—prevention & control—congresses. 5. Hostility—congresses.
WG 100 A587 1983]
RC669.A54   1985   616.1'08   84-25348
ISBN 0-89116-393-X
ISSN 8756-467X

Contents

Contributors		*ix*
Foreword		*xi*
Preface		*xiii*

I
DEFINITIONS AND ASSESSMENT

1 **The Experience and Expression of Anger: Construction and Validation of an Anger Expression Scale** 5
Charles D. Spielberger, Ernest H. Johnson, Stephen F. Russell, Rosario J. Crane, Gerard A. Jacobs, and Timothy J. Worden

Anger, Hostility, and Aggression: The AHA! Syndrome	7
The Expression of Anger	11
Development and Validation of the Anger Expression (AX) Scale	14
Conclusions	28
References	28

2 **The Dynamics of Aggression and Their Application to Cardiovascular Disorders** 31
Edwin I. Megargee

Overview	32
The Algebra of Aggression	33
Instigation to Aggression	36
Habit Strength	42
Inhibitions against Aggression	45
Situational Factors	49
Response Competition	52
Implications of the Dynamics of Aggression for Research on Cardiovascular Disorders	52
References	55

3 **The Measurement of Anger as a Multidimensional Construct** 59
Judith M. Siegel

Scale Development	64
Responses to the Multidimensional Anger Inventory (MAI)	67
References	76
Appendix 1	78
Appendix 2	80

	Appendix 3	80
	Appendix 4	81
4	**A Microsocial Analysis of Anger and Irritable Behavior** *G. R. Patterson*	83
	A Social Interaction Perspective	86
	Microsocial Analyses: Search for a Mother-Child Pattern	88
	Negative Attributions, Affect, and Anger	92
	Negative Affect and Aggressive Behavior	95
	Discussion	96
	References	98

II
HEALTH CONSEQUENCES

5	**Health Consequences of Anger and Implications for Treatment** *Ray H. Rosenman*	103
	Some Relationships of Anger Dimensions with Blood Pressure and Cardiovascular Responsiveness	103
	Relationships of Stressors to Neurohormonal Responses and Blood Pressure	104
	Relationships of Type A Hostility and Anger Dimensions to CHD	107
	Genetic, Evolutionary, and Environmental Factors in Hostility and Anger Dimensions	111
	Sex Differences in Aggressiveness, Anger Dimensions, and Cardiovascular Responsiveness	114
	Some Relationships of Emotions to CNS Receptors	116
	Implications for Therapeutic Approaches	117
	References	119
6	**Suppressed Anger in Hypertension: Facts and Problems** *Stevo Julius, Robert Schneider, and Brent Egan*	127
	Hemodynamic and Pharmacologic Evidence	127
	Psychobehavioral Evidence	130
	Does Abnormal Behavior Lead to Neurogenic Hypertension?	132
	References	135
7	**Relationship of Anger-Coping Styles and Blood Pressure among Black Americans** *W. Doyle Gentry*	139
	Suppressed Anger and Hypertension	139
	Suppressed Anger among Black Americans	141
	Suppressed Anger and Hypertension in Black Americans	142
	Future Research Issues	144
	References	145
	Reference Notes	147

8 Behavioral Factors in Hypertension: Cardiovascular Responsivity, Anger, and Social Competence 149
Stephen B. Manuck, Randall L. Morrison, Alan S. Bellack, and Joanna M. Polefrone

Personality Factors in Hypertension 150
Hypertension, Familial Risk for Hypertension, and Behaviorally-Induced Cardiovascular Reactivity 153
A Model of Idiosyncratic Cardiovascular Reactivity 157
Hypertension and Social Competence 162
References 167
Reference Notes 172

9 The Health Consequences of Hostility 173
Redford B. Williams, Jr., John C. Barefoot, and Richard B. Shekelle

Health Correlates of Hostility 174
Hostility: Pathophysiological Mechanisms 181
References 184
Reference Notes 185

10 An Animal Model of Coronary-Prone Behavior 187
Stephen B. Manuck, Jay R. Kaplan, and Thomas B. Clarkson

Experimental Procedures 189
Behavioral Observations 190
Pathologic Observations 191
Individual Differences in Cardiac Responsivity to Stress 193
Concluding Comments 195
References 195

III
INTERVENTIONS

11 Anger and Its Therapeutic Regulation 203
Raymond W. Novaco

Factors Curtailing Research on Anger/Aggression Modification 204
Anger and Aggression 208
Research on the Modification of Anger and Aggression 214
Overview of Intervention Studies and Prevailing Issues 221
References 222

12 On the Diagnosis and Treatment of Chronically Hostile Individuals 227
Michael H. L. Hecker and Donald T. Lunde

Typology of Chronic Hostility 229
Goals and Methods of Treatment 234
References 239

13 A Social Interactional Approach to Child Abuse: Risk, Prevention, and Treatment 241
John B. Reid and Kate Kavanagh

Prevalence of Abuse and Physical Coercion of Children by Their Parents	241
Factors Associated with Abuse: A Conceptual Framework	242
Implications for the Treatment/Prevention of Child Abuse	243
Treatment of Child Abuse	244
Systematic Parent Training for Abusive Families	245
General Implications	254
References	255

14 The Possible Effects of Beta-Adrenergic Blocking Drugs on Behavioral and Psychological Concomitants of Anger 259
Lynn A. Durel and David S. Krantz

Evidence that Peripheral Sympathetic Responses Can Influence Anger and Aggression	260
Assessment of Type A Behavior: Dissecting Attitudinal and Stylistic Components	261
Physiological Correlates of Type A Behavior	262
Behavioral Effects of Beta-Blockers: Peripheral Views of Emotion Revisited	267
Central versus Peripheral Actions of Beta-Blockers: Issues and Cautions	270
Further Evidence for Effects of Adrenergic Blockers on Anger and Aggression	271
Concluding Comments	272
Summary	273
References	273

15 Anger and Hostility: Future Implications for Behavioral Medicine 277
Margaret A. Chesney

Anger: Defining the Target Behavior	277
Behavioral Assessment of Anger	278
Intervention	283
Conclusion	287
References	288
Reference Note	290

Index 291

Contributors

John C. Barefoot   Duke University Medical Center, Durham, North Carolina
Alan S. Bellack   The Medical College of Pennsylvania, Philadelphia
Margaret A. Chesney   SRI International, Menlo Park, California
Thomas B. Clarkson   Wake Forest University, Winston-Salem, North Carolina
Rosario J. Crane   University of South Florida, Tampa
Lynn A. Durel   Uniformed Services, University of the Health Sciences, Bethesda, Maryland
Brent Egan   University of Michigan Medical School, Ann Arbor
W. Doyle Gentry   University of Virginia, Charlottesville
Michael H. L. Hecker   SRI International, Menlo Park, California
Gerard A. Jacobs   University of South Florida, Tampa
Ernest H. Johnson   University of South Florida, Tampa
Stevo Julius   University of Michigan Medical School, Ann Arbor
Jay R. Kaplan   Wake Forest University, Winston-Salem, North Carolina
Kate Kavanagh   Oregon Social Learning Center, Eugene
David S. Krantz   Uniformed Services, University of the Health Sciences, Bethesda, Maryland
Donald T. Lunde   Stanford University Medical Center, Palo Alto, California
Stephen B. Manuck   University of Pittsburgh, Pennsylvania
Edwin I. Megargee   Florida State University, Tallahassee
Randall L. Morrison   The Medical College of Pennsylvania, Philadelphia
Raymond W. Novaco   University of California, Irvine
G. R. Patterson   Oregon Social Learning Center, Eugene
Joanna M. Polefrone   University of Pittsburgh, Pennsylvania
John B. Reid   Oregon Social Learning Center, Eugene
Ray H. Rosenman   SRI International, Menlo Park, California
Stephen F. Russell   University of South Florida, Tampa
Robert Schneider   University of Michigan Medical School, Ann Arbor
Richard B. Shekelle   University of Texas Health Center, Houston
Judith M. Siegel   University of California, Los Angeles
Charles D. Spielberger   University of South Florida, Tampa
Redford B. Williams, Jr.   Duke University Medical Center, Durham, North Carolina
Timothy J. Worden   University of South Florida, Tampa

Foreword

Medical literature has long suggested that anger and hostility have adverse health consequences. However, it was the Type A, or coronary prone, behavior pattern described by Rosenman and Friedman, with behavioral attributes of time urgency, competitiveness, and hostility, that brought substance to these early observations. Prospective studies of the Western Collaborative Group in California and of the Framingham Heart Study in Massachusetts have confirmed that Type A behavior is a strong and independent risk factor for ischemic heart disease. The dynamic evolution from patient observation to prospective study is presented in this book, which describes the development of Type A behavior as a consequence of social learning, perhaps interacting with genetic predisposition, and views competitiveness leading to habitual rushed pace, and enhanced hostility and anger, as its key coronary behaviors.

A further link between anger and cardiovascular disease was documented approximately 10 years ago. With Esler, Julius, and Harburg, in a study of young white males with high renin hypertension, we found that plasma norepinephrine coexisted with suppressed hostility. Harburg had previously used a self-report scale of anger and found that the elevated blood pressure of inner city blacks was related to their "anger in;" in other words, suppressed anger. Subsequently, Sullivan and I used the same scales in a California sample of men and women, both black and white. We found that hypertensives had an increased prevalence of "anger-in," associated with increased plasma and spinal fluid norepinephrine. Despite predictable limitations with this scale, we were in awe that in three separate populations it could tie a behavioral trait to cardiovascular disease. Sullivan and I personally completed this questionnaire, and we were relieved to find that we were "anger out," a contributing factor, perhaps, for our normotensive status.

"Is the sympathetic nervous sytem the biochemical link between anger and hostility and certain cardiovascular diseases? Do the catecholamines, which are so vital in protecting us in acute situations of fight or flight, become cardiovascular poisons in response to excessive stress?" Rage, an extreme of anger, is impressively associated with adrenomedullary discharge. This is mediated by the hypothalamus and associated with increased blood pressure and heart rate. Langer, Vincent, Brown, and others have pointed out that, while epinephrine has long been known to raise heart rate and perhaps lower diastolic blood pressure acutely, recent experiments show that its chronic infusion releases norepinephrine and increases peripheral vascular resistance, hence diastolic blood pressure.

Presuming that it is important to weed out inappropriate anger and hostility from our perception and cognition, can we decrease this behavior in order to reduce our cardiovascular risk? It may be too late for those of us born in the 1930s and 1940s. The work ethic that helped us overcome a depression and a world war, that taught such phrases as "idle hands are in the devil's workshop," "a stitch in time saves nine," "nice guys finish last," appears to have emphasized a competitive edge and, on the other hand, guilt when we pursue more recreational pastimes. Many of us may have already passed or taught these traits to our offspring, and why not? Is it not a tough world out there?

This book is an "Olympic torch" in search of answers to these and your own questions. The authors have found a critical mass of data that characterize anger and hostility as risk factors in hypertension, in premature coronary heart disease, and other illnesses. Since the early studies of Rosenman, Friedman, Harburg, and others, there have been refinements in the definitions and assessments of anger, and the dynamics of its consequences. Herein, Megargee discusses the intensity, direction, intentionality, and form of anger. Spielberger, with improved scales to quantitate the measurement of these dimensions, demonstrates the importance of the distinction between the expression and suppression of anger. Siegel, using elaborate self-report instruments, independently derives similar conclusions. Patterson emphasizes that the study of anger requires examination of social interaction in the natural environment. Julius voices a cautionary note—that suppressed hostility seems to be a feature of milder, but not necessarily sustained, hypertension. Gentry views suppressed anger as a powerful factor that may play a role in the higher prevalence of hypertension among black compared to white Americans, an intriguing hypothesis that requires further investigation. Manuck presents evidence linking anger and its expression to the cardiovascular responses to stress. Williams reviews the findings that link Type A hostility/anger dimensions to coronary heart disease, and Manuck studies an animal model that links hostility to atherosclerotic vascular disease.

The book closes on an upbeat note. Novaco finds reduction of anger after patients were taught skills to reduce anger arousal and to help them deal with conflicts. Similarly, Hecker and Lunde use assertive training, cognitive reappraisal, and relaxation to reduce chronic hostility. Reid and Kavanagh demonstrate that teaching social skills can prevent the escalation of social interactions into aggression and violence. As an alternative, Durel and Krantz present the rationale and evidence for pharmacologic treatment of anger and hostility. In the final chapter, Chesney synthesizes the theories of anger and hostility, and articulates issues important to the determination of health consequences, and the assessment, prevention, and treatment of anger and hostility.

Thus, the contributions of these authors light the way toward "the inner smile." This book is a passport to that quest and to a cardiovascular system in turmoil.

Vincent de Quattro, M.D.
Chief, Hypertension Service
School of Medicine
University of Southern California
Los Angeles

Preface

Anger and hostility have long been considered a threat to the communal and individual quality of life. Recently, studies from laboratories have converged independently on anger and hostility as potential risk factors in cardiovascular and behavioral disorders. Despite the recognition that anger and hostility are relevant to health, research and intervention have been handicapped by the fragmented state of knowledge regarding the definition, measurement, health consequences, and treatment of anger and hostility.

In this context, Stephen E. Goldston, Director of the Office of Prevention at the National Institute of Mental Health (NIMH), saw a need for research on anger and hostility as part of the developing national prevention program. With Dr. Goldston's support, we organized a working conference on anger assessment, health consequences, and treatment or intervention. Our objective was to provide a forum for an open exchange of ideas and research findings and for a discussion of their implications for future basic and applied programs of study. To achieve this objective, we brought together scientists who were studying anger and hostility from diverse perspectives, including cardiology and cardiovascular physiology, behavioral medicine, psychiatry, behavioral assessment, and biobehavioral treatment. The result was a research planning workshop, "Prevention Research on the Assessment, Health Correlates and Treatment of Disabling Anger," held in January 1983 at Menlo Park, California, the proceedings of which form the basis of this volume.

The three sections of this volume focus respectively on assessment, health consequences, and intervention. Specifically, the first section addresses issues of definition and measurement of anger, thereby providing a foundation for the topics discussed in the subsequent sections. In the second section, the emphasis is on new evidence documenting the relationship of anger, hostility, and aggressiveness to cardiovascular disease. In the third section, alternative approaches to anger management are presented from the perspective of their applicability to behavioral medicine and cardiovascular risk reduction. The final chapter turns to the future and raises questions that must be addressed by the behavioral and medical communities interested in interventions for anger and hostility. As these questions are presented, the interdependence among the issues of assessment, health consequences, and intervention is demonstrated.

We are deeply indebted to Drs. Stephen M. Weiss and Katrina Johnson of the Behavioral Medicine Branch of the National Heart, Lung, and Blood Institute, and to Dr. Goldston of NIMH, which cosponsored the conference on which this work is based. In particular, we would like to acknowledge Dr. Goldston for his support, guidance, and foresight. In his assignments at NIMH, he has been a pioneer in recognizing public health needs, assembling scientists, and initiating the work necessary to address these needs. The conference and book are a direct result of his perceptive awareness of the emergence of anger and hostility as significant risk factors for cardiovascular and behavioral disorders, and of the potential opportunity to prevent these disorders through biobehavioral intervention.

Margaret A. Chesney
Ray H. Rosenman

Anger and Hostility in Cardiovascular and Behavioral Disorders

I

DEFINITIONS AND ASSESSMENT

Anger and hostility have recently emerged as potential risk factors for cardiovascular and behavioral disorders. However, research and intervention to explore these factors have been hampered by the lack of consensus definitions and techniques for their measurement. This first section includes chapters that address issues of definition and measurement, and, by doing so, provides a foundation for the issues discussed in the subsequent sections of the book, as well as a point of departure for future research. Each of the four chapters defines anger, hostility and related constructs from different perspectives. This absence of consensus reflects the "state of the science" and the fact that determining the distinctions between anger, hostility and aggression is an issue awaiting resolution. Despite the differences, common themes emerge across the chapters in this section.

In the first chapter, "The Experience and Expression of Anger," Charles Spielberger and his associates review the mounting evidence of the influence of anger, hostility, and aggression in the etiology of cardiovascular disease. The concept of the "AHA Syndrome" is introduced to point out that anger, hostility, and aggression have been used interchangeably, obscuring conceptual differences between them. Spielberger et al. make a major contribution to resolving the ambiguity and confusion as to how these variables should be measured by providing working definitions. They propose that "anger" be used to refer to an emotional state varying in intensity from mild irritation to fury and rage. "Hostility" is defined as a complex set of attitudes that motivate aggressive behavior. These hostile attitudes include animosity, resentment, and the major component of chronic anger. "Aggression" is used to refer to destructive or punitive behaviors directed toward other persons or objects.

Recognizing the central role of anger in the general syndrome of anger, hostility, and aggression, Spielberger and his colleagues describe a comprehensive research program for developing scales to assess the experience and expression of anger. The construction and validation of the State-Trait Anger Scale, a psychometric instrument for assessing the intensity of anger as an emotional state and individual differences in anger proneness, is briefly described. The major focus of the chapter is on the construction of the Anger Expression Scale, which measures the extent to which responders express and suppress the anger they experience. Findings from recent investigations are presented by Spielberger that demonstrate relationships between suppressed and expressed anger and blood pressure.

In "The Dynamics of Aggression and Their Application to Cardiovascular Disorders," Edwin Megargee warns newcomers to the study of anger, aggression, and hostility about past pitfalls in measurement and presents a detailed account of the conceptual framework he developed to describe aggressive behavior. This conceptual framework, termed the algebra of aggression, grew out of clinical work with violent offenders and takes into account such determining factors as intensity, direction, intentionality, and form. Megargee illustrates the robust nature of the system by highlighting the parallels to behavioral medicine, and introduces the reader to the concept that the instigation to aggress is checked more or less successfully by inhibitions, such as cultural norms and mores. Megargee further highlights the distinction between intrinsic and instrumental instigation. In the former, the subject experiences anger and may engage in an aggressive act when the path to achieving a goal is frustrated or blocked. The relevance of this dynamic pattern to the anger observed in the Type A coronary-prone behavior pattern is pointed out, and Megargee also emphasizes the importance of situational factors in determining anger and aggression in Type A individuals.

In a position similar to that held by Spielberger, Megargee designated "anger" to refer to a transitory *state* of instigation, whereas, "hostility" refers to a longer lasting *trait* or predisposition to intrinsic instigation. Factors such as the duration, intensity, and situation not only determine the response, they suggest appropriate preventive interventions. Among these are intervention strategies for Type A individuals focusing on avoiding anger expression by reducing instigation through such means as cognitive restructuring or redefinition of the perceived situation.

Megargee's "Algebra of Aggression" not only presents a model by which anger and aggression are elicited or instigated, it documents the manner in which these negative behaviors are systematically reinforced or strengthened by our culture. This model is applied to behavioral medicine with relevant examples describing potential intervention strategies, including modification of situational factors to reduce the anger/aggression habit once it has been acquired and reinforced. The need to develop and validate measurement tools for anger, aggression, and related constructs is also noted by Megargee, who cautions medical and behavioral scientists to appreciate the complexity of the dynamics of aggression.

The final two chapters in this section reflect two markedly different approaches to the assessment of anger in specific research contexts. Judith Siegel sought a tool to measure multiple dimensions of anger as a potential risk factor for cardiovascular disease. To set the stage for developing this new instrument she summarizes the data (a) relating anger to elevated blood pressure, (b) implicating anger as a major component of Type A behavior, and (c) demonstrating associations between anger and atherosclerosis. From this literature, Siegel defines those dimensions of anger that she believes are most relevant to hypertension and coronary heart disease, including frequency of occurrence, duration, magnitude, and mode of anger expression. In her chapter, Siegel describes the preliminary psychometric work on the Multidimensional Anger Inventory, a self-report scale, and compares findings with this scale to other available anger inventories. From the perspective of self-reports of anger, the results of studies with college students and adult factory workers suggest that two major factors are involved: (1) a general anger factor encompassing the dimensions of frequency, duration, and magnitude, and (2) an anger expression factor containing two dimensions— anger-in and anger-out. Thus, in independent research with a self-report instrument designed for use in studies of anger and cardiovascular disease, Siegel's findings concur with the conceptual distinctions proposed by Spielberger regarding the experience of anger as an emotional state and individual differences in anger expression.

The last chapter in this section, while departing from the previous emphasis on the individual, and self-report in the assessment of anger, strikes common chords regarding dimensions of anger and its expression. In "A Microsocial Analysis of Anger and Irritable Behavior," Gerald Patterson points out that anger often arises or is expressed in the context of social interaction, and that the study of anger should include a focus upon social interaction sequences assessed as they occur in the natural environment. This chapter describes one approach that has been found useful in studying anger as it is elicited and expressed in aggressive families, and indicates how background factors influence the experience of anger and how patterns of social interaction determine the nature and magnitude of anger expression. Thus, a naturalistic approach to anger assessment distinguishes between anger as an emotional state and anger expression, while indicating the complexity of factors that determine behavioral consequences of anger.

1
The Experience and Expression of Anger: Construction and Validation of an Anger Expression Scale

Charles D. Spielberger, Ernest H. Johnson,
Stephen F. Russell, Rosario J. Crane,
Gerard A. Jacobs, and Timothy J. Worden,
University of South Florida, Tampa

Anger, hostility and aggression have long been regarded as important factors in the etiology of essential hypertension and coronary heart disease (Diamond, 1982; Friedman & Rosenman, 1974). As early as 1939, Franz Alexander postulated that hypertensives struggled against their feelings of anger and had difficulty expressing them. Alexander theorized that the angry feelings of hypertensives were suppressed because of their anxiety about the consequences of expressing anger, and that the hypertensives' strenuous efforts to control their anger led to chronic activation of the autonomic and cardiovascular systems, and, eventually, to fixed elevations in blood pressure.

Flanders Dunbar (1943), a pioneer in psychosomatic medicine, described patients with coronary heart disease (CHD) as ambitious, hard-driving and strongly aggressive. On the basis of her clinical observations of CHD patients, Dunbar postulated a "coronary personality," which was characterized by aggressiveness, compulsive striving, self-discipline, and a strong need for achievement and success. Although Dunbar's views have been criticized by other investigators (e.g., Miles, Waldfogel, Barrabee, & Cable, 1954), her work has nevertheless stimulated a great deal of research on the relationship between anger, hostility and aggression, and the occurrence of CHD (e.g., Cleveland & Johnson, 1962; Gildea, 1949; Miles et al., 1954; Miller, 1965).

Competitive drive and hostility are also major components of the Type-A Behavior Pattern (TABP), which was identified by Friedman and Rosenman (1959) on the basis of their extensive research and clinical treatment of CHD patients. The TABP refers to an action-emotion syndrome characterized by competitiveness, aggressiveness, achievement striving, impatience, and an extreme

---

Research described in this chapter was supported, in part, by grants from the National Institutes of Health, U.S. Public Health Services (BSRG-No. SO7RR07121-03) and R. J. Reynolds, Inc. We would like to express our appeciation to the Hillsborough County (Florida) Health Department and Public Schools for their assistance in obtaining the personality test data and blood pressure measures for the high school students who participated in our studies.

sense of time urgency. Because of their excessive competitive drive, according to Friedman and Rosenman: "Persons possessing this pattern are quite prone to exhibit a free floating but extraordinarily well-rationalized hostility..." (1974, p. 67), and they may often display "... easily aroused hostility, which was likely to flare up under very diverse conditions" (1974, p. 59).

The most impressive evidence linking the TABP to CHD comes from the Western Collaborative Group Study (WCGS), a large-scale prospective investigation of more than 3500 middle-aged men employed in eleven large companies in the San Francisco Bay area (Rosenman, Friedman, Straus, Wurm, Kositchek, Hahn, & Werthessen, 1964). The WCGS findings indicated that men classified as Type A at the time they entered the study were more than twice as likely to develop CHD as those classified as Type B (Rosenman, Brand, Jenkins, Friedman, Straus, & Wurm, 1975). Moreover, the relative risk remained even after statistically adjusting for other major CHD risk factors such as age, blood pressure, serum cholesterol, and cigarette smoking (Brand, 1978).

Evidence of a strong association between CHD and anger-hostility as a component of the TABP was reported by Matthews, Glass, Rosenman, and Bortner (1977), based on the reanalysis of a subset of the WCGS data. These investigators evaluated ratings of tape-recorded answers given by 186 men to the structured interview on the basis of which of these men were classified as Type A or Type B in the WCGS study. The extent to which Type A behavior was reflected in each of 44 different variables was rated on a 5-point scale. Item analyses indicated that clinical CHD cases were rated higher than age-matched healthy controls on the following seven variables: "Potential for hostility"; "Anger directed outward"; "Subject gets angry more than once a week"; "Irritation at waiting in lines"; "Subject's answers are vigorous"; "Explosive voice modulation"; "Competitive in games with peers." Four of the seven significant items were directly related to anger; the other three could be motivated by anger. Thus, anger and hostility would seem to be critical components of the TABP in contributing to the etiology of CHD.

The results of several recent studies of the relationship between hostility and coronary artery disease (CAD) provide further evidence of the contributions of anger-hostility to CHD. Williams (see Chapter 9) reviews several studies in which scores on an MMPI measure of hostility and cynicism were found to be related to the presence of clinically significant CAD, as well as the angiographically demonstrated severity of disease. A recent finding by Dembroski, MacDougall, Williams, and Haney (1984) that potential for hostility was associated with severity of atherosclerosis for patients who suppress anger (anger-in) documents the importance of assessing how anger-hostility is expressed as well as how often it is experienced.

Although evidence of an association between anger-hostility and CHD is mounting, there is considerable ambiguity and inconsistency with regard to how these constructs are defined and even less agreement on how they should be measured. Our primary goal in this chapter is to describe the construction and preliminary validation of the Anger Expression (AX) Scale. Prior to describing this scale, however, the concepts of anger, hostility, and aggression will be examined and working definitions of these constructs will be proposed. The State-Trait Anger Scale, a new psychometric instrument for assessing the intensity of anger as an emotional state and individual differences in anger proneness as a personality trait, will also be briefly described.

ANGER, HOSTILITY, AND AGGRESSION: THE AHA! SYNDROME

The research literature on anger, hostility, and aggression reveals a great deal of conceptual ambiguity and confusion. These terms are defined in different and often contradictory ways by different investigators, and are sometimes used interchangeably (Berkowitz, 1962; Buss, 1961). Moreover, the conceptual ambiguity is reflected in a diversity of measurement operations of questionable validity (Biaggio, Supplee, & Curtis, 1981; Spielberger, Jacobs, Russell, & Crane, 1983). Given the overlap in the conceptual definitions of anger, hostility, and aggression, and the variety of operational procedures that have been used to assess these constructs, we will refer to them collectively as the AHA! Syndrome.

Progress in research on the role of anger and hostility in the etiology of essential hypertension and CHD urgently requires conceptual clarification of the components of the AHA! Syndrome as well as the construction of objective, reliable, and valid measures of each component. Megargee and his colleagues (Megargee & Mendelsohn, 1962; Megargee & Menzies, 1971) have previously reviewed research on the psychological assessment and correlates of aggression and violence, and this analysis has been recently extended to the concepts of anger and hostility (see Chapter 2). Spielberger, Jacobs, Russell, and Crane (1983) have also examined the research literature on anger, hostility and aggression, and have proposed the following working definitions of these constructs:

> Anger is generally considered to be a simpler concept than hostility or aggression. The concept of anger usually refers to an emotional state that consists of feelings that vary in intensity, from mild irritation or annoyance to fury and rage. Although hostility usually involves angry feelings, this concept has the connotation of a complex set of attitudes that motivate aggressive behaviors directed toward destroying objects or injuring other people.
> While anger and hostility refer to feelings and attitudes, the concept of aggression generally implies destructive or punitive behavior directed towards other persons or objects. It should be noted, however, that aggression and hostility are often used interchangeably. A useful convention for distinguishing between these concepts is the distinction between hostility and instrumental aggression. Whereas hostile aggression refers to behavior motivated by anger, instrumental aggression refers to aggressive behavior directed toward removing or circumventing an obstacle that stands between an aggressor and a goal, when such behavior is not motivated by angry feelings (1983, p. 16).

From the foregoing analysis, it is apparent that anger is at the core of the AHA! Syndrome, but different aspects of this emotion have been emphasized in various definitions. For example, Buss (1961) includes facial-skeletal and autonomic components in his definition of anger reactions, and Feshbach (1964) conceptualizes anger as an undifferentiated state of emotional arousal. Kaufman (1970) encompasses intentionality as well as physiological arousal in defining anger as " ... an emotion that involves a physiological arousal state coexisting with fantasized or intended acts culminating in harmful effects on another person" (p. 12). Schacter (1970) and Novaco (1975) also emphasize physiological and cognitive factors in their definitions of anger as an emotional state or reaction.

The effects of anger-provoking situations on physiological measures of autonomic arousal, for example pulse rate, blood pressure, and behavioral manifestations and correlates of aggression, have been investigated in numerous studies. The earliest efforts to assess anger and hostility were based on clinical interviews, behavioral observations, and projective techniques such as the Rorschach Inkblots and the Thematic Apperception Test. Beginning in the 1950's, a number of self-report psychometric scales were developed for assessing anger and hostility (e.g., Buss & Durkee, 1957; Caine, Foulds, & Hope, 1967; Cook & Medley, 1954; Schultz, 1954; Siegel, 1956), but the phenomenological experience of anger, that is, angry feelings, has been largely neglected in psychological research. Apparently, recognition of the importance of distinguishing between anger and hostility occurred in the early 1970's, as reflected by the appearance in the psychological literature of three anger scales. The major characteristics of these scales are briefly described in the following section.

The Assessment of Anger

The Reaction Inventory (RI) was developed by Evans and Stangeland (1971) to assess the extent to which anger was evoked in a number of specific situations (e.g., "People pushing into line"). In responding to the RI, subjects are instructed to report the amount of anger they believe they would experience in each situation by rating themselves on a five-point scale, from "Not at all" to "Very much." Since the RI was developed primarily for use in clinical assessment, its potential as a research instrument has not been extensively explored. However, moderate positive correlations ($r = .52$, .57) between "Degree of Anger" as measured by the RI and Total scores on the Buss-Durkee (1957) Hostility Inventory (BDHI) provide evidence of the concurrent validity of the RI as a measure of hostility (Evans & Stangeland, 1971).

Similar in conception and format to the RI, Novaco's (1975) Anger Inventory (AI) consists of 90 statements that describe anger-provoking incidents ("Being called a liar"; "Someone spits at you"). Subjects report the degree to which each incident would anger or provoke them, by rating themselves on a five-point scale, from "Not at all" to "Very much." Novaco (1975) reported high internal consistency for the original AI (Cronbach Alpha = .96), but a test-retest reliability coefficient of only .17 was reported by Biaggio, Supplee, and Curtis (1981) for a revised 80-item version of the AI (Novaco, 1977). Moreover, Biaggio et al. (1981) failed to find any significant correlations between AI scores and self-report ratings of anger in provocative imaginal and role-play laboratory situations, nor with the number of anger-provoking incidents experienced during a two-week period.

Zelin, Alder, and Meyerson (1972) designed the Anger Self Report (ASR) to assess both the experience and the expression of anger. The ASR is comprised of seven subscales: "Awareness of Anger"; three separate subscales for measuring different modes of "Anger Expression" (General, Physical, and Verbal); "Condemnation of Anger"; "Mistrust"; and "Guilt." Zelin et al. (1972) reported that:

(1) ASR scores of psychiatric patients correlated significantly with psychiatrists' ratings; and (2) the ASR "Awareness of Anger" scores of college students correlated significantly with peer ratings of the extent that acquaintances "feel anger." While early research findings with the ASR were promising, the scale has been used infrequently by other investigators, and its predictive and construct validity are yet to be firmly established.

The BDHI and the three anger scales described above were evaluated and compared by Biaggio et al. (1981), who concluded that evidence of the validity of these measures was fragmentary and limited. Biaggio (1980) has also reported the results of a factor analysis based on the total scores for the four measures, plus the 15 BDHI and ASR subscales. Of the five factors that were identified, one of these ("Anger-provoking incidents") was defined entirely by high loadings of the RI and AI Total Scores. The BDHI and the ASR were both factorially complex, each with subscales loading on the other four factors, which Biaggio labelled: "Willingness to experience and express anger"; "Overt anger expression"; "Resentment, mistrust, and guilt"; and "Negativism." However, the eigenvalues for two of Biaggio's factors were less than 1.00, which raises serious questions about the legitimacy of her five-factor solution.

Empirical efforts to assess anger as distinguished from the concepts of hostility and aggression reflect an important theoretical development in research on the AHA! Syndrome, but there are several inherent limitations in using the scales described above to assess anger as a psychological construct. For example, none of these scales adequately distinguishes between anger as an emotional state (angry feelings) and individual differences in anger-proneness as a personality trait. Moreover, in inquiring about presumed anger reactions to hypothetical provocative situations, the RI and the AI confound angry feelings with situational determinants of anger reactions. While some of these issues are addressed by Siegel (see Chapter 3), the multidimensional scale she has constructed does not appear to evaluate the intensity of angry feelings and only indirectly assesses how often they occur. In measuring the fundamental properties of anger, it seems essential to assess the intensity of angry feelings at a particular time, the frequency that anger is experienced, and whether anger is held in (suppressed) or expressed toward other persons or objects in the environment.

The State-Trait Anger Scale

The *State-Trait Anger Scale* (*STAS*) was designed to assess the intensity of anger as an emotional state and individual differences in anger proneness as a personality trait (Spielberger, 1980; Spielberger et al., 1983). A rational-empirical approach was employed in developing the STAS, which is analagous in conception and similar in format to the *State-Trait Anxiety Inventory* (Spielberger, 1983; Spielberger, Gorsuch, & Lushene, 1970).

Trait anger (T-Anger) was conceptually defined in terms of individual differences in the disposition to experience anger, which would be reflected in the *frequency* that State anger (S-Anger) was experienced over time. Persons high in T-Anger were expected to perceive a wider range of situations as anger provoking (e.g., annoying, irritating, frustrating) than individuals low in T-Anger, and to respond to such situations with elevations in S-Anger. High T-Anger individuals were also expected to experience more intense elevations in S-Anger whenever annoying or frustrating conditions were encountered.

On the basis of these working definitions of S-Anger and T-Anger as psychological constructs, a pool of items was assembled to assess the intensity of angry feelings and individual differences in anger-proneness. Examples of the S-Anger items are: "I am furious;" "I feel angry;" "I feel irritated;" "I am burned up." Subjects respond to these items by indicating the intensity of their angry feelings, "right now," by rating themselves on the following four-point scale: "Not at all;" "Somewhat;" "Moderately so;" "Very much so." Examples of T-Anger items are: "I have a fiery temper;" "I am a hotheaded person;" "It makes me furious when I am criticized in front of others." In responding to the T-Anger items, subjects indicate how they generally feel by rating themselves on the following four-point scale: "Almost never;" "Sometimes;" "Often;" "Almost always."

A preliminary form of the *STAS* was administered to samples of college students and Navy recruits (Barker, 1979; Westberry, 1980). Those items with the best psychometric properties, and the highest internal consistency as reflected in item-remainder correlations, were retained for the final form of the scale, which consists of two 15-item subscales for measuring S-Anger and T-Anger. Detailed information about the psychometric properties of the S-Anger and T-Anger scales are reported by Spielberger et al. (1983), and in the Preliminary *STAS* Test Manual (Spielberger, 1980).

The concurrent validity of the T-Anger scale was investigated by Westberry (1980), who found correlations with *BDHI* Total Scores ranging from .66 to .73 for college students and Navy recruits. She also factored the T-Anger items and found that it was comprised of two subscales, which were labeled Angry Temperament ("I am a hotheaded person") and Angry Reaction ("I feel infuriated when I do a good job and get a poor evaluation"). Barker (1979) tested Navy recruits when they first reported for training, and found that those subsequently discharged as unsuitable for military service had significantly higher S-Anger scores.

Crane (1981) compared the *STAS* Scores of male hypertensive patients with a control group of general medical patients who had no history of hypertension and/or heart disease. The hypertensives scored significantly higher than the controls on the *STAS* S-Anger and T-Anger scales, but the differences in T-Anger were due almost entirely to the hypertensives' higher scores on the Angry Reaction subscale, especially, on the individual items that reflected a strong disposition to experience intense anger when criticized in interpersonal situations. Although the hypertensives reported experiencing more intense angry feelings than the controls, they appeared to suppress these feelings in interpersonal situations, which resulted in less overt aggressive behavior.

On the basis of our research with the *STAS* in assessing experiences of anger, the importance of measuring the extent to which people express or suppress their anger has become increasingly apparent. Research on anger expression and the procedures employed in constructing and validating the *Anger Expression (AX) Scale* are described in the following section.

THE EXPRESSION OF ANGER

The expression of anger must be distinguished conceptually and empirically from the experience of anger as an emotional state (S-Anger) and individual differences in anger as a personality trait (T-Anger). In research on anger expression, individuals are typically classified as "anger in" if they tend to suppress their anger or direct it inward toward the ego or self (Averill, 1982; Funkenstein, King, & Drolette, 1954; Tavris, 1982). They are classified as "anger out" if they express anger toward other persons or the environment. Thus, "anger out" generally involves both the experience of S-Anger and manifestations of aggressive behavior.

When anger is held in (suppressed), it is subjectively experienced as an emotional state, S-Anger, which varies in intensity and may fluctuate over time as a function of the provoking circumstances and the individual's level of T-Anger. The psychoanalytic conception of anger turned inward toward the ego or self (Alexander, 1939, 1948) implies that feelings of guilt and depression will be experienced (Alexander & French, 1948), though thoughts and memories relating to the anger provoking situation and the feelings of anger themselves may be repressed and, thus, not directly experienced.

Anger directed outward may be expressed in physical acts such as assaulting other persons, destroying objects, and slamming doors. The outward expression of anger may also take the behavioral form of criticism, insult, verbal threats, or the extreme use of profanity. Moreover, both physical and verbal manifestations of anger may be expressed directly toward the source of provocation or frustration, or indirectly toward persons or objects closely associated with, and thus, symbolic of the provoking agent.

When the anger expressed in aggressive behavior is motivated by animosity and hateful-destructive attitudes, it may properly be labled as hostility. The fact that aggressive behavior is not always motivated by anger, however, provides the basis for an important conceptual distinction between hostile attitudes, and *hostile* and *instrumental* aggressive behavior (Buss, 1961). Hostile aggression specifically denotes aggressive behaviors that are motivated by angry feelings. In instrumental aggression, the aggressive behavior is directed toward removing or circumventing an obstacle which stands between the aggressor and a desired goal, but is not motivated by anger. Using explosives in mining or road construction are examples of instrumental aggression.

Research on Anger Expression

The conceptual distinction between "anger in" and "anger out" was introduced by Funkenstein et al. (1954) in their classic studies of the effects of anger expression on the cardiovascular system. Pulse rate and blood pressure were measured in healthy college students exposed to stress-inducing laboratory situations. In post-stress interviews, the students were divided into "anger out," "anger in," and "anxiety" groups on the basis of the feelings they reported experiencing during the experiment. Students were classified as "anger out" if they directed anger toward the experimenter; they were classified as "anger in" if they reported feeling irritated or annoyed with themselves, rather than with the experimenter; those who reported feeling "anxious, apprehensive, or frightened" were assigned to the "anxiety" subgroup.

The increase in pulse rate for the "anger in" group was three times greater than for the "anger out" group; significant differences between these groups were also found for three other ballistocardiograph measures. In contrast, the "anger in" and "anger out" groups did not differ in systolic and diastolic blood pressure. The pattern of physiological changes for the "anxiety" group were quite similar to those found for the "anger in" group. While differences between the "anger out" and "anxiety" groups were similar to those found in the comparison of the "anger in" and "anger out" groups, systolic blood pressure for the "anxiety" group was significantly higher than for the "anger out" group. It should be noted, however, that "anger in" and "anger out" strategies were not stable and consistent—the direction of anger expression changed frequently and seemed to be influenced by situational factors.

Relationships between "anger in," "anger out" and blood pressure were investigated in a major research program on hypertension by Harburg and his associates (Harburg, Blakelock, & Roeper, 1979; Harburg, Erfurt, Hauenstein, Chape, Schull, & Schork, 1973; Harburg & Hauenstein, 1980; Harburg, Schull, Erfurt, & Schork, 1970). These concepts were operationally defined on the basis of subjects' responses to a self-report questionnaire that described several hypothetical anger-provoking situations, such as being verbally abused by a police officer or landlord. Persons who reported they would either not get angry, or would get annoyed, angry, or mad but keep it in, were classified as "anger in." Persons who reported they would get angry or mad, and show it, were classified "anger out." The questionnaire also included items for assessing the amount of guilt that would result from expressing anger in each situation.

Harburg and his colleagues observed that persons residing in high stress areas who used "anger in/guilt" coping styles, which they labeled "suppressed hostility," had significantly higher diastolic blood pressure and a greater incidence of hypertension than men with "Anger out/no guilt" coping styles, labeled "expressed hostility." Moreover, black males residing in high stress areas had higher blood pressure than any other group. These high stress black males also reported more "anger in" and guilt in responding to the hypothetical situations involving verbal abuse by a policeman or landlord. A similar pattern of results was found for white males residing in high and low stress areas: Higher blood pressure levels were associated with "anger in" and guilt.

Gentry (1972) and his colleagues (Gentry, Chesney, Hall, & Harburg, 1981; Gentry, Chesney, Gary, Hall, & Harburg, 1982) have reported findings that clarify the effects of race, sex, socio-ecological stress, and habitual-anger coping styles on blood pressure and the risk of hypertension. In a more intensive analysis of Harburg's (1973) data, subjects were first classified as "anger in" or "anger out" on the basis of their responses to each of five different hypothetical, anger-provoking interpersonal situations, and were then classified as low, medium, or high in anger expression by determining the proportion of their "anger out" responses. Black subjects of both sexes had significantly higher systolic (SBP) and diastolic blood pressure (DBP) levels (adjusted for age and weight) than whites. Both blacks and whites classified as high in anger expression ("anger out") had lower DBP than subjects classified as medium or low in expressed anger, and there was a tendency for the high "anger out" subjects to have lower SBP than those in the medium or low categories. The odds for being diagnosed as hypertensive were greater for blacks, males, persons residing in high stress areas, and subjects who reported low levels of "anger out."

The findings of Harburg, Gentry, and their colleagues clearly demonstrate the importance of the "anger in" and "anger out" distinction, and show that elevated blood pressure and hypertension are associated with holding anger in rather than expressing it in anger-provoking situations. There are, however, a number of problems in the procedures they employed in the assessment of anger expression that make it difficult to interpret their findings and limit the extension of their procedures to other populations. For example, the hypothetical anger-provoking situations that comprised Harburg's questionnaire were designed to assess anger expression in adults residing in a large city and may not be appropriate for other populations. Moreover, they inquired about subjects' reactions to hypothetical situations that many had never actually experienced and failed to take into account the frequency of occurrence of reactions to the same or similar situations.

Another major limitation of the Harburg assessment procedure is that subjects are classified into dichotomous groups on the basis of their responses to only two hypothetical situations. A much larger number of situations would be needed to establish the ecological validity of this classification and it would be desirable to have a continuous measure of the degree of "anger in" and "anger out" expression. While the procedures employed by Gentry are based on five hypothetical anger-provoking situations, and subjects are classified into low, medium, and high "anger out" groups, the ecological validity of their situations is still questionable, and there are only three categories, rather than a continuous measure of anger expression.

The procedure used by Harburg and Gentry of categorizing persons as "anger in" who report they do *not* feel angry in a particular anger-provoking situation also seems highly questionable. This procedure seems to equate individuals who do not experience anger or guilt with those who experience S-Anger and suppress it, or who turn anger in and feel guilty. Rosenzweig (1976, 1978) attributes very different personality dynamics to "impunitive" persons who regard anger-provoking situations as unavoidable, and "intropunitive" persons who turn anger in because they blame themselves for provoking anger in others.

The problem of distinguishing between the absence of anger, the suppression of anger, and guilt can be resolved by using measures of S-Anger to assess the intensity of the experience of anger at a particular time, and by developing separate scales to measure anger suppression ("anger in") and guilt. The problem of ecological validity in measuring anger expression can be easily bypassed by assessing the frequency that people hold anger in, or engage in aggressive behavior when they feel angry or furious. This approach has proved useful in constructing reliable and valid measures of anxiety and anger as personality traits (Spielberger, 1983; Spielberger, Jacobs, Russell, & Crane, 1983).

Anger expression is implicitly defined by Funkenstein et al. (1954), Harburg et al. (1973), and Gentry et al. (1982) as a unidimensional construct. In developing a scale to assess this construct, low scores should indicate extreme "anger in," resulting from marked suppression and inhibition of anger, and high scores should indicate extreme "anger out" which may be reflected in a variety of aggressive behaviors. Our efforts to construct a unidimensional self-report rating scale to assess anger expression as a personality trait are described in the following section.

DEVELOPMENT AND VALIDATION OF THE ANGER EXPRESSION (AX) SCALE

A working definition of anger expression was formulated as a first step in constructing the *AX Scale*. In formulating this definition, it was deemed essential to distinguish between anger as an emotional state (S-Anger), how often angry feelings were experienced (T-Anger), and the behaviors that people engage in when they feel angry or furious. On the basis of previous research, it was assumed that anger expression could be most meaningfully defined in terms of a single bipolar dimension, for which the behaviors ranged from strong inhibition or suppression of angry feelings to the extreme expression of anger toward other persons or the environment.

Another important factor that influenced the procedures used in developing the AX Scale was to try to assess individual differences in anger expression as a personality trait, rather than the intensity of the expression of anger at a particular moment in time. Two main considerations motivated us to construct a "trait anger-expression" scale: (a) Our general interest in investigating the role of anger in the etiology of heart disease; and (b) Previous research findings in which individual differences in the direction of anger expression were found to be associated with elevated blood pressure and hypertension (e.g., Harburg et al., 1973; Gentry et al., 1982). It was our goal, however, to build a continuous measure for assessing individual differences in the direction and extent to which anger was held in, or expressed, in contrast to the procedures used in the Harburg and Gentry studies of assigning subjects to dichotomous "anger in" and "anger out" categories, or dividing them into low, medium, and high "anger out" groups.

Consistent with our working definition of anger expression as a personality trait, anger-in refers to how often angry feelings are experienced but not expressed. The decision to define anger-in in terms of suppressed anger, rather than the psychoanalytic construct of anger turned against the ego, was based on three important considerations: (a) This definition was consistent with the approach followed by Harburg and Gentry; (b) Our conviction that the mechanisms mediating suppressed anger and guilt were quite different; and (c) The fact that a number of measures of guilt were already available. Our concept of anger-out is reasonably straight-forward, as previously defined, that is, anger-out refers to the extent that an individual engages in aggressive behaviors when motivated by angry feelings.

Construction of the AX Scale

To assess individual differences in anger expression as a personality trait, a pool of 33 items was assembled in accordance with our working definition of the anger-expression dimension, as described above. Some of these items were adapted from the Zelin et al. (1972) Anger Self-Report Scale and the Buss-

Durkee Hostility Inventory (1957); others were based on a brief self-report instrument developed by Baer, Collins, Bourianoff, and Ketchel (1979) to measure personality factors in essential hypertension. In addition, a number of entirely new items were written to assess different points along the anger-expression dimension.

In constructing the items for the AX Scale, a rating-scale format was employed, which was essentially the same as the procedures used in the assessment of T-Anxiety and T-Anger (Spielberger, 1983; Spielberger et al., 1970, 1983). The instructions for the AX Scale differed considerably, however, from those used with other trait measures. Rather than requiring subjects to respond to the individual AX items according to how they generally feel, the instructions directed them to indicate how *often* they *behaved* in a particular manner (e.g., "I say nasty things"; "I lose my temper"; "I boil inside, but I don't show it") when they feel "*angry*" or *furious*" by rating themselves in terms of the frequency of occurrence of these behaviors on the following four-point scale: (1) Almost never; (2) Sometimes; (3) Often, (4) Almost always.

The 33-item preliminary version of the AX Scale was administered to 1114 high school students (634 males, 480 females) enrolled in Health Science courses during regular class periods, as part of a study of the relationship between personality factors and blood pressure. Three items were subsequently discarded because they had poor psychometric properties, or were judged to be ambiguous on the basis of frequent questions raised by the students during the administration of the scale.

In order to verify that the remaining AX items measured a unitary psychological construct, item-remainder correlations for each of the 30 AX items were computed. The students' responses to the 30 AX items were also factored, separately for males and females, to determine if meaningful subscales could be identified. Initial factor extraction was by the principal components method, utilizing iterations of squared multiple correlations as communality estimates (Nie, Hull, Jenkins, Steinbrenner, & Bent, 1975). The following criteria were utilized for ascertaining the number of factors to be extracted: (a) Guttman's (1954) latent roots greater than 1.00; (b) Cliff and Hamburger's (1967) "breaks" criterion; and, most important, (c) the "psychological meaningfulness" of the resulting factor solutions. Kaiser's (1958) Varimax procedure was used to facilitate orthogonal rotation to simple sturcture of the factors to be extracted.

The latent roots criterion indicated that six factors could be extracted for males and eight factors for females; the "breaks" criterion suggested that a two-factor solution was optimal for both sexes. Given this discrepancy, successive rotations of 6, 5, 4, 3, and 2 factors were carried out. Inspection of these solutions revealed that the 3, 4, 5, and 6 factor solutions were either lacking in simple structure, or were somewhat different for males and females. The factors identified in the two-factor solution, which were relatively invariant for males and females and came closest to satisfying the multiple criteria, were labeled Anger/In and Anger/Out on the basis of the content of the items loading each factor.

Although we originally intended to develop a unidimensional, bipolar measure of anger expression, the results of the statistical analyses suggested that the *AX* items were tapping two relatively independent underlying dimensions. This was most clearly reflected in the finding that the eigenvalues for the first two factors extracted by the principal components method were almost equal in size (4.40, 4.01 for females; 4.66, 3.76 for males), and much larger than the eigenvalues for the remaining factors (all less than 2.00). Moreover, a majority of the items had strong loadings on either the first or the second factor, with negligible loadings on the other. Thus, rather than assessing a single, continuous bipolar anger-in/anger-out scale, the AX items seemed to define two relatively independent anger-in and anger-out dimensions.

Given the clarity and strength of the Anger/In and Anger/Out factors, the striking similarity (invariance) of these factors in the separate analyses for males and females, and the large samples on which the statistical analyses of the *AX* items were based, we decided to develop separate subscales for measuring anger-in and anger-out as independent dimensions, along with a scale to measure the extent of total anger expression, irrespective of its direction. In modifying our test construction strategy to achieve these goals, further analyses were undertaken to identify homogeneous subsets of items for defining Anger/In and Anger/Out subscales. Of the 30 AX items on which the identification of Anger/In and Anger/Out factors was based, 8 items had relatively low loadings (below .35) on both the Anger/In and Anger/out factors, for either males or females. These items were eliminated and separate item-remainder correlations were computed for males and females for the remaining 22 items. Two additional items with relatively low item-remainders for the females were eliminated, reducing the number of items in the final version of the AX Scale to 20.

The selection of the items for the AX Anger/In and Anger/Out subscales was based on separate factor analyses for male and females of the 20 AX items, using the same procedures and factor extraction criteria described above. The two-factor solutions were again optimal in terms of simple structure and invariance for males and females; the Anger/In and Anger/Out factors that were identified in these analyses were clearer than in the previous analysis which was based on 30 AX items. The item content and loadings on the Anger/In and Anger/Out factors for males and females are reported in Table 1, along with the eigenvalues for these factors. Individual items with the highest loadings on the Anger/in and Anger/Out factors are grouped according to their respective loadings on these factors. The column at the extreme left of the table indicates the order in which each item appears in the AX Scale.

Eight items with uniformly high loadings for both sexes on the Anger/In factor and negligible loadings on Anger/Out were selected for the Anger/In subscale, comprising the first subset if items in Table 1. The loadings of these items on the Anger/In factor ranged from .58 to .72 (median = .665); the loadings on Anger/Out ranged from −.16 to .17 (median = −.045). Similarly, eight items were selected for the Anger/Out subscale that had uniformly high loadings for both sexes on the Anger/Out factor, and negligible loadings on Anger/In. As can be seen in the second subset of items in Table 1, these loadings ranged from .44 to .72 on the Anger/Out factor (median = .59), and from −.12 to .17 (median = −.01) on Anger/In.

The final subset of items in Table 1 includes an additional Anger/Out item ("Make threats") with weaker psychometric properties than the items selected for the Anger/Out subscale, and three times with substantial loadings on both Anger/In and Anger/Out. The content of these items ("Control my temper;" "Keep my cool;" "Calm down faster") appears to be related to the control of

Table 1 Factor loadings, item-remainder correlations, and alpha coefficients for the Anger EXpression scale and its Anger/In and Anger/Out subscales for high school students

AX No.	Item content	Factor loadings Anger/In M	F	Anger/Out M	F	Item-remainder correlations AX/EX M	F	AX/In M	F	AX/Out M	F
6.	Withdraw from people	.72	.68	−.05	−.04	.48	.38	.63	.57		
5.	Pout or sulk	.72	.65	.04	−.10	.48	.32	.63	.53		
15.	Angrier than willing to admit	.69	.63	−.11	−.12	.43	.31	.59	.52		
14.	Secretly critical of others	.69	.58	−.04	−.02	.46	.34	.59	.47		
10.	Boil inside	.68	.66	.09	.17	.52	.49	.56	.51		
12.	Harbor grudges	.67	.71	−.06	−.12	.43	.36	.58	.60		
3.	Keep things in	.61	.61	.11	.08	.46	.40	.49	.50		
18.	Irritated more than people are aware	.60	.60	−.13	−.16	.34	.27	.50	.50		
9.	Slam doors	.04	−.01	.65	.58	.30	.28			.47	.41
17.	Say nasty things	.04	−.11	.64	.67	.30	.28			.49	.53
7.	Make sarcastic remarks to others	.00	−.12	.63	.55	.27	.21			.46	.41
11.	Argue with others	.06	.06	.61	.59	.31	.34			.46	.45
19.	Lose my temper	−.04	−.01	.59	.72	.22	.37			.42	.57
13.	Strike out at whatever infuriates me	−.05	−.10	.53	.49	.19	.19			.39	.37
2.	Express my anger	.15	.17	.49	.48	.32	.34			.37	.37
20.	If someone annoys me I tell them how I feel	−.05	−.11	.44	.68	.15	.31			.32	.48
1.	Control my temper	.52	.44	.43	.50	.56	.53				
8.	Keep my cool	.48	.41	.39	.41	.50	.45				
16.	Calm down faster	.46	.37	.17	.32	.38	.37				
4.	Make threats	−.02	−.15	.44	.46	.17	.14				
	Eigen values	4.53	3.97	3.13	3.55						
	Alpha coefficients					.80	.77	.84	.81	.73	.75

anger, which logically cuts across both modes of anger expression. In the factor analyses of the 30 *AX* items previously reported, these same items had salient loadings on a third factor, which included items with content suggesting anger control and/or resistance to becoming angry (e.g., "Patient with others;" "Cover up personal opinion of others;" "Don't let unimportant things irritate me"). In a study in which the AX Scale was administered to college students, Pollans (1983) found evidence of an "anger control" factor for males, but not for females for whom the anger control and Anger/Out items loaded on the same factor. The latter finding suggested that college women who overtly express anger have stronger control over their angry feelings.

The internal consistency of the 20-item Anger Expression (AX/EX) Scale and the 8-item Anger/In and Anger/Out subscales were evaluated by computing alpha coefficients and item-remainder correlations, which are also reported in Table 1. The item-remainder correlations for the AX/EX scale were based on all 20 items; the AX/In and AX/Out item-remainder correlations were based only on the items comprising these subscales. The alphas ranged from .73 to .84, and were highest for the AX/In subscale. Although somewhat lower, the alphas for the AX/Out subscale were nevertheless reasonably satisfactory for a brief 8-item inventory.

The item-remainders for the AX/EX items were heterogeneous, ranging from .14 to .56, with a median of only .33. This was not surprising, however, considering the fact that the AX/EX scale was comprised of two relatively independent subscales. In contrast, the item-remainder correlations for the Anger/In items were surprisingly large (median = .53), and those for the Anger/Out Subscale, though somewhat lower than for the AX/In items, were quite satisfactory (median = .435). For both 8-item subscales, all but one of the item-remainder correlations were .37 or greater, and all but two of the AX/In item remainders were .50 or higher.

The mean scores of the high school males and females on the AX/EX, AX/In, and AX/Out scales, and the correlations among these scales, are reported in Table 2. Gender differences were evaluated in analyses of variance (ANOVA's); the F-ratios obtained in these analyses are also reported in Table 2. The highly

Table 2 Means and standard deviations for the Anger EXpression scale, the Ax/In and AX/Out subscales, and correlations between these scales for high school students

	AX/EX		AX/In		AX/Out	
Scales	M (634)	F (480)	M (634)	F (480)	M (634)	F (480)
Mean	46.30	48.05	18.92	18.04	16.64	16.75
SD	9.07	8.33	5.93	5.28	4.18	4.38
F-ratio	10.72***		6.50**		.20	
Correlations						
AX/In	−.83***	−.70***				
AX/Out	.58***	.64***	−.07	.04		

*$p < .05$.
**$p < .01$.
***$p < .001$.

significant F-ratios for the AX/EX and AX/In scales indicated that the females had substantially higher total anger expression scores than the males, whereas the males scored higher on anger-in. No differences were found in the AX/Out subscale scores, which were similar for males and females.

The AX/In and AX/Out subscales were moderately to highly correlated with AX/EX scores, which would be expected, of course, given the overlap of the subscale items with the total anger expression scores. The finding that the AX/In correlated more highly with the AX/EX for both sexes indicated that suppressed anger contributed more to the total anger expression scores than expressed anger. Perhaps the most interesting findings in these analyses were the correlations between the AX/In and AX/Out subscales which were essentially zero for both males and females. Thus, the Anger/In and Anger/Out subscales are empirically independent, as well as factorially orthogonal. Clearly, the Anger/In and Anger/Out subscales assess two independent anger-expression dimensions.

Convergent and Divergent Validity of the AX Scale

A modified form of the Harburg et al. (1973) questionnaire was developed and administered by Johnson (1984) during the same testing sessions in which the high school students responded to the AX Scale. The original Harburg questionnaire was designed to measure "coping patterns and suppressed hostility" on the basis of subjects' responses to a series of vignettes relating to injustices perpetrated by authority figures such as a police officer, a landlord, and an angry boss. A modified version of the Harburg procedures, developed by Johnson to classify high school students according to their anger coping styles, consisted of two vignettes that required the students to report how they would feel in the anger-provoking situations described below:

Angry Teacher: Imagine that you were at school and your teacher got angry and blew up at you for something that wasn't your fault. How would you feel?

Movie Line: Someone cuts in front of you at the movie and gets the last ticket. How would you feel?

In responding to these vignettes, the students were required to rate themselves according to the amount of anger they would experience in each situation, and whether or not they would express or suppress their anger. Students were classified as "anger out" if they responded to the vignettes by indicating that they would "get angry or mad and show it" or "get annoyed and show it." They were classified as "anger in" if they reported they would get angry, mad, or annoyed but would keep it in.

Table 3 reports the means and standard deviations (SDs) for the AX/EX, AX/In and AX/Out scales for students classified as "anger in" or "anger out" on the basis of their responses to the "Angry Teacher" and "Movie Line" vignettes. The percentage of males and females classified as "anger in" or "anger out" for each vignette is indicated in the bottom line of the Table. Although approximately equal numbers of the males and females were assigned to the "anger in" and "anger out" categories, it should be noted that some students who were classified as "anger in" on the basis of their responses to the Angry Teacher

Table 3 Means and standard deviations for the Anger EXpression scales for students classified as Anger/In or Anger/Out in two anger-provoking situations

	Angry teacher				Movie line			
	Anger/In		Anger/Out		Anger/In		Anger/Out	
AX scales	M	F	M	F	M	F	M	F
AX/EX								
$\bar{X}$	42.39	43.87	50.58	52.05	41.56	44.42	50.41	51.31
SD	9.17	7.88	6.77	6.54	9.15	8.32	6.73	6.82
AX/IN								
$\bar{X}$	20.94	19.72	16.68	16.42	21.57	19.50	16.61	16.72
SD	6.43	6.02	4.34	3.80	6.52	6.10	4.18	3.98
AX/OUT								
$\bar{X}$	15.60	15.14	17.75	18.29	15.55	15.41	17.57	17.96
SD	3.72	3.57	4.38	4.51	3.67	3.56	4.38	4.69
N	329	232	299	247	294	224	335	254
%	52	48	48	52	47	47	53	53

vignette were classified as "anger out" on the basis of their reactions to the Movie Line vignette, and vice versa.

Differences in the AX scores of students classified as "anger in" or "anger out" according to the Harburg criteria were evaluated in 2 × 2 factorial ANOVA's, in which Anger in/out and gender were the independent variables and scores on the AX scales were the dependent measures. The results of the separate ANOVA's of the AX scores based on the classification of students according to their responses to each vignette are reported in Table 4. In all six analyses, the highly significant F-ratios for the Anger in/out variable indicated that students classified as "anger out" on the basis of how they indicated they would cope with the anger-provoking situations described in the vignettes had substantially higher AX/Out and AX/EX total anger-expression scores, and substantially lower scores on the AX/In subscale, than students classified as "anger in."

Significant gender effects were found for the AX/EX and the AX/In scores; females had somewhat higher AX/EX total anger-expression scores than males, and somewhat lower scores on the AX/In subscale. Significant anger by sex interactions were also found for the AX/EX and the AX/In scores when students were classified according to their reactions to the "Movie Line" situation, but not for the Angry Teacher situation. Females who were classified as "anger in" in the Movie situation had higher AX/EX and lower AX/In scores than males, whereas the AX/EX and AX/In scores for males and females classified as "anger out" in this situation were quite similar. Although there were no gender effects on the AX/Out scores for either vignette, the anger by sex interaction was significant for the Angry Teacher situation. Females classified as "anger out" in this situation had relatively higher AX/Out scores than males.

The analysis of the AX scores of students classified as "anger in" and "anger out" on the basis of the modified Harburg procedure provides evidence of the concurrent and construct validity of the AX and its subscales. Differences in the AX scores of males and females classified as "anger in" and "anger out" according to the Harburg criteria, especially, the Anger by Sex interactions, suggest that males and females may respond differently to different types of anger-provoking situations. These results provide evidence that the classification of a person as "anger in" or "anger out" on the basis of the Harburg procedure will depend on the subject's gender and the particular situations that are used in making these classifications. Since the AX scales assess how often subjects respond in a particular manner, rather than how they respond to a particular situation, scores on these scales provide an index of the frequency that an individual expresses or suppresses anger across a variety of anger-provoking situations that are typically encountered in daily life.

Further evidence of the convergent and divergent validity of the AX and its subscales is presented in Table 5, which reports correlations with other anger and personality measures. The biserial correlations of the AX scales with the dichotomous classification of students as "anger in" and "anger out" on the basis of their responses to the Teacher and Movie situations were consistent with the findings in the ANOVA's reported in the preceding analyses. The negative correlations with AX/In and the positive correlations with AX/Out were consistent with the assignment of scores of "1" for subjects classified as "anger in" and "2" for subjects classified as "anger out." The findings that the correlations of the anger-in/out classifications with the AX/EX total anger-expression scores were somewhat larger than with the AX/In and AX/Out subscales suggested that the results of the dichotomous classification were influenced by both "anger in" and "anger out."

It is interesting to note that the AX/In and AX/Out subscales correlated more

Table 4 Summary of the ANOVAs for scores on the Anger EXpression scales as a function of gender and classification as Anger/In or Anger/Out in two anger-provoking situations

Source	df	Angry teacher		Movie line	
		MS	F	MS	F
AX/EX					
Anger in/out	1	18095.25	300.25***	16619.34	272.80***
Sex	1	573.93	9.52**	944.57	15.51***
Anger × sex	1	.63	.01	230.60	3.79*
Error	1115	60.27		60.92	
AX/IN					
Anger in/out	1	3888.26	138.35***	4019.84	145.24***
Sex	1	145.45	5.18*	259.55	9.38**
Anger × sex	1	60.91	2.17	306.72	11.08***
Error	1115	28.11		27.68	
AX/OUT					
Anger in/out	1	1906.48	115.51***	1418.57	83.68***
Sex	1	.47	.03	4.42	.26
Anger × sex	1	72.10	4.37*	19.16	1.13
Error	1115	16.51		16.95	

*$p < .05$.
**$p < .01$.
***$p < .001$.

Table 5 Correlations of the Anger EXpression scales with the STPI scales and Anger-In/Out classification in two anger-provoking situations

	AX/EX		AX/In		AX/Out	
	M	F	M	F	M	F
Anger-provoking situations						
Angry teacher	.46***	.49***	−.36***	−.31***	.26***	.36***
Movie line	.49***	.41***	−.42***	−.26***	.24***	.29***
STPI scales						
Trait anger	.14***	.20***	.24***	.29***	.52***	.58***
T-anger/R	−.13**	−.04	.34***	.33***	.24***	.30***
T-anger/T	.21***	.25***	.12**	.16***	.47***	.50***
State anger	−.11**	−.12**	.23***	.24***	.10*	.09*
Trait anxiety	.00	−.01	.24***	.30***	.26***	.26***
State anxiety	−.12**	−.14**	.27***	.28***	.10*	.07
Trait curiosity	−.03	−.03	−.03	−.01	.02	.00
State curiosity	−.07	−.08	.03	.06	−.02	.00

*$p < .05$.
**$p < .01$.
***$p < .001$.

highly with the STPI anger measures than did the AX/EX total anger expression scores. The moderately high correlations of the AX/Out scores with the STPI T-Anger and T-Anger/T scores suggested that expressing anger was associated with the more frequent experience of anger as a personality trait. While the STPI T-Anger/T scale correlated more highly with the AX/Out scale than with AX/In, correlations of the same magnitude were obtained between the T-Anger/R scale and the AX subscales. These findings suggested that people who experience angry reactions are equally likely to express or suppress their anger, whereas persons who experience anger more often because they have angry temperament are more likely to express their anger outward, i.e., toward other persons and objects in the environment.

Although the correlations of the AX scales with the STPI state anger measures were relatively small, the finding that these correlations were slightly higher with the AX/In subscale suggested that students who suppressed their anger felt somewhat more angry in the testing situation than students low in anger suppression. Finally, it is interesting to note that the AX/In and AX/Out subscales were both more highly correlated with the STPI anger scales than was the AX/EX total anger expression scale, whereas the opposite was true for the correlations based on the dichotomous classification of students as "anger in" or "anger out" in terms of their reactions to the Teacher and Movie situations. This complex pattern of correlations suggested that the Harburg procedure for classifying subjects as "anger in" or "anger out" was more sensitive to total anger expression than to how often anger was either directed outward or suppressed.

The correlations with the STPI anxiety and curiosity measures provide evidence of the divergent validity of the AX scales. The correlations for all three AX measures with the STPI Trait and State Curiosity scales were essentially zero. The small but highly significant correlations of the AX subscales with trait anxiety suggested that persons who were high in anger expression or suppression were more likely to experience anxiety than persons with low scores on these measures. The correlations of the AX scales with state anxiety, like those with state anger, suggested that students who tended to suppress their anger were somewhat more anxious in the testing situation.

The Relation of Anger Expression to Blood Pressure

A major reason for constructing the AX Scale was to investigate the role of anger expression in the etiology of hypertension and coronary heart disease. Harburg et al. (1973, 1979) and Gentry et al. (1981, 1982) have reported that persons who tend to suppress anger have higher systolic and diastolic blood pressure, as was previously noted, and Williams et al. (1980; see Chapter 9) found that patients with scores above a certain level on an MMPI hostility scale were more likely to have coronary atherosclerosis. Similarly, in a more recent study, Dembroski et al. (1984) found that high ratings of potential for hostility and "anger in" were significantly and positively associated with angiographically documented severity of coronary artheroslerosis.

In our first study of the relationship between anger expression and blood pressure (BP), Johnson (1984) obtained systolic (SBP) and diastolic (DPB) measures for the 1114 high school students who were tested in the construction and validation of the AX scales during the same class period in which these students responded to the psychological tests. An automatic BP monitor, manufactured by Sears (Model 8-2153), which consisted of a microphone located within the BP cuff to pick up Korotkoff sounds, was used to measure blood pressure. The cuff was attached to the right forearm, above the eblow and just under the bicep muscle, with the microphone positioned over the brachial artery. Immediately after the cuff was deflated, SBP, DBP, and pulse rate were displayed on a digital readout and recorded by the experimenter.

Two blood pressure measures were obtained while each student was seated in an unpadded chair. The first was taken immediately after the student's height and weight were measured. The second BP measurement was taken approximately 30 seconds after the first was completed. The Pearson product-moment correlations between the first and second SBP measures were .90 and .83 for males and females, respectively; the corresponding correlations for the DBP measures were .86 and .88. Although these correlations were high, indicating that the rank-order of the BP measures was relatively stable, the initial SBP and DBP measures were significantly higher than the second measures, suggesting that the testing situation may have been stressful for some of the students. Since we were interested in the relationship between anger expression and basal (resting) blood pressure measures, rather than the effects of stress on BP reactivity, the second set of BP measures was used in all of the analyses reported below in which the relationships between anger expression and blood pressure were examined.

Pearson product-moment correlations of the AX/EX, AX/In and AX/Out scales with the SBP and DBP measures are reported separately for males and females in Table 6. The correlations between the AX/EX scores and the BP measures were negative and highly significant; these correlations were consistently higher with SBP than DBP for both sexes. The correlations of the AX/EX Scale with the blood pressure measures were also consistently larger for the males than for the females.

Positive correlations were found between AX/In scores and the two blood pressure measures for both males and females, as can be seen in Table 6. Though opposite in sign, these correlations were similar in magnitude to the correlations obtained between the AX/EX total anger expression measure and blood pressure. Since the correlations between the AX/Out scale and the BP measures were quite small, the overall pattern of correlations for the three AX scales with blood pressure indicated that holding anger in was associated with higher blood

Table 6 Correlations of the anger and control measures with systolic and diastolic blood pressure

AX scales	Males		Females	
	SBP	DBP	SBP	DBP
AX/EX	−.45***	−.27***	−.30***	−.16***
AX/In	.47***	.29***	.27***	.16***
AX/Out	−.13**	−.09*	−.13**	.05

*$p < .05$.
**$p < .01$.
***$p < .001$.

pressure, especially with higher SBP, and that the total amount of expressed anger, as reflected in AX/EX scores, has relatively little influence on blood pressure beyond the effect attributable to suppressed anger alone.

While the magnitude of the linear relationships between anger and blood pressure is reflected in the Pearson correlations reported in Table 6, it is possible that these relationships may actually be curvilinear, that is moderate levels of anger expression may have no more influence on BP than low levels, whereas high levels of anger expression, especially holding anger in, may have a strong impact on BP. Therefore, in an effort to clarify the nature of the relationship between anger-in and BP, the students were divided into five subgroups on the basis of their AX/In scores.

Since the number of males greatly exceeded the number of females, and it was considered desirable to use the same cut-off scores for both sexes, the females were divided into five subgroups, using an unbiased "counting off" procedure, in which the extreme groups were as nearly equal in size as possible. The same cut-off scores were then used in defining comparable anger-in subgroups for the males. The AX/In cut-off scores for the five female subgroups, and the number of students in each of the groups were: 8-13 (N = 86); 14-15 (N = 88); 16-18 (N = 127); 19-22 (N = 87); 23-32 (N = 90). Using the same cut-off scores for the males, the number of students in the five anger-in subgroups were: 103, 105, 135, 107, and 169. Figure 1 reports mean SBP in millimeters of mercury (mm/Hg) for the five subgroups of male and female students defined as a function of increasing AX/In scores.

Differences in SBP for males and females in the five anger-in groups were evaluated by a 5 × 2 factorial ANOVA, in which Anger/In and gender were the independent variables. In this analysis, which is summarized in the upper part of Table 7, the main effects of Anger/In and Sex, and the Anger/In by Sex interaction, were statistically significant. The larger Anger/In effect reflected the finding that SBP was substantially higher for the groups of students of both sexes who had the highest Anger/In scores, than for students who were low on anger-in, as can be seen in Figure 1. The Sex main effect indicated that the SBP for males was consistently higher than for the females at every level of the anger-in variable, as can be seen in Figure 1. The AX/In by Sex interaction resulted from the finding that the SBP for the males began to increase at a lower level of anger-in than for the females, and was approximately 8 mm/Hg higher for the two highest AX/In groups, whereas the SBP of the males was only 2 to 4 points higher than the females in the three groups with lower AX/In scores.

Using a similar procedure to evaluate differences in SBP as a function of anger-out, the female students were divided into five anger-out subgroups on the basis of their AX/Out scores and the same cut-off scores were used to define comparable anger-out subgroups for the males. The range of AX/Out scores for each of the five subgroups were: 8-13, 14-15, 16-17, 18-21, and 22-32. The number of males and females and the mean SBP for each of the five anger-out subgroups are reported in Figure 2; the results of the 5 × 2 ANOVA by which differences in SBP were evaluated are summarized in Table 7. The Anger/Out and Sex main effects were highly significant, but the AX/Out by Sex interaction was not significant in this analysis. These results indicated that the SBP for the males was substantially higher than for the females, as was found in the analyses of anger-in effects, and that there was a trend for students with higher AX/Out

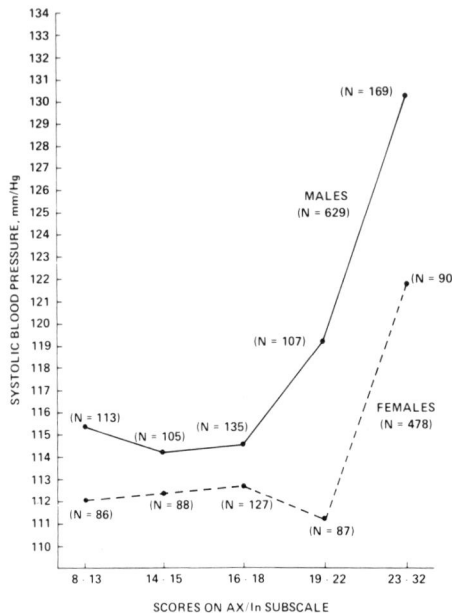

Figure 1 Mean systolic blood perssure for five groups of male and female high school students defined on the basis of increasing scores on the AX/In subscale

scores to have lower SBP. The absence of an AX/Out by Sex interaction seems to indicate that the SBP for the males was uniformly higher than for the females at every level of the anger-out variable.

The results of the analyses of the relationship between anger expression and DBP were generally similar to the findings for SBP, and will be only briefly summarized here. Higher DBP was associated with high AX/In scores for both sexes, and there was also a trend for lower DBP to be associated with higher AX/Out scores. However, in contrast to the finding that males were consistently higher then females in SBP, the females were consistently higher than the males in DBP.

Table 7 Summary of the analyses of variance of the systolic blood pressure of males and females as a function of anger EXpression (AX) scores

Source	df	MS	F
Anger/In	4	6677.68	49.19*
Sex	1	5897.23	43.44*
AX/In by sex	4	602.74	4.44*
Error	1097	135.75	
Anger/Out	4	891.88	5.48*
Sex	1	8459.89	51.98*
AX/Out by sex	4	140.97	.87
Error	1100	162.75	

*$p < .001$.

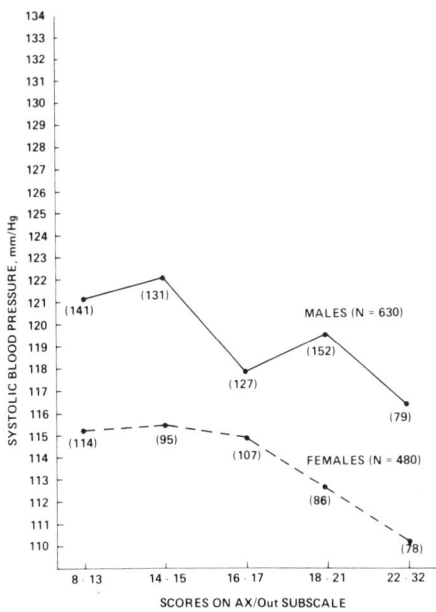

Figure 2 Mean systolic blood pressure for five groups of male and female students defined on the basis of increasing scores on the AX/Out subscale.

The analyses of the combined effects of anger-in and anger-out on SBP and DBP yielded somewhat different results for males and females. While high AX/In scores were associated with higher SBP for both sexes, there was a trend for SBP to be lower for females with high Anger/Out scores which was not found for males. Males with very high Anger/Out scores were somewhat lower in DBP than were males with low Anger/Out scores. For females, a significant AX/In by AX/Out interaction was found for DBP, reflecting higher DBP for females with high AX/In and low AX/Out scores, and somewhat lower DBP for females with high AX/Out and low AX/In scores.

Further analyses of the relationship between anger expression and BP were carried out by Johnson (1984), taking into account the influence of a number of control measures such as height, weight, dietary factors (salt intake), racial differences, and family history of hypertension and CHD. Although significant correlations were found between most of these measures and BP, Anger/In scores were positively and significantly associated with elevated SBP and DBP after partialling out the influence of the control variables in covariance and regression analyses. Johnson also found that black males and black females were higher in SBP, and had higher AX/In scores than their white counterparts. Moreover, in separate multiple regression analyses, the Anger/In scores were found to be better predictors of blood pressure than any other measure for white males and black males and females; that is, the AX/In scores were first to enter step-wise multiple discriminant equations for these groups. Higher Anger/In scores were also associated with higher SBP for the white females, but weight was the dominant variable in predicting SBP for this group, which was markedly lower in blood pressure than the other groups.

CONCLUSIONS

There is a great deal of conceptual ambiguity and confusion in current theoretical interpretations of anger, hostility, and aggression, and in the methods by which they are measured. On the basis of a review of the research literature, it was concluded that these constructs refer to overlapping phenomena, which we have collectively labelled the AHA! Syndrome. Mounting evidence that implicates the AHA! Syndrome in the etiology and pathogenesis of essential hypertension and coronary heart disease calls attention to the critical need to develop objective, reliable, and valid measures of this Syndrome.

Anger is most often defined as an emotional state that consists of feelings of irritation, annoyance, fury and rage, and heightened activation or arousal of the autonomic nervous system. Hostility also involves angry feelings, but this concept is much broader, usually having the connotation of negative destructive attitudes such as hatred, animosity and resentment, as well as chronic anger. Aggression generally refers to destructive punitive behaviors directed toward other persons or objects in the environment.

Since the concept of anger subsumes phenomena that are both more fundamental and simpler than the phenomena of hostility and aggression, anger is at the core of the AHA! Syndrome. Therefore, in measuring the components of the AHA! Syndrome, it would seem essential to begin with anger. As a first step in the assessment of anger, it is imperative to distinguish conceptually and empirically between the intensity of the experience of anger as an emotional state (S-Anger) and individual differences in anger-proneness as a personality trait (T-Anger). It is also essential to differentiate between angry feelings and how these feelings are expressed.

Three scales for assessing anger that were reported in the literature in the early 1970's were briefly reviewed and critically evaluated. The construction and validation of a scale for assessing angry feelings, the *State-Trait Anger Scale,* was also described. After examining the research on anger expression, the procedures employed in constructing and validating a new psychometric instrument, the *Anger EXpression (AX) Scale,* were described. A major part of the chapter was devoted to discussing the psychometric properties and evidence of the concurrent, convergent and divergent validity of the AX scale, and its subscales for measuring suppressed anger (anger-in) and anger expressed toward other people and the environment (anger-out). Finally, the results of a recent investigation of the relationship between anger-expression and systolic and diastolic blood pressure were reported.

REFERENCES

Alexander, F. G. Emotional factors in hypertension. In F. Alexander & T. M. French (Eds.), *Studies in psychosomatic medicine: An approach to the cause and treatment of vegetative disturbances.* New York: Ronald, 1948. (Originally published, 1939.)

Alexander, F. G. Emotional factors in essential hypertension: Presentation of a tentative hypothesis. *Psychosomatic Medicine,* 1939, *1,* 175–179.

Alexander, F. G., & French, T. M. (Eds.). *Studies in psychosomatic medicine: An approach to the cause and treatment of vegetative disturbances.* New York: Ronald, 1948.

Averill, J. R. *Anger and aggression: An essay on emotion.* New York: Springer-Verlag, 1982.

Baer, P. E., Collins, F. H., Bourianoff, G. G., & Ketchell, M. Assessing personality factors in essential hypertension with a brief self-report instrument. *Psychosomatic Medicine,* 1979, *41,* 321–331.

Barker, L. R. *Personality variables as determinants of performance problems of recruits in the U.S. armed forces.* Unpublished master's thesis, University of South Florida, 1979.
Berkowitz, L. *Aggression: A social psychological analysis.* New York: McGraw-Hill, 1962.
Biaggio, M. K., Supplee, K., & Curtis, N. Reliability and validity of four anger scales. *Journal of Personality Assessment,* 1981, *45,* 639-648.
Brand, R. J. Coronary-prone behavior as an independent risk factor for coronary heart disease. In T. M. Dembroski, S. M. Weiss, J. L. Shields, S. G. Haynes, & M. Feinleib (Eds.), *Coronary-prone behavior.* New York: Springer-Verlag, 1978.
Buss, A. H. *The psychology of aggression.* New York: Wiley, 1961.
Buss, A. H., & Durkee, A. An inventory for assessing different kinds of hostility. *Journal of Consulting Psychology,* 1957, *21,* 343-349.
Caine, T. M., Foulds, G. A., & Hope, K. *Manual of the hostility and direction of hostility questionnaire (HDHQ).* London: University of London Press, 1967.
Cleveland, S. E., & Johnson, D. L. Personality patterns in young males with coronary heart disease. *Psychosomatic Medicine,* 1962, *24,* 600-610.
Cliff, N., & Hamburger, C. D. The study of sampling errors in factor analysis by means of artificial experiments. *Psychological Bulletin,* 1967, *68,* 430-455.
Cook, W. W., & Medley, D. M. Proposed hostility and pharisaic-virtue scales for the MMPI. *The Journal of Applied Psychology,* 1954, *38,* 414-418.
Crane, R. *The role of anger, hostility and aggression in essential hypertension.* Unpublished doctoral dissertation, University of South Florida, 1981.
Dembroski, T. M., MacDougall, J. M., Williams, R. B., & Honey, T. L. Components of Type A, hostility, and anger-in: Relationship to angiographic findings. *Psychosomatic Medicine,* in press.
Diamond, E. L. The role of anger and hostility in essential hypertension and coronary heart disease. *Psychological Bulletin,* 1982, *92,* 410-433.
Dunbar, H. F. Hypertensive cardiovascular disease. In H. F. Dunbar (Ed.), *Psychosomatic diagnosis.* New York: Hoeber, 1943.
Evans, D. R., & Strangeland, M. Development of the reaction inventory to measure anger. *Psychological Reports,* 1971, *29,* 412-414.
Feshbach, S. The function of aggression and regulation of aggressive drive. *Psychological Review,* 1964, *71,* 257-272.
Friedman, M., & Rosenman, R. H. Association of specific overt behavior pattern with blood and cardiovascular findings. *Journal of the American Medical Association,* 1959, *169,* 1286-1296.
Friedman, M., & Rosenman, R. H. *Type-A behavior and your heart.* Greenwich, Conn.: Fawcett, 1974.
Funkenstein, D. H., King, S. H., & Drolette, M. E. The direction of anger during a laboratory stress-inducing situation. *Psychosomatic Medicine,* 1954, *16,* 404-413.
Gentry, W. D. Biracial aggression: I. Effect of verbal attack and sex of victim. *The Journal of Social Psychology,* 1972, *88,* 75-82.
Gentry, W. D., Chesney, A. P., Hall, R. P., & Garburg, E. Effect of habitual anger-coping pattern on blood pressure in black/white, high/low stress area respondents. *Psychosomatic Medicine,* 1981, *43,* 88.
Gentry, W. D., Chesney, A. P., Gary, H. G., Hall, R. P., & Harburg, E. Habitual anger-coping styles: I. Effect on mean blood pressure and risk for essential hypertension. *Psychosomatic Medicine,* 1982, *44,* 195-202.
Gildea, E. Special features of personality which are common to certain psychosomatic disorders. *Psychosomatic Medicine,* 1949, *11,* 273-281.
Guttman, L. Some necessary conditions for common-factor analyses. *Psychometrika,* 1954, *19,* 149-161.
Harburg, E., Blakelock, E. H., & Roeper, P. J. Resentful and reflective coping with arbitrary authority and blood pressure: Detroit. *Psychosomatic Medicine,* 1979, *3,* 189-202.
Harburg, E., Erfurt, J. C., Hauenstein, L. S., Chape, C., Schull, W. J., & Schork, M. A. Socio-ecological stress, suppressed hostility, skin color, and black-white male blood pressure: Detroit. *Psychosomatic Medicine,* 1973, *35,* 276-296.
Harburg, E., & Hauenstein, L. Parity and blood pressure among four race-stress groups of females in Detroit. *American Journal of Epidemiology,* 1980, *111,* 356-366.
Harburg, E., Schull, W. J., Erfurt, J. C., & Schork, M. A. A family set method for estimating heredity and stress–I. *Journal of Chronic Diseases,* 1970, *23,* 69-81.

Johnson, E. H. *Anger and anxiety as determinants of elevated blood pressure in adolescents.* Unpublished doctoral dissertation, University of South Florida, 1984.

Kaiser, H. F. The varimax criterion for analytic rotation in factor analysis. *Psychometrika,* 1958, *23,* 187-200.

Kaufman, H. *Aggression and altruism.* New York: Holt, 1970.

Matthews, K. A., Glass, D. C., Rosenman, R. H., & Bortner, R. W. Competitive drive, Pattern A, and coronary heart disease: A further analysis of some data from the Western Collaborative Group Study. *Journal of Chronic Diseases,* 1977, *30,* 489-498.

Megargee, E. I., & Mendelsohn, G. A. A cross-validation of 12 MMPI indices of hostility and control. *Journal of Abnormal and Social Psychology,* 1962, *65,* 431-438.

Megargee, E. I., & Menzies, E. The assessment and dynamics of aggression. In P. Reynolds (Ed.), *Advances in psychological assessment* (Vol. 2). Palo Alto: Science and Behavior, 1971.

Miles, H. W., Waldfogel, S., Barrabee, E. L., & Cable, S. Psychosomatic study of 46 young men with coronary artery disease. *Psychosomatic Medicine,* 1954, *16,* 455.

Miller, C. K. Psychological correlates of coronary artery disease. *Psychosomatic Medicine,* 1965, *25,* 257.

Nie, N. H., Hull, C. H., Jenkins, J. G., Steinbrenner, K., & Bent, D. H. *Statistical package for the social sciences.* New York: McGraw-Hill, 1975.

Novaco, R. W. *Anger control: The development and evaluation of an experimental treatment.* Lexington, Mass.: D.C. Heath, 1975.

Pollans, C. H. *The psychometric properties and factor structure of the Anger EXpression Scale.* Unpublished master's thesis, University of South Florida, 1983.

Rosenman, R. H., Brand, R. J., Jenkins, C. D., Friedman, M., Straus, R., & Wurm, M. Coronary heart disease in the Western Collaborative Group Study: Final follow-up experience of 8½ years. *Journal of the American Medical Association,* 1975, *233,* 872-877.

Rosenman, R. H., Friedman, M., Strauss, R., Wurm, M., Kositchek, R., Hahn, W., & Werthessen, N. T. A predictive study of coronary heart disease: The Western Collaborative Group Study. *Journal of the American Medical Association,* 1964, *189,* 15-22.

Rosenzweig, S. Aggressive behavior and the Rosenzweig picture frustration study. *Journal of Clinical Psychology,* 1976, *32,* 885-891.

Rosenzweig, S. *The Rosenzweig Picture-Frustration (P-F) Study basic manual and adult form supplement.* St. Louis: Rana, 1978.

Schacter, S. *Emotions, obesity and crime.* New York: Academic, 1971.

Schultz, S. D. A differentiation of several forms of hostility by scales empirically constructed from significant items on the MMPI. *Dissertation Abstracts,* 1954, *17,* 717-720.

Siegel, S. The relationship of hostility to authoritarianism. *Journal of Abnormal and Social Psychology,* 1956, *52,* 368-373.

Spielberger, C. D. *Preliminary manual for the State-Trait Anger Scale (STAS).* Tampa, Fla.: University of South Florida Human Resources Institute, 1980.

Spielberger, C. D. *Manual for the State-Trait Anxiety Inventory.* Palo Alto, Calif.: Consulting Psychologists, 1983.

Spielberger, C. D., Gorsuch, R. L., & Lushene, R. E. *Manual for the State-Trait Anxiety Inventory.* Palo Alto, Calif.: Consulting Psychologists, 1970.

Spielberger, C. D., Jacobs, G., Russell, S., & Crane, R. Assessment of anger: The State-Trait Anger Scale. In J. N. Butcher & C. D. Spielberger (Eds.), *Advances in personality assessment* (Vol. 2). Hillsdale, N.J.: LEA, 1983.

Tavris, C. *Anger, the misunderstood emotion.* New York: Simon & Schuster, 1982.

Westberry, L. G. *Concurrent validation of the Trait-Anger Scale and its correlation with other personality measures.* Unpublished master's thesis, University of South Florida, 1980.

Williams, R. B., Haney, T. L., Lee, K. L., Kong, Y., Blumenthal, J., and Whalen, R. E. Type A behavior, hostility, and coronary atherosclerosis. *Psychosomatic Medicine,* 1980, *42,* 539-549.

Zelin, M. L., Adler, G., & Myerson, P. G. Anger self-report: An objective questionnaire for the measurement of aggression. *Journal of Consulting and Clinical Psychology,* 1972, *39,* 340.

2
The Dynamics of Aggression and Their Application to Cardiovascular Disorders

Edwin I. Megargee
Florida State University

After decades of focusing on the psychophysiological effects of anxiety, physicians and psychologists are rediscovering the importance of animosity and aggression as etiological factors in physical as well as emotional disorders. Such concepts as anger, hostility, and aggression are increasingly being investigated in that branch of behavioral medicine concerned with cardiovascular disorders.

Although sophisticated in the assessment of physiological disorders, many researchers who are experts on coronary heart disease (CHD) are unaware of the extensive body of research that has accumulated on aggressive and agonistic behaviors, attitudes and emotions. Much of this literature has developed in fields far removed from medicine such as social psychology (Geen & Donnerstein, 1983a; b) and criminology (Wolfgang & Weiner, 1982).

Those of us who have concentrated on aggressive behavior have made many false starts and entered numerous blind alleys. Measurement problems have abounded, and it has become customary to begin books on aggressive behavior with a section analyzing the impossibility of adequately defining aggression either semantically or operationally (cf. Baron, 1977; Johnson, 1972). Nevertheless, often through trial and error, some progress has been made.

Unfortunately, some medical researchers who are attempting to relate animosity to cardiovascular functioning appear to be repeating our mistakes and reentering these same blind alleys. Some fail to differentiate aggression (behavior which delivers noxious stimulation to a goal object) from anger [an emotional state that occasionally precedes aggression (Buss, 1961)]. Others use concepts such as "annoyance" and "irritability" interchangeably with rage, hate and fury, despite the differences in emotional intensity and duration that these terms denote. Some constructs,[1] such as "anger," are being operationally defined by a confusing array of dissimilar techniques, including direct self-reports on face-valid paper-and-pencil checklists, scores on empirically derived personality scales,

---

[1] A *"construct"* is an hypothesed inner trait that is not directly measurable, such as hostility. *"Construct validity"* refers to whether or not an assessment device measures the trait that it is supposed to measure; for example, does the Cook and Medley Hostility Scale actually measure hostility? This question is answered by validational studies determining whether the scale correlates with other measures it should relate to, such as ratings of aggressive behavior, and does not correlate with measures it should not assess, such as ratings of physical attractiveness.

observations of ongoing behavior in both structured and unstructured situations, and ratings of case histories. Other researchers have used autonomic indicators of arousal, such as blood pressure and heart rate to study anger indirectly (Hokanson, 1970).

Most social psychologists and personality theorists who have studied agonistic behavior have found it necessary to distinguish among attitudes, emotions, and behaviors. Other distinctions are also important. Direction is one of these. It is important to note whether the aggressive behavior or attitudes are directed outward (extrapunitive) or inward (intropunitive), or are so diffuse that they lack any focus. Intensity is another important distinction. Violence is not the same as milder forms of aggression, and criminal violence differs from legally sanctioned forms (Megargee, 1982). Moreover, it is often important to note whether aggression is overt or covert, direct or indirect, intentional and unintentional, real or symbolic, verbal or physical.

The importance of these conceptual distinctions may not be immediately obvious to researchers new to the field of agonistic behavior. Without some forewarning, it is easy to reinvent the wheel, or, worse yet, the flat tire. Oversimplification of the dynamics involved is more likely to lead to errors than to enlightenment. To cope with these complexities, this author has evolved a conceptual frame of reference, shamelessly stolen from Hullian learning theory, that has proved useful in such disparate activities as attempting to predict dangerous behavior, designing and interpreting research studies on aggression, and training Secret Service agents to identify potential assassins. The purpose of the present chapter is to present this framework, termed the "algebra of aggression," to investigators in behavioral medicine studying aggressive behavior, attitudes, and emotions. Although it will not cut this Gordian knot of aggression, it might help unravel it a bit.[2]

OVERVIEW

The algebra of aggression grew out of clinical work with violent offenders. Although the academic view of the violent individual in the early 1960s was of a sociopathic person who was "all id with no lid," clinical practice indicated that not all violent criminals fell into this category. My first breakthrough was the empirical demonstration that, in addition to this widely recognized Undercontrolled Assaultive Type, there was also a Chronically Overcontrolled Type characterized by excessive inhibitions. Prevented from the normal discharge of aggressive instigation, the response was an uncharacteristic act of extreme violence in a normally mild-mannered, self-effacing individual (Megargee, 1966).

Although this hypothesis drew strong criticism at the time, it now seems obvious to maintain that more than one type of person can commit an act of violence. Other studies in this country and abroad have contributed data supporting the existence of the overcontrolled type (cf. Blackburn, 1968; Davis & Sines, 1971; Fine, 1972; Fredericksen, 1975; Gamble, 1972; Haven, 1972; Molof, 1967; Quinsey, Maguire & Varney, 1983; Stein, 1967; Wenk & Emrich,

---

[2] Readers who wish to explore the literature on aggressive behavior more thoroughly are referred to Baron (1977), Geen and Donnerstein (1983a, b), Johnson (1972), Megargee (1969), and Wolfgang and Weiner (1982).

1972). In 1978, Lane published an annotated bibliography of studies that supported the validity of the typology and of the MMPI O-H (Overcontrolled-Hostility) scale (Megargee, Cook & Mendelsohn, 1967) that identifies this type. Moreover, clinical evidence suggests the existence of at least five other types of violent people including normal individuals who have experienced strong provocation (often in conjunction with intoxication), offenders with organic or functional psychopathology, people with high instigation stemming from chronic frustration or oppression, and "instrumentally" motivated offenders who use violence to achieve personal, political or religious goals (Megargee, 1982).

What is the significance of this taxonomy of violent criminals for researchers in behavioral medicine? Often extreme forms of behavior shed light on behavior in the normal range. Just as studies of starvation and obesity can contribute to our understanding of normal hunger and nutrition, research on criminal violence can help classify the factors involved in everyday anger and aggression. For example, we tend to attribute aggression to anger or hostility, but the study of professional "hit men," assassins, bank robbers, and arsonists shows that other motives, like greed or power, can also lead to aggressive behavior. The paradoxical assaultiveness of the overcontrolled person illustrates the importance of inhibitions as well as instigation. Violence on the part of those committed to a violent lifestyle, as is true of many undercontrolled offenders, demonstrates the role of aggressive habits. The variations in aggressive behavior by people in all these categories illustrate the importance of situational factors.

Although the variables included in the algebra of aggression were derived from the study of criminal violence, they are also important in less extreme types of aggressive behavior. It is their interaction that determines whether or not an aggressive act can take place and, if so, its characteristics and severity. Indeed, from the standpoint of behavioral medicine, (as opposed to the study of criminal violence), it is probably those instances in which overt aggression is suppressed or inhibited that are of primary concern. In either case, this conceptual framework helps one to understand the dynamics that are involved.

THE ALGEBRA OF AGGRESSION

Most behavior, including aggressive behavior, takes place in a smooth-flowing, almost automatic sequence, with little time spent in reflection or conscious decision-making. As responses follow one another, it is easy to lose sight of their complex determinants. If we analyze a single response, however, we can see that each act results from the interaction of many factors and from dozens of implicit decisions.

How do we choose among the various possibilities? Typically, we select the response that appears to offer the subject the most satisfaction and the least dissatisfaction in a particular situation. This response is selected through a rapid but complex internal bargaining process in which the capacity of any response to fulfill many different drives and motives is weighed, often subconsciously, against the pain that might also result from performing that response, as well as any discomfort stemming from postponing the satisfaction of other competing drives. For example, a person who feels unfairly criticized by a supervisor could lash back angrily at the risk of losing his or her job. Backing down and suppressing an aggressive counter-response would preserve the position at the expense of diminished self-esteem. By means of this internal algebra, which occurs so rapidly that a person is often unaware of it, the net strength of each possible response is calculated, compared to all other responses, and the strongest is selected.

What determines the reaction potential of a response? In the case of aggressive responses, we can isolate four broad factors that interact to determine response strength. (See Figure 1.) The first of these is *instigation to aggression,* the sum of all the internal factors which motivate a person to behave aggressively. This not only includes any desire to injure the victim (angry instigation) but also any wish for other outcomes which an aggressive act might result in (instrumental instigation). The second variable is *habit strength,* the degree to which aggressive behavior has been reinforced in the past. The more a given aggressive response has been rewarded or successful, the more likely that it will be chosen again. The third major construct is *inhibitions against aggression,* the sum of all internal factors opposing a particular aggressive act directed at a given target. These include moral prohibitions such as conscience or "superego," learned taboos, bonds of empathy with the victim, and utilitarian concerns. The fourth variable consists of *situational factors* that may either facilitate or impede the overt expression of aggression.

At any given time, for any particular aggressive act directed at any given target, the interaction of these four variables will determine whether that act against that target is possible. If the inhibiting factors outweigh the motivating ones, that particular act will be blocked. (See Case 1, Figure 2). On the other hand, if the motivations exceed the inhibitions, that particular act at that given target is possible, but this does not mean that it will necessarily occur. At any given time, several different aggressive responses aimed at various targets may be possible in the sense that the motivating factors outweigh the inhibitions. Before any one can occur, they have to compete with one another and with any possible nonaggressive responses as well. In this response competition, the alternative affording the greatest satisfaction with the least cost should be chosen.

Imagine a Madison Avenue advertising agent who has been censured by his boss for losing a major account to a rival agency. When he blamed the loss on his rival's unfair tactics, the vice-president replied that she wanted results, not excuses, and would fire the agent for any further difficulties. In a nearby lounge after work, the agent pours out resentment as he pours in martinis. He describes his rival's chicanery to a sympathetic secretary, announcing that he will punch

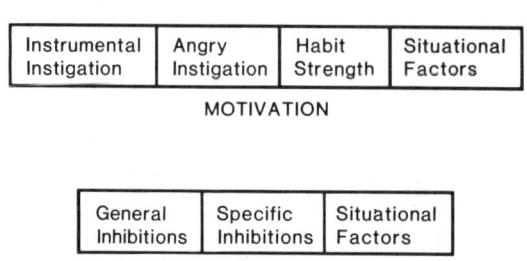

Figure 1 Motivating and inhibiting variables in the algebra of aggression.

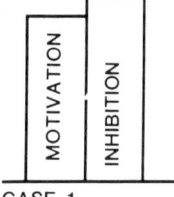

CASE 1
Inhibition exceeds Motivation:
Violent response is blocked

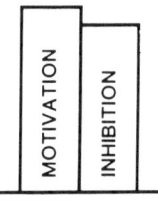

CASE 2
Motivation exceeds Inhibition:
Violent response is possible

Figure 2   Possible outcomes of the algebra of aggression.

out the other agent the next time he sees the SOB. She helpfully points out that his rival is in a nearby booth with his fellow account executives, apparently celebrating his triumph. What will our agent do?

Despite his anger over losing the account and being criticized, inhibitions would no doubt block extreme violence such as an immediate homicidal attack. Indeed, the vice president's threat to fire him for *any* further difficulties might inhibit any direct confrontation. (Case 1, Figure 2). If so, he might content himself with further muttering. However, a burst of laughter from the other table, further goading by the secretary, or additional alcohol might change the balance so that more direct and overt aggressive responses become possible (Case 2, Figure 2). These might include loudly remarking that it is easy to be successful if you don't have any ethics, going to the other table and accusing the rival of unprofessional conduct, or, perhaps, even physical action such as throwing a drink in the other man's face.

In this response competition, our hero would choose the act likely to offer him the most satisfaction at the least cost. Indeed, even though a moderately aggressive response might be possible, in the sense that motivations exceed inhibitions, he might, instead, select a non-aggressive alternative offering greater satisfactions by saying to his companion, "I'd rather make love than war; let's go someplace where we can get better acquainted."

In the pages which follow, we will examine each of these variables—*instigation, habit strength, inhibitions,* and *situational factors*—more closely, inquiring into their causes and their consequences. Where do instigation or inhibitions come from? How are they diminished once acquired? What are the implications? Although detailed or definitive answers are beyond the scope of this chapter, this exposition should serve to illustrate the utility of this conceptual framework and some of its applications to behavioral medicine.

INSTIGATION TO AGGRESSION

When analyzing any aggressive or violent act, the first factor most people consider is motivation. If we ask why John Hinckley shot President Reagan, we are not usually asking for a complex analysis of all the various factors involved; we simply want to know what inner needs, drives or desires motivated Hinckley to attack the president.

The technical term for such motivation is *instigation to aggression.* There are two types of instigation: *intrinsic* or *angry* instigation, and *extrinsic* or *instrumental* instigation. Intrinsic instigation refers to the desire or drive to hurt or injure someone. It commonly goes by such names as anger, rage, or hostility. The question, "Why did Hinckley want to hurt the President?" addresses this intrinsic type of motivation. Extrinsic instigation refers to aggression which is used by the aggressor as a means to an end. "What did Hinckley hope to accomplish by shooting President Reagan?" focuses on extrinsic motivation. We shall discuss intrinsic and extrinsic motivation separately.

Intrinsic (Angry) Instigation

Intrinsic (angry) instigation refers to the conscious or unconscious desire to injure someone's person, property, or reputation in some fashion, ranging from inflicting mild discomfort up to engaging in homicidal violence. The common denominator of all the varied manifestations of this motivational state is that, in the absence of punishment, the angry person finds the aggressive act intrinsically reinforcing or gratifying.

Although it took personality theorists decades to differentiate between "trait" and "state" anxiety (cf. Spielberger, 1966), differences in the duration and intensity of intrinsic instigation have long been firmly entrenched in the English language. (See Figure 3). "Anger" refers to a transitory state of moderate instigation; "hostility" to a longer lasting trait or predisposition. Similar state-trait distinctions can be made between rage and hatred, and between annoyance and grouchiness. In the present chapter anger will be used as a shorthand for all these subtypes of intrinsic instigation.

Origins of Intrinsic (Angry) Instigation

What are the sources of anger? On a purely *a priori* basis it would seem logical to divide the causes into two broad categories, physical and psychological. The physical category includes any innate or genetically based instigation, as well as anger or hostility resulting from CNS pathology, endocrinological and hormonal

	INTENSITY		
	LOW	MED.	HIGH
DURATION SHORT	ANNOYANCE	ANGER	RAGE
LONG	GROUCHINESS	HOSTILITY	HATRED

Figure 3 Types of intrinsic instigation.

factors, or physical illness. The psychological includes instigation resulting from environmental sources and life experiences.

Physical Sources

Ethologists such as Lorenz (1966) contend that instigation to aggression is an innate characteristic of the human species; Freud (1920) maintained that aggression, or the "death instinct," was one of the two central drives motivating all human behavior. Although many scientists are profoundly skeptical of such innate explanations, there is no denying the fact that selective breeding has produced strains of fighting bulls, dogs, chickens, and fish that are characterized by extraordinary aggressiveness. Moreover, the role of hormones in aggressive behavior has been well known for centuries to animal husbandrymen who castrate bulls and stallions to render them more docile. Although testosterone is the hormone most often linked to aggressive behavior, thyroid disorders can also lead to irritability, and the so-called "premenstrual syndrome" resulting from hormonal imbalances has even been advanced as a defense in a murder trial (Press, 1982).

A large body of research on the brain-correlates of aggressive behavior has accumulated, and cerebral centers for rage reactions and predatory attacks have been identified in cats, primates and even humans (Johnson, 1972; Mark & Ervin, 1970). Certain drugs and toxic substances have been linked with aggression and violence. Although detailed discussion of all these possible sources of instigation is far beyond the scope of this chapter, researchers, theorists and clinicians should be alert to physical as well as psychological causes of angry instigation.

Psychological Origins

Frustration, defined as interference with a goal-directed response, is the most thoroughly established cause of angry instigation. This stems directly from the influence of the "Yale group" (Dollard, Doob, Miller, Mowrer, and Sears), who hypothesized ... "that *aggression is always a consequence of frustration.* More specifically the proposition is that the occurrence of aggressive behavior always presupposes the existence of frustration and, contrariwise, that the existence of frustration always leads to some form of aggression" (1939, p. 1, italics in original).

Research quickly accumulated testing this unambiguous hypothesis. It soon became clear that frustration did not inevitably lead to overt aggressive behavior. Miller revised the original proposition to read, "Frustration produces instigation to a number of different types of responses, one of which is an instigation to some form of aggression" (Miller, 1941, p. 338). Other factors, such as inhibitions and situational variables, determine whether or not this instigation results in overt aggressive behavior. (The astute reader will detect the origins of this author's algebra of aggression in Miller's revised formulation.)

The Yale theorists proposed that anger varies directly with frustration, and suggested several factors that determine how much frustration people will experience in various situations. Since the clinical picture of the so-called type A individual suggests a person who often experiences frustration as a result of perceived interferences with ongoing goal-directed behavior, this formulation should be particularly interesting to cardiovascular researchers.

The first determinant of anger is the strength of the frustrated drive. If you are turned away from a restaurant because you failed to get a reservation, the hungrier you are the greater will be your frustration. Type A people are often described as being exceptionally achievement and goal-oriented. If their drive strength is indeed greater (if they are more motivated to have their way), they should experience more frustration and anger than their Type B counterparts in a situation in which they are blocked from achieving a selected goal.

The second determinant is the degree of interference. If you can't get seated at your favorite restaurant, you should be less frustrated if there are tables available in other equally desirable eating places nearby. At first this appears to be a situational circumstance that would affect Type A and non-Type A people equally. However, the flip side of the dominance, autonomy and need for control found among Type A people (Chesney et al., 1981; Glass, 1978) is likely to be a lack of flexibility and an unwillingness to alter plans once they are made. If so, Type A people may experience greater interference when their initial path is blocked. Instead of going to another restaurant, Type A people may persist in their attempts to secure a table at the original one, perhaps demanding to see the manager or offering the captain a large tip for preferential treatment.

If they persevere in this fashion, then the Yale group's third principle might come into play. Dollard et al. (1939) maintained that the frustrations engendered by a number of different goal-blocking experiences can summate to produce more instigation to aggression than would be expected from any one. In the above scenario, if a Type A person persisted to no avail, the frustrations engendered by each successive failure would accumulate. This process might accelerate as needs for self-esteem and importance, as well as food, became frustrated. Recollections of previous rejections, as well as residual resentment from other frustrations experienced that day, could add more fuel to the fire, resulting in the Type A person becoming enraged over an apparently trivial incident.

If this scenario correctly describes the Type A person's behavior, perhaps researchers could fruitfully investigate whether such people are, indeed, more persistent in striving to overcome obstacles, less flexible in accepting reasonable alternatives, more likely to view any setback as a humiliating personal rejection, and more prone to summation of frustrations. To the extent that these hypotheses are supported, it would suggest therapeutic strategies that might lessen the frustrations and anger Type A people experience. For example, rational and cognitive approaches helping Type A people to anticipate possible sources of frustration and put setbacks in perspective might prove helpful.

In addition to the three principles enunciated by the Yale group, Pastore (1952) suggested that the arbitrariness of the frustration is also a factor. According to this principle, people are less angry if a reasonable explanation is offered for the goal-blocking. However, Type A people may reject such "excuses" and thereby experience most frustrations as being arbitrary. If so they would be more likely to become angry than their Type B counterparts.

Expectations and adaptation level are also important determinants of frustration. It is more frustrating to lose a tennis match to a ten-year old novice than to the current Wimbledon champion. An American businessman who expects punctuality and efficiency is less able to tolerate delays and ceremonial circumlocutions than a person raised in a culture where these are routine. By changing cognitive expectancies, it may be possible to lessen some frustrations. A major reappraisal of life goals often takes place during the so-called "mid-life crisis," but the hard-driving achievement orientation associated with some Type A people might make it more difficult for them to alter their goals and thereby avoid some frustrations.

One of the more frivolous controversies in aggression literature was the long debate over whether frustration was the *only* antecedent of instigation to aggression. Those who steadfastly held this position generally had to redefine frustration so that it lost any semblance of its original meaning. Conceding that an overt physical attack could cause someone to become angry, frustration-aggression purists maintained that this was because getting punched in the nose frustrated one's need for autonomy or self-esteem (Berkowitz, 1962; 1969). This author prefers to include attacks, both physical and verbal, with jealousy and revenge as additional causes of instigation, and leave the original definition of frustration unchanged (Megargee, 1969, 1982).

Diminishing Intrinsic (Angry) Instigation

It is possible to discern three broad ways of reducing angry instigation. The first is through direct aggressive behavior, or catharsis, in those cases where the motivational forces outweigh the inhibitions. (See Figure 2, Case 2). If the primary aggressive response toward a target is blocked, it is still possible to discharge instigation by means of response substitution (resorting to other alternative responses), or by displacement (expressing aggression toward some alternate target). As a steelworker reported, " ... all day I wanted to go tell my foreman to go fuck himself, but I can't. So I find a guy in a tavern. To tell him that. And he tells me too ... He's punching me and I'm punching him because we actually want to punch someone else" (Terkel, 1974, p. xxxiii).

"Vicarious expression of aggression" has been touted as another means for reducing instigation; this is the classic response of the little boy who gets his big brother to beat up on the neighborhood bully. Media replete with violence maintain that they are performing a public service by draining the public's instigation. Who knows how much violence we all would be engaging in if we didn't have our nightly dose of televised vicarious aggression.

Although many social psychologists have investigated these phenomena, it is not surprising, considering the complexity of the algebra of aggression and the simplicity of the measures typically used, that studies of catharsis have produced mixed findings (Baron, 1977). Aggressing against someone might decrease one's instigation, but, if successful, it could also simultaneously increase habit strength and lower inhibitions. But how can these constructs be measured?

Hokanson and his colleagues (1970) assessed the effect of counter-aggression on autonomic indices of arousal. If blood pressure and heart rate are valid indicators of arousal associated with anger, Hokanson's research suggests that it depends on one's reinforcement history whether aggressive behavior reduces such instigation. If one has learned that aggressive behavior prevents further attacks, arousal level is likely to decrease, but this is not true if aggression has not "worked" in the past.

It is clear that catharsis, displacement, and similar mechanisms are quite complex and their effectiveness in reducing instigation is hardly clearcut or unequivocal. Before prescribing pillow-beating sessions to hostile patients, recall the algebra of aggression and ask if you are draining instigation, reducing inhibitions, strengthening aggressive habits, or, perhaps, doing all of the above. As noted at the outset, complicated problems rarely have simple solutions.

A second method of reducing angry instigation is through need satisfaction. This should be particularly effective in diminishing frustration-induced instigation. When a hungry diner is finally ushered to a table, or if a member of a minority group is no longer treated as a second class citizen, the frustration and instigation thereby engendered should stop accumulating and may even decrease, although there is likely to be some lingering resentment.

Recently, my studies of presidential assassins have suggested another related instigation-reducing mechanism, "substitute satisfaction." Academically, vocationally, familially, and interpersonally, most domestic assassins have failed in everything they have ever attempted (with the possible exception of the actual assassination attempt). This suggested that for most people some areas of successful coping can alleviate the frustration and anger engendered in other realms. For example, if a person who is trapped in a miserable unfulfilling job has a warm and satisfying family life, a rewarding hobby or avocation, or a fulfilling community activity, these outlets may compensate for vocational dissatisfactions and thereby decrease job-induced instigation.

Unfortunately, the clinical description of the Type A personality suggests a person who is afflicted with psychological tunnel vision, particularly in the area of vocational achievement. To the extent that Type A people are competitive and achievement-oriented, regarding any non-work-related activities as a "waste of time," they will be less able to use substitute satisfactions to compensate for job-related frustrations.[3] As Lorenz noted, "Human beings of today are attacked by so-called *manager diseases,* high blood pressure, renal atrophy, gastric ulcers and torturing neuroses: they succumb to barbarism because they have no more time for cultural interests" (1966, p. 38, italics in original).

The third method for reducing instigation is through cognitive redefinition. Suppose that someone jostles you while you are standing on a street corner. Turning, you see she is blind. Your anger will probably disappear as you redefine the situation as an accident rather than an affront. Cognitive expectancies play a central role in Novaco's (1979) model in which affective reactions such as anger are conceptualized as stemming from external stimuli impinging on cognitive appraisals and expectancies.

Laughter may be the single most effective technique for redefining situations to alleviate tension. As Seneca[4] wisely stated nineteen centuries ago, "It better befits a man to laugh at life than to lament over it." When things are going

---

[3] Of course, when Type A people do get involved in community activities, they are apt to bring to them their basic competitiveness. They want their Little League team to win the national championship, their service club to set a new record for raising money for the United Fund. Consider this description of a hard-driving, extremely competitive N.F.L. coach "relaxing" on a hunting trip: "He jerks with the kick of his Browning automatic, again and again, and birds drop like thick precipitation. The other hunters in his party finally stop, sore and tired, but when Vermeil is happy with the hurt in his right shoulder, he switches the shotgun to his left and goes on and on" (Smith, 1983, p. 74).

[4] All quotations without specific dates or page references have been drawn from Morley and Everett (1948), Peter (1977), or Tripp (1970), with the exception of Willie Sutton, who is quoted from memory.

wrong, a person who can view the resulting frustrations as part of the essentially ridiculous human situation, who can laugh rather than fume, will experience less stress (Baron, 1977). Most assassins take themselves very seriously. Lawrence, Booth, Czolgosz, Oswald, Moore, Fromme, Hinckley ... whatever else they had in common it was certainly not a good sense of humor. Perhaps this is also true of the Type A person. In our search for what Type A people have in common, let us not overlook what they may lack in common, that is, an objective viewpoint that enables them to laugh at the world in general and themselves in particular.

Implications for Prevention and Treatment

Much of the current literature on cardiovascular disorders focuses on the role of personality characteristics, especially animosity. Intrinsic instigation to aggression, defined by a variety of methods, and variously referred to as anger, hostility, rage, and fury, has been implicated in such disorders. Note that the coronary-prone Type A personality is frequently referred to as angry, hostile, and impatient.

Research on aggressive behavior, particularly on the etiology of intrinsic instigation and the methods whereby it may be dissipated, has important implications for the management of these patients. Although some maintain that instigation is at least partly innate or stems from physical conditions, it is also clear that much is also environmentally caused. In the absence of effective mechanisms for its dissipation, instigation can accumulate with possibly adverse consequences.

Much more research is needed on the nature of the association between intrinsic instigation and cardiovascular disorders. Many investigators implicitly or explicitly assume a direct causal link. If we accept the frustration-aggression hypothesis, then the causal chain would be:

$$\text{Frustration} \rightarrow \begin{array}{c} \text{Instigation to} \\ \text{Aggression (Anger)} \end{array} \rightarrow \begin{array}{c} \text{Cardiovascular} \\ \text{Disorders} \end{array}$$

One implication of this admittedly plausible sequence would be for clinicians to teach patients constructive ways to cope with anger. If residual, unexpressed, instigation causes cardiovascular problems, then effective ways of discharging such instigation should be identified and prescribed.

However, there are other possible causal sequences with different implications. It is well established that frustration causes instigation to aggression; perhaps it also leads directly to cardiovascular diseases. If so:

$$\text{Frustration} \begin{array}{c} \nearrow \text{Instigation to Aggression} \\ \\ \searrow \text{Cardiovascular Disorders} \end{array}$$

If this is the case, any attempts to deal with the instigation, once aroused, would have little impact on the cardiovascular disorders. Instead, interventions should be focused on eliminating the frustrations that cause both conditions.

Patient, painstaking research is needed to untangle these causal mechanisms; until such studies have been performed, investigators must remain open to a variety of alternatives and not sieze on premature, superficial, or simplistic explanations.

Extrinsic (Instrumental) Instigation

Although most researchers concentrate on intrinsically-motivated (angry) aggression, the study of such violent crimes as robbery, arson, terrorism and kidnapping, shows that not all aggression stems from anger or hostility. Among the motives for violent crime are the acquisition of property; the enhancement of the self-concept; a search for excitement, affection, respect, or power; removal of threats, problems, or impediments; and acquistion or maintenance of one's position in a group. As Al Capone explained, "You can get much farther with a kind word and a gun than you can with a kind word alone."

Turning from criminal violence to less extreme forms of aggression increases the possible range of extrinsic goals that aggression might be instrumental in achieving. The vice-president who criticized the account executive was probably motivated more by a desire to improve his performance (and thereby the success of her division) than by hostility toward her subordinate.

Of course, both intrinsic and extrinsic motivation can operate simultaneously. President Harry S Truman fired General-of-the-Army Douglas McArthur because Truman felt it was in the best interest of national policy, but it is no secret that Truman was infuriated by MacArthur's perceived insubordination and arrogance. Parents disciplining children may be expressing anger as well as attempting to modify the children's behavior.

People prone to coronary and vascular disorders are often described as aggressive, abrasive, and assertive, as they ruthlessly and relentlessly pursue their goals. Is it the aggressive behavior these people engage in, or the intensity of their pursuit (their conviction that ends justify means), that leads to the cardiovascular disorders? Or is there a third factor, perhaps intrinsic instigation, that causes both?

Researchers exploring the relation between CHD and intrinsic (angry) instigation need to be sensitive to instrumental motivation as well. If they use case histories or other observations of overt aggressive behavior to measure anger or hostility, they may obtain inconsistent or inconclusive results by including extrinsically motivated subjects in their samples.

HABIT STRENGTH

People learn from experience. In any given situation, we are more likely to repeat an action that has worked for us in the past than some other behavior that has been less successful. This is the essence of Thorndike's classic "Law of Effect" which states that success, or "positive reinforcement," strengthens habits whereas failure diminishes them.

Aggressive behavior is no exception. Other things being equal, aggressive acts that have been positively reinforced will be chosen more often. Our second major construct, habit strength, incorporates the degree to which an individual has been reinforced for previous aggressive behavior into the algebra of aggression. As with all of our variables, habit strength varies from act to act and from target to target.

The rewards for aggressive behavior depend on the motivation. Angry aggression is reinforced by injury to the victim, instrumental aggression by the attainment of the extrinsic goal that was sought. However, we must be alert to additional unanticipated or secondary rewards that can also strengthen aggressive habits. When asked why he robbed banks, Willie (The Actor) Sutton was (erroneously) quoted as replying, "Because that is where the money is," implying only extrinsic motivation. However, another, less famous, bank robber of my acquaintance confided that he found he enjoyed the "adrenaline high," the gratifying sense of power he obtained from holding a lobby full of people at bay with a machine gun and the thrills and excitement of high speed chases, as much as the actual money he stole.

A detailed comparison of bank robbers with businessmen is beyond the scope of this chapter, but it is safe to assume that many chief executive officers are also motivated by more than mere financial incentives. After all, as Hobart Brown noted, "Money doesn't always bring happiness. People with ten million dollars are no happier than people with nine million dollars." Although seeking a fortune might have been the initial incentive to enter the business world, in the upper brackets money has often become a way of keeping score in a game that has no final whistle. In other fields the chips may be publications, trophies, or newspaper clippings, but the principle is the same. Thoreau might well have been addressing a modern Type A person when he inquired, "Why should we be in such desperate haste to succeed, and in such desperate circumstances?" Many driven people find aggression is one way to achieve success in their chosen fields of endeavor.

Acquisition of Aggressive Habit Strength

Aggressive habits are acquired according to the basic principles of operant learning. Not only can they develop from direct experience, but also indirectly through observation and modeling.

Direct Acquisition

Although the Christian ethic prescribes nonviolence, most parents in our culture prefer to raise their children, especially the boys, to "take care of themselves" and not "let anyone push them around." Peers, too, often reinforce aggressive behavior. A "bully" gets more respect than a "wimp," and children raised in our society are exposed to many contingencies conducive to developing aggressive habits. The assertive or aggressive child who shoves to the head of the line, who can extort candy from smaller children, who grabs the largest portion at the table, and who appropriates the most desirable toy learns that "nice guys finish last." Although the meek may eventually inherit the earth, it apparently takes an interminable time for the estate to be probated, and immediate rewards are far more potent than those which are long deferred.

When a person successfully performs an aggressive act and is rewarded by injury to the victim or by attainment of some desired goal, or both, this reinforcement serves to increase the habit strength for this particular response in this situation. In addition, through the phenomenon of *response generalization*, the habit strength of other aggressive responses is also increased somewhat.

Consider this scenario: A Little League ballplayer dashing from third base to home is called out in a close play at the plate, thereby ending the game and snuffing out a last-inning rally. Enraged, the player jumps up and down, addressing a number of uncharitable remarks to the unfortunate adult officiating the game. Teammates and their parents join in, supporting the protest. Since the game is over, the umpire stalks away rather than risk escalating the confrontation by attempting to punish the player.

In addition to the direct reinforcement stemming from overt expression of angry instigation, the tantrum has succeeded in diverting the blame for the botched play from the player's poor base running to the umpire's poor eyesight. The support and encouragement of friends and fans has provided further reinforcement. What will be the consequences?

One outcome will be an increase in the likelihood that the player will argue with umpires in the future. This tendency will be strongest toward the umpire who tolerated the tirade, but it should generalize to other officials as well. Moreover, the habit strength generalized from this incident should increase the likelihood of aggressive outbursts toward other adult authorities such as coaches, teachers, and even parents.

Indirect Acquisition

Even in the absence of direct reinforcement for aggressive behavior, habit strength can be acquired indirectly through observation and imitation. Our Little League ballplayer's outburst might have stemmed in part from observing models such as outspoken major league manager Billy Martin and the leather-lunged Little League parents who often abuse umpires.

Western culture affords us many opportunities to acquire aggressive habits indirectly. Our media are replete with violence, both actual and fictional, and frequently depict aggression and violence as the most effective means to a variety of ends. From "High Noon" to "Superman II," film makers have portrayed pacifists as people who must learn that only violence can counteract evil. Cross-cultural comparisons of such diverse cultures as the head-hunting Iatmul and the pacifist Hutterites vividly demonstrate the influence of direct and indirect social learning on habit strength; whereas Iatmul society is replete with interpersonal aggression, such behavior is virtually unknown among the Hutterites (Bandura & Walters, 1963).

Decreasing Aggressive Habit Strength

As anyone who has tried to give up smoking can testify, habits are much easier to acquire than to lose. Studies of learning and conditioning in species ranging from planaria to people have demonstrated that extinction (a sustained absence of any reinforcement) is the only sure way to eliminate habits once they have been formed. But how is one to arrange the contingencies or circumstances so as to eliminate any rewards for aggressive behavior? By definition, intrinsically motivated (angry) aggressive behavior is rewarding. Even if the umpire or a coach had punished the Little League player who protested so vehemently, the immediate satisfaction of expressing anger would have reinforced the behavior and thereby increased the player's habit strength; any subsequent punishment would only have increased the inhibitions against aggressive behavior somewhat.

Turning to extrinsic motivation, once aggression has been effective in achieving desired goals, it is virtually impossible in our culture to manipulate the environment so that a person will no longer be rewarded for aggressive behavior. Extinction of aggressive habits requires a person to perform aggressive acts over and over again without receiving any reinforcement whatsoever. This is very difficult to accomplish, and if some of these acts do get rewarded, we have instituted a "partial reward schedule" which, paradoxically, makes for even more persistent habits.[5]

Implications for Prevention and Treatment

To prevent the development of aggressive habit strength, one must eliminate, or at least minimize, the rewards for aggressive behavior. Swift intervention is necessary to prevent completion of intrinsically motivated (angry) aggressive behavior sequences, thereby blocking the reinforcement. (Although this will constitute a frustration and therefore increase instigation, anger is a transitory state, whereas habit strength persists.) In children, a "time-out" procedure is apt to be particularly effective in blocking the primary reinforcement of expressing instigation or the secondary reinforcement of obtaining attention; it is also aversive enough to serve as a punishment without the disadvantage of furnishing an aggressive model.

Similarly, one also needs to minimize the extrinsic rewards for aggressive behavior. One tactic is to use reinforcement to increase the habit strength of competing nonaggressive responses. A child who has learned that socially appropriate behavior is more effective than aggression in obtaining attention should choose the more strongly reinforced nonaggressive alternative when different possible responses are being evaluated (Brown & Elliot, 1965). Similar strategies can be applied to adults. Although it is more difficult to alter life-long behavior patterns, and although reinforcements in most adults' lives are harder to control, with more mature people verbalizing the contingencies helps to save time. Sometimes this works; other times it does not, as any cardiologist who has told CHD patients to stop smoking, if they want to survive, can testify.

Once aggressive habits have been formed, they are difficult to eliminate, especially in a society that admires and reinforces aggression. Aggressive habits are rarely totally extinguished, but minimizing reinforcement and strengthening alternative responses may prevent any further increases in habit strength.

INHIBITIONS AGAINST AGGRESSION

Inhibitions against aggression are all those internal factors that operate to oppose the performance of aggressive behavior, in general, as well as the specific concerns that restrain a particular aggressive response. Most people have broad

---

[5] For a succinct summary of the principles governing acquisition and extinction of habits, including the paradoxical persistance of partially reinforced patterns, readers unfamiliar with these phenomena should consult the chapter on operant conditioning in any current basic text on general psychology.

general inhibitions against certain classes of aggressive behavior, such as homicide, or against aggressive behavior directed at certain classes of targets, such as parents. In addition, there are specific inhibitions against particular acts toward certain targets in well-defined circumstances. Like instigation, inhibitions can vary over time, and, as we shall see, it is often possible to suspend them.

Acquisition of Inhibitions

As with instigation, it is possible to differentiate physical and physiological sources of inhibitions from psychological and environmental sources.

Physical Sources of Inhibitions

Although ethologists such as Lorenz (1966) maintain that inhibitions against aggression are innate, there is no rigorous evidence for their genetic basis. Nevertheless, the monks of the Swiss Hospice of St. Bernard succeeded in producing exceptional docility in the large dogs they bred to assist snow-stranded travelers. Moreover, physiologists have identified brain centers that inhibit aggressive attacks.

While genetic factors and inhibiting brain centers are of theoretical significance, in actual clinical practice the psychoactive drugs that have been developed to control antisocial behavior and violence are the most important physical source of inhibitions. More than any other single factor, these drugs have made possible the community treatment and maintenance of many patients formerly deemed too dangerous to be allowed in society.

Psychological Sources of Inhibitions

Surveying the empirical and theoretical literature, this author recently identified "... four broad, somewhat overlapping determinants of inhibitions against aggression: (1) anxiety or conditioned fear of punishment; (2) learned values and attitudes; (3) empathy or identification with the potential victim; and (4) utilitarian concerns" (Megargee, 1982, p. 149).

Anxiety or conditioned fear of punishment. Punishing aggression produces anxiety or fear which forms the basis for inhibitions against such behavior. The Yale Group "... stated that the *strength of inhibition of any act of aggression varies positively with the amount of punishment anticipated to be a consequence of that act...*" (Dollard et al., 1939, p. 33, italics in the original).

Since punishment depends upon external authorities who may not always be present, most children learn to discriminate those situations in which punishment is likely from those in which they can aggress with impunity. The overall effectiveness of punishment is further complicated by the fact that, being frustrating, it can also increase instigation. Moreover, physically punitive parents serve as aggressive models for their children.

Learned values and attitudes. Every culture, subculture, and family has evolved its own implicit and explicit set of rules governing aggressive behavior. As we are socialized, we learn what aggressive acts are permitted, under what circumstances, toward which targets. We may strike back when hit by a peer, but not when spanked by a parent. Wrestling may be allowed, but strangling is taboo. Free-for-alls permitted in the yard are prohibited in the parlor. Whatever the specific code of ethics, the more stable, warm, and nurturant the family, the more likely the child is to introject its value system.

Empathy with the victim. Most of us feel bonds of empathy and compassion towards other humans, especially those with whom we identify because of their similarity, familiarity, or proximity. The greater this empathy, the more reluctant we are to injure them (Baron, 1977).

Utilitarian concerns. Two closely related practical considerations can also increase inhibitions—the likelihood of retaliation and the probability of success. If it appears that aggression will result in bad things happening to the aggressor, or that the attack will fail in accomplishing its intrinsic or extrinsic objective, these cost-benefit considerations can increase inhibitions.

Decreasing Inhibitions

Inhibitions that took years to acquire can often be offset in a matter of minutes. This is generally discouraging for those of us dealing with criminal behavior; except for the unusual case of the Chronically Overcontrolled Assaultive Type (Megargee, 1966), we are generally attempting to foster rather than diminish inhibitions, especially among potential assassins.

Clinicians might have different goals for nonviolent patients suffering from cardiovascular disorders. If blocked instigation is an etiological factor in CHD or other physical disorders, reducing inhibitions in order to facilitate socially appropriate expression of instigation might be therapeutic.

Physical Mechanisms for Reducing Inhibitions

Obviously, chemically-induced inhibitions can be diminished by withdrawing the tranquilizing medication. Learned inhibitions against aggression, including those stemming from anticipation of punishment, introjected societal values and bonds of empathy with the victim, can all be decreased by the ingestion of substances which anesthetize the cortex (most notably alcohol). As Seneca noted, "Drunkenness does not create vices, but it brings them to the fore." Because of alcohol's inhibition-lowering effects, no drug, with the possible exception of phencyclidine (PCP), is more closely linked with aggression and violence.

Psychological Mechanisms for Reducing Inhibitions

Some inhibitions stem from the anticipation of punishment. If, despite their fears, people engage in aggressive behavior and the anticipated punishment is not forthcoming, then these conditioned inhibitions will decrease. Observing others aggress with impunity will also lower inhibitions. The children who observed the irate Little Leaguer successfully act out against an adult probably had their inhibitions against criticizing authorities decreased somewhat by the incident.

Inhibitions based on moral prohibitions or values can be overcome by rationalization and neutralization techniques (Sykes & Matza, 1957). We use rationalization to convince ourselves that our case is an exception to the general rule; 250 years before Freud, Moliere wrote, "There's nothing people can't contrive to praise or condemn and find justification for doing so, according to their age and inclinations."

Conflicting values, as manifested by some appeal to a higher authority, assist in neutralizing inhibitions against aggression. A father who beat his eight year old son with a baseball bat after the child performed poorly during a ballgame asserted, "As with any normal parent there comes a time when you . . . discipline the child." ("Man beats son," 1983). One reason we have instituted independent panels of peers to review our research proposals is that investigations such as Milgram's (1965) have demonstrated how easily we can convince ourselves that the benefits of our particular study justify the stress or pain we may inflict on our human or animal subjects.

Compartmentalization is another effective neutralization technique. The notion that we should be altruistic and love our neighbors is fine for church on Sunday, but not for the office on Monday. As Charles Dickens noted in *Martin Chuzzlewit,* " 'Do other men for they would do you.' That's the true business precept."

Tactics which decrease the aggressor's individual responsibility and humanity can also lessen inhibitions. If a white man is part of a mob and his identity is hidden by a white robe and hood, it is easier for him to participate in lynching a black person. Inhibitions against aggression can also be lowered by decreasing any empathy felt toward the potential target. This can be done by isolating victims or adversaries, minimizing communications with them, and emphasizing their differences (Baron, 1977). These principles apply in circumstances ranging from hostage-taking situations to labor-management negotiations.

Implications for Prevention and Treatment

There is a great need for research on the relation of inhibitions to health. Inhibitions determine whether instigation is suppressed or expressed, directly or indirectly, turned outward or inward. Is the hard driving competitiveness of the Type A personality a manifestation of the achievement motive or sublimated instigation to aggression whose direct expression has been blocked by inhibitions? Have inhibitions displaced the target of aggression from parents to competitors? What are the physical consequences of suppressing versus expressing annoyance, anger, or rage?

Such research will be complicated by the fact that inhibitions are more difficult to assess than either instigation or habit strength (Megargee, 1983). [A nonaggressive behavior pattern is not sufficient evidence of strong inhibitions since such a pattern could also stem from low instigation. Some psychological test measures have been developed, but most are indirect at best (Megargee, 1967; 1971)].

Even if these measurement problems are solved, it seems unlikely that research will yield any simple solutions. In addition to physiological and psychological consequences of different ways of dealing with animosity, clinicians will also need to consider the social consequences for each individual. Aggression is, by necessity, an interpersonal interaction, and the overall effects of encouraging or discouraging aggression by increasing or decreasing inhibitions can not be considered in isolation. Such behavior will have an impact on others whose behavior will, in turn, influence the individual. Thus, even with a sounder empirical understanding of the health consequences of inhibiting aggressive behavior, it is most unlikely we will arrive at any simple solutions or universal panaceas.

SITUATIONAL FACTORS

Situational factors that can either facilitate or impede the overt expression of aggression are the final variables to be considered in the algebra of aggression. If we recall the case of the aggressive advertising agent, the fact that his adversary was with a table full of friends was a situational factor inhibiting a physical attack. On the other hand, in the case of the belligerent ballplayer, the chorus of protests by fellow players and their parents facilitated the verbal expression of aggression.

Monahan and Klassen (1982) recently delineated several issues that must be considered in evaluating the influence of situational factors: "They are (1) the definition of a situation or environment, (2) the size of the environmental unit to be employed, (3) the perceived versus the actual situation, and (4) the interactive nature of persons and situations." We shall discuss each in turn.

Defining Situational Factors

There is general agreement that all behavior is a function of the interaction of personality and situational factors [$B = f(P \cdot S)$], but this consensus rapidly breaks down when one asks people to define what they mean by "personal" or "situational." We shall adopt Monahan and Klassen's crude but common sense demarkation, "The boundary line used here appears to be the person's skin: Within the skin is the 'person,' outside the skin is the 'environment'" (1982, p. 293).[6]

Size of the Environmental Unit

Environments, settings, situations, and stimuli are often used interchangably in the ecological literature, but this author will arbitrarily treat these terms as points marking a rough continuum from extremely broad and pervasive influences (environments) to quite narrow and specific ones (stimuli). Analyses at each level are potentially informative.

Environments

This means pervasive influences such as the culture ("When in Rome do as the Romans do"), the climate, and the state of the economy. Being in midtown Manhattan in the 20th century during a recession were environmental factors contributing to our advertising agent's inhibitions against challenging his rival to a duel or resigning after being criticized.

Settings

Settings are various realms we find ourselves in as we go about our daily activities; these include family, work, recreation, social and religious settings. Some settings are private, others public; some are in our home territory and others are away; in some we can control events and in others we must respond

---

[6] In adopting this definition we will not tolerate any quibbling over such sophistries as whether a bullet is transformed from a situational to a personal variable when it hits a person in the shoulder and fails to exit.

to them. Part of our advertising agent's embarrassment stemmed from attempting to deal with commercial issues in a social setting and from abruptly having to shift from his semiprivate world of aggressive fantasy to the public realm of external reality.

Situations

These are somewhat narrower sets of circumstances that are immediately present. For violence to occur, there must be an aggressor and a victim in close proximity. The behavior of bystanders, who might intervene or incite violence, and the availability of weapons are important factors. In our example, the physical characteristics and ambience of the lounge and the behavior of the potential victim and various bystanders could strongly influence the course of events.

Stimuli

Stimuli are very specific events. If the secretary said, "If you're really man enough to hit him, he's over there," this challenging statement would have constituted a *stimulus*. In an aggressive interaction, stimuli and responses often follow one another in rapid succession.

All these levels, from environments to stimuli, can be informative in analyzing the distant and proximate causes of aggression. Different investigators naturally focus on the level that is most germane to their interests and relevant to their research. In their laboratories, experimental social psychologists typically examine stimuli, whereas, in the field, cultural anthropologists are more likely to study environments or settings. Unfortunately, there is a tendency for researchers to fixate on the level which they have chosen to analyze and ignore those which are broader or narrower.

Perceived Versus Actual Situations

Some researchers study the actual characteristics of settings such as population density, the amount of space available, or ambient temperature (Megargee, 1977). Others focus on their subjects' *perceptions* of the environment, such as whether they *feel* crowded or hot. Novaco (1979), for example, maintains that it is cognitive apprasials and expectancies that determine whether or not a person will experience a stimulus as frustrating.

Person-Situation Interactions

The fact that we have chosen to "freeze the action" and focus on the dynamics associated with a particular aggressive response at a single point in time should not blind us to the fact that aggressive behavior typically involves an ongoing interpersonal interaction in which each person influences the other. Many incidents of violence stem from complex scenarios in which it is not at all certain who will eventually be the perpetrator or the victim (Luckenbill & Sanders, 1977; Toch, 1969). Indeed, Wolfgang (1957) demonstrated that many homicides can be classified as victim-precipitated. Less extreme aggressive interactions can also be complex, involving give-and-take by both parties, as any labor-management arbitrator or marital counselor can testify.

One approach to studying situations is to investigate their demand characteristics. Bem and Funder (1978) suggested that assessment and prediction of behavior would be improved by examining how different types of settings influence different types of people, then basing the prediction on the person-setting match.

Some social ecologists overlook the fact that there is a two-way interaction between people and settings (Monahan & Klassen, 1982). It is true that people behave differently in a church than they do in a stadium, but we must not overlook the fact that they chose whether to attend religious services or a football game. By choosing to repair to a public place apparently frequented by advertising people instead of going home or working late, our account executive consciously or unconsciously increased the risk of encountering his rival. W. C. Fields acknowledged the influence of personal choices on situations when he wryly admitted, "I always keep a supply of stimulant handy in case I see a snake—which I also keep handy."

This interactive nature of situations and personality patterns is evident in the life-style of the Type A person. Many suffer from chronic stress stemming from multiple commitments, short deadlines, and intense pressure to achieve high personal goals. Yet clinical and experimental research indicates that the Type A person creates this lifestyle with ever-expanding goals and efforts to achieve more and more in less and less time (Chesney & Rosenman, 1983).

Would changing the setting alter their behavior significantly? Probably not. This author recently played golf with a vacationing attorney. Even though the attorney was 3000 miles from his office and had no commitments or demands on his time, he became very upset, pounding the ground with his driver, when the foursome ahead halted play to conduct a leisurely search for a lost ball. Later, at the resort's video game room, he discovered a new challenge, PacMan; the rest of his vacation was spent attempting to set a new record for the game.

Implications for Prevention and Treatment

Using situations to make behavioral predictions involves answering three basic questions (Bem & Funder, 1978; Monahan & Klassen, 1982):

1) What are the characteristics of the situations in which the person has engaged in this behavior in the past? If we are discussing the competitiveness and drive that characterize the Type A person, this means analyzing the settings and situations which elicited these Type A behavior patterns. This approach can also be applied to cardiovascular symptoms such as angina or high blood pressure.

2) What are the characteristics of the situations the person will be facing in the future?

3) How similar are the situations the person will face in the future to those which elicited the stress, competitiveness, or symptomatic reactions in the past?

If this situational analysis suggests that the behavior in question has a high probability of recurring, then one approach may lie in attempting to innoculate the individual, influencing expectations or cognitions so as to lessen the stress (Monahan & Klassen, 1982; Novaco, 1979). Another would be to intervene at the situational level, altering the contingencies or demands so as to make them less stressful for the person in question.

RESPONSE COMPETITION

Response competition is the final element in the algebra of aggression. The algebraic sum of instigation, habit strength, inhibitions, and situational factors facilitating and impeding a particular aggressive act directed at a given target determines its "reaction potential." If the reaction potential is greater than zero—if the forces favoring the aggressive response outweigh those opposing it—then the act is possible. Before it can actually be performed it must compete with other possible responses—some aggressive, others nonaggressive—that may lead to greater satisfactions with fewer costs.

The phenomenon of response competition complicates the interpretation of research findings. If a subject makes an aggressive response, the experimenter can conclude that the factors favoring an aggressive response outweighed those inhibiting it. The reverse is not true. Failure to act aggressively does not necessarily mean that inhibitory factors blocked the excitatory ones; it could be that some other response was selected that yielded more satisfactions.

IMPLICATIONS OF THE DYNAMICS OF AGGRESSION FOR RESEARCH ON CARDIOVASCULAR DISORDERS

H. L. Mencken could have been describing many current theories on the role of aggression in the etiology of cardiovascular disorders when he wrote, "There's always an easy solution to every human problem—neat, plausible and wrong." The primary goal of the present chapter has been to emphasize the complexity of the dynamics of aggression and to present a conceptual framework that should make it easier for medical researchers to cope with that complexity.

A major problem in investigating the relationship between cardiovascular disorders and aggressive emotions, attitudes and behavior is obtaining reliable and valid measures of the various unobservable constructs that enter into the algebra of aggression.[7] Unfortunately, people do not come supplied with dipsticks in their skulls which we can use to check their instigation or inhibition levels.

Surveying the literature on the assessment of animosity and aggression, Megargee and Menzies (1971, p. 156) concluded:

> The eagerness of psychologists to invent new techniques has prevented premature fixation on a particular approach, but too many workers... have too little regard for empirically establishing their reliability, validity, and generality... Too many investigations, involving thousands of man hours and dollars, have been crippled by the use of an unvalidated, hastily constructed "test" as the independent or dependent measure...
>
> More studies are needed to determine the interrelationships and redundancy of existing tests and to make recommendations as to those that should be used in future

---

[7] *Reliability* refers to the consistency of measures; *validity* indicates whether they measure what they are supposed to. Practical validity refers to whether a scale can accurately assess or can predict some observable criterion, such as the occurence of CHD. *Construct* validity, as noted in Footnote 1, refers to whether a scale actually assesses the unobservable trait (construct) that it is supposed to measure.

research (Megargee & Cook, 1967). The next logical step is to find how these measures relate to different criteria of aggression in various populations.

Our review ... also showed that most tests are based on an oversimplified concept of aggression. The need is for a new generation of sophisticated instruments that will assess inhibitions and instigation as a function of situational events and stimuli, along with studies of how these factors interact to produce overt aggression, displacement, response substitution, and the like.

A dozen years later, test authors are more concerned about establishing the psychometric properties of their instruments, but the other conclusions still apply. Researchers investigating the relationship of intrinsic instigation to cardiovascular disorders can choose from a number of competing measures of anger and hostility, some newly derived and others adopted from scales developed earlier; we must establish how these scales relate to one another. In contrast, there is a dearth of measures assessing other relevant constructs, such as inhibitions, habit strength, and situational or ecological factors.

Establishing the construct validity of existing scales is of the utmost importance. Recent research using Cook and Medley's (1954) Hostility (*Ho*) scale illustrates the problem of interpreting data derived using insufficiently validated scales. Williams et al. (1980) have demonstrated noteworthy concurrent associations between *Ho* scale scores and the occurrence of coronary occlusions. If it is established that *Ho* can predict as well as postdict such disorders, then the scale can be of enormous *practical* value in helping to identify those people who are most likely to develop coronary artery disease. However, until the construct validity of the *Ho* scale is established, until we can be sure it actually assesses hostility, such associations tell us nothing about the role of hostility in cardiovascular disorders.

One way of evaluating a scale is to examine the procedures used in deriving it. The *Ho* scale was constructed by comparing the MMPI scores of Minnesota teachers who scored in the top and bottom 8% on yet another paper-and-pencil test, the Minnesota Teacher Aptitude Inventory. The MMPI items that characterized the poor teachers were identified through empirical item analyses; there was no cross-validation to eliminate those that might have appeared significant by chance alone. These items were next submitted to five judges who sorted them into two scales, "hostility" and "pharisaic virtue." The latter scale has lapsed into well-deserved obscurity; *Ho* has not.

What evidence is there that *Ho* actually measures hostility? The manifest content cited by Williams et al. (1980) could reflect hostility, but one could just as easily argue that the items assess rigidity or authoritarianism, especially since 94% of them are keyed "true." Schless, Mendels, Kipperman, and Cochrane (1974) administered the *Ho* scale, along with a number of other measures, to 37 clinically depressed patients. Factor analyzing the results, they reported that *Ho* loaded on the factor they interpreted as reflecting suspiciousness and resentment rather than the factor they felt indicated overt hostility. Snoke (1955) found college students with high *Ho* scores were more apt to miss appointments, and McGee (1954) noted high scorers were more apt to attribute hostility to pictures of mental patients in the Szondi test. None of these findings is sufficient to convince us of the scale's construct validity.

Pallis and Birtchnell (1976) found no overall differences among large samples of men and women who (a) attempted suicide, (b) thought about suicide, or

(c) had no suicidal activity. However, in a subsequent study these authors reported that patients who made a non-serious suicide attempt had significantly higher *Ho* scores than samples of patients who had made serious attempts or who had never been suicidal. The mean *Ho* scores of the latter two groups were virtually identical. Thus *Ho* did not have a consistent or predictable relationship with suicidal behavior.

Most distressing is the failure of *Ho* to detect differences in overt hostility or aggression. Shipman (1965) reported that *Ho* failed to correlate significantly with reliable ratings of a) verbal hostility, b) physical hostility, and c) hostile attitudes in a sample of 120 psychiatric outpatients. In two independent studies the present writer and his colleagues failed to find any systematic or significant relationship between *Ho* scale scores and criminal violence (Megargee & Mendelsohn, 1962; Megargee, Cook, & Mendelsohn, 1967), but Deiker (1974) found that property offenders had significantly *higher* Hostility scale scores than criminals who a) threatened violence, b) assaulted people inflicting injuries, or c) committed homicide.

All in all, the evidence for the construct validity of the *Ho* scale is minimal. Thirty years after its derivation it is difficult to say with any confidence what *Ho* measures.

What about the newer measures? Are they assessing intrinsic instigation? If so, is it anger or hostility, rage or hate? Or are they detecting some generalized propensity toward aggression, a mixture of intrinsic and extrinsic instigation, inhibitions and habit strength? Answering these questions should be given high priority.

Much more needs to be known about the interrelationships among the various measures being used in behavioral medicine research. What are their strengths and weaknesses? Can they predict behavior or disease, or do they only reflect what is already known about the patient?[8] Above all, their construct validity needs to be established. Until this is done, researchers would do well to risk redundancy and use several scales in each study. The time and expense involved in administering "too many" tests is usually miniscule compared with the cost of obtaining other data, especially in longitudinal investigations. If the primary test or measure later proves invalid, the extra testing may salvage an expensive research program.

The development and validation of improved assessment techniques will obviously not resolve all the difficult challenges confronting behavioral medicine research. Improved experimental methods with more precise measures of other relevant variables, additional longitudinal and predictive studies using better sampling methods, and an integration of human with infrahuman research as well as laboratory with clinical studies are all needed. But failure to appreciate the complexity of the dynamics of aggression and the associated measurement problems will "occlude" progress in research and may even lead to fatal errors. Moreover, there is no way to bypass this type of blockage. The basic measurement problems must be faced and solved.

---

[8] In technical terms, do they have predictive as well as concurrent validity? The former is obviously much more useful but also much more difficult to establish. The power of the Type A personality syndrome as assessed by the Structured Interview is that it can forecast future occurrences of CHD (i.e., has predictive validity). Assessment of present CHD (concurrent validity) can obviously be done more accurately and simply by using direct medical measures of CHD.

REFERENCES

Bandura, A., & Walters, R. H. *Adolescent aggression.* New York: Ronald, 1959.
Baron, R. A. *Human aggression.* New York: Plenum, 1977.
Bem, D., & Funder, D. Predicting more of the people more of the time: Assessing the personality of situations. *Psychological Review,* 1978, *85,* 485-501.
Berkowitz, L. *Aggression: A social psychological analysis.* New York: McGraw-Hill, 1962.
Berkowitz, L. (Ed.). *Roots of aggression: A reexamination of the frustration-aggression hypothesis.* New York: Atherton, 1969.
Blackburn, R. Personality in relation to extreme aggression in psychiatric offenders. *British Journal of Psychiatry,* 1968, *114,* 821-828.
Brown, P., & Elliott, R. Control of aggression in nursery school class. *Journal of Experimental Child Psychology,* 1965, *2,* 103-107.
Buss, A. H. *The psychology of aggression.* New York: Wiley, 1961.
Chesney, M. A., Black, G. W., Chadwick, J. H., & Rosenman, R. H. Physiological correlates of the Type A behavior pattern. *Journal of Behavioral Medicine,* 1981, *4,* 217-229.
Chesney, M. A. & Rosenman, R. H. Specificity in stress models: Examples drawn from Type A behavior. In C. Cooper (Ed.) *Stress Research,* London: Wiley, 1983.
Cook, W. W., & Medley, D. M. Proposed hostility and pharisaic virtue scales for the MMPI. *Journal of Applied Psychology,* 1954, *38,* 414-418.
Davis, K. R., & Sines, J. O. Antisocial behavior pattern associated with a specific MMPI profile. *Journal of Consulting and Clinical Psychology,* 1971, *36,* 229-234.
Deiker, T. E. A cross-validation of MMPI scales of aggression on male criminal criterion groups. *Journal of Consulting and Clinical Psychology,* 1974, *42,* 196-202.
Dollard, J., Doob, L. W., Miller, N. E., Mowrer, O. H., & Sears, R. R. *Frustration and aggression.* New Haven, Conn., Yale University Press, 1939.
Fine, B. J. Field-dependent introvert and neuroticism: Eysenck and Witkin united. *Psychological Reports,* 1972, *31*(3), 936-939.
Frederiksen, S. J. *A comparison of selected personality and history variables in highly violent, mildly violent, and nonviolent female offenders.* Unpublished doctoral dissertation, University of Minnesota, 1975.
Freud, S. Beyond the pleasure principle. In J. Strachey (Ed.), *The standard edition of the complete psychological works of Sigmund Freud* (Vol. 18). London: Hogarth, 1955. (Originally published, 1920.)
Gamble, K. R. The Holtzman inkblot technique: A review. *Psychological Bulletin,* 1972, *77,* 172-194.
Geen, R. G., & Donnerstein, E. I. (Eds.). *Aggression: Theoretical and empirical reviews, Vol. 1: Theoretical and methodological issues.* New York: Academic, 1983a.
Geen, R. G., & Donnerstein, E. I. (Eds.). *Aggression: Theoretical and empirical reviews, Vol. 2: Issues in research.* New York: Academic, 1983b.
Glass, D. C. *Behavior patterns, stress, and coronary heart disease.* Hillsdale, N.J.: Erlbaum, 1977.
Haven, H. J. Descriptive and developmental characteristics of chronically overcontrolled hostile prisoners. *FCI Research Reports,* 1972, *4*(6), 1-40.
Hokanson, J. E. Psychophysiological evaluation of the catharsis hypothesis. In E. I. Megargee & J. E. Hokanson (Eds.), *The dynamics of aggression: Individual, group, and international analyses.* New York: Harper & Row, 1970.
Johnson, R. N. *Aggression in man and animals.* Philadelphia: Saunders, 1972.
Lane, P. J. Annotated bibliography of the overcontrolled-undercontrolled assaultive personality literature and the overcontrolled-hostility (O-H) scale of the MMPI. JSAS *Catalog of Selected Documents in Psychology,* 1978, *8,* (Ms. No. 1760)
Lorenz, K. [*On aggression*] (trans. by M. K. Wilson). New York: Bantam, 1966.
Luckenbill, D. F., & Sanders, W. B. Criminal violence. In E. Sagarin & F. Montanino (Eds.), *Deviants: Voluntary actors in a hostile world.* Morristown, N.J.: General Learning, 1977.
Man beats son with baseball bat after youth doesn't hustle in game. *Tallahassee Democrat,* April 26, 1983, p. 1.
Mark, V. H. & Ervin S. R. *Violence and the brain.* New York: Harper & Row, 1970.
Megargee, E. I. Undercontrolled and overcontrolled personality types in extreme antisocial aggression. *Psychological Monographs,* 1966, *80,* (3, Whole No. 611).

Megargee, E. I. Hostility on the TAT as a function of defensive inhibition and stimulus situation. *Journal of Projective Techniques and Personality Assessment*, 1967, *31*(4), 73-79.

Megargee, E. I. The psychology of violence: A critical review of theories of violence. In D. J. Mulvihill & M. M. Tumin (Eds.), *Crimes of violence: A staff report to the National Commission on the Causes and Prevention of Violence. NCCPV Staff Report Series* (Vol. 13). Washington, D.C.: U.S. Government Printing Office, 1969.

Megargee, E. I. The prediction of violence with psychological tests. In C. D. Spielberger (Ed.), *Current topics in clinical and community psychology* (Vol. 2). New York: Academic, 1970.

Megargee, E. I. The role of inhibition in the assessment and understanding of violence. In J. E. Singer (Ed.), *The control of aggression and violence: Cognitive and physiological factors*. New York: Academic, 1971.

Megargee, E. I. The association of population density, reduced space and uncomfortable temperatures with misconduct in a prison community. *American Journal of Community Psychology*, 1977, *5*, 289-298.

Megargee, E. I. Psychological correlates and determinants of criminal violence. In M. E. Wolfgang & N. Weiner (Eds.) *Criminal violence*. Beverly Hills, Calif.: Sage, 1982.

Megargee, E. I., Aggression and violence. In H. Adams & P. Sutker, (Eds.), *Comprehensive handbook of psychopathology*. New York: Plenum, 1983.

Megargee, E. I., & Cook, P. E. The relation of TAT and inkblot aggressive content scales with each other and with criteria of overt aggressiveness in juvenile delinquents. *Journal of Projective Techniques and Personality Assessment*, 1967, *31*(1), 48-60.

Megargee, E. I., Cook, P. E., & Mendelsohn, G. A. The development and validation of an MMPI scale of assaultiveness in overcontrolled individuals. *Journal of Abnormal Psychology*, 1967, *72*, 519-528.

Megargee, E. I., & Mendelsohn, G. A. A cross-validation of 12 MMPI indices of hostility and control. *Journal of Abnormal and Social Psychology*, 1962, *65*, 431-438.

Megargee, E. I., & Menzies, E. The assessment and dynamics of aggression. In P. McReynolds (Ed.), *Advances in psychological assessment* (Vol. 2). Palo Alto, Calif.: Science and Behavior, 1971.

Milgram, S. Some conditions of obedience and disobedience to authority. In I. D. Steiner & M. Fishbine (Eds.), *Current studies in social psychology*. New York: Holt, 1965.

Miller, N. E. The frustration-aggression hypothesis. *Psychological Review*, 1941, *48*, 337-342.

Molof, M. J. *Differences between assaultive and nonassaultive juvenile offenders in the California Youth Authority*. Research report No. 51, Division of Research, State of California, Department of Youth Authority, February, 1967.

Monahan, J., & Klassen, D. Situational approaches to understanding and predicting individual violent behavior. In M. E. Wolfgang & N. A. Weiner (Eds.), *Criminal violence*. Beverly Hills, Calif.: Sage, 1982.

Morley, C., & Everett, L. D. (Eds.). *Familiar quotations by John Bartlett* (12th ed.). Boston: Little, Brown, 1948.

Novaco, R. The cognitive regulation of anger and stress. In P. Kendall & S. Hollon (Eds.), *Cognitive-behavioral interventions: Theory, research, and procedures*. New York: Academic, 1979.

Pallis, D. J., & Birtchnell, J. Personality and suicidal history in psychiatric patients. *Journal of Clinical Psychology*, 1976, *32*, 246-253.

Pallis, D. J., & Birtchnell, J. Seriousness of suicide attempt in relation to personality. *British Journal of Psychiatry*, 1977, *130*, 253-259.

Pastore, N. The role of arbitrariness in the frustration-aggression hypothesis. *Journal of abnormal and Social Psychology*, 1952, *47*, 728-731.

Pastore, N. The role of arbitrariness in the frustration-aggression hypothesis. *Journal of Abnormal and Social Psychology*, 1952, *47*, 728-731.

Peter, L. J. *Peter's quotations: Ideas for our time*. New York: Morrow, 1977.

Press, A. Not guilty because of PMS? *Newsweek*, November 8, 1982, p. 111.

Quinsey, V. L., Maguire, A., & Varney, G. Assertion and overcontrolled hostility among mentally disordered murderers. *Journal of Consulting and Clinical Psychology*, 1983, *51*, 550-556.

Schless, A. P., Mendels, M. D., Kipperman, A., & Cochrane, C. Depression hostility. *Journal of Nervous and Mental Diseases*. 1974, *159*, 91-100.

Shipman, W. G. The validity of MMPI hostility scales. *Journal of Clinical Psychology*, 1965, *21*, 186-190.

Smith, A. A new life. *Sports Illustrated*, March 28, 1983, *58*, p. 74.

Snoke, M. L. *A study in the behavior of men students of high and low measured hostility under two conditions of goal clarity.* Unpublished doctoral dissertation, University of Minnesota, 1955.
Spielberger, C. D. Theory and research on anxiety. C. D. Spielberger (Ed.), *Anxiety and behavior.* New York: Academic, 1966.
Stein, K. B. Correlates of the ideational preference dimension among prison inmates. *Psychological Reports,* 1967, *21,* 553-562.
Sykes, G. M., & Matza, D. Techniques of neutralization: A theory of delinquency. *American Sociological Review,* 1957, *22,* 664-670.
Terkel, S. *Working.* New York: Pantheon, 1974.
Toch, H. *Violent men.* Chicago: Aldine, 1969.
Tripp, R. T. (Ed.). *The international thesaurus of quotations.* New York: Crowell, 1970.
Wenk, E. A., & Emrich, R. L. Assaultive youth: An exploratory study of the assaultive experience and assaultive potential of California Youth Authority wards. *Journal of Research in Crime and Delinquency,* 1972, *9*(2), 171-176.
Williams, R. B., Haney, T. L., Lee, K. L., Kong, Y., Blumenthal, J. A., & Whalen, R. E. Type A behavior, hostility and coronary atherosclerosis. *Psychosomatic Medicine,* 1980, *42,* 539-549.
Wolfgang, M. E. Victim-precipitated criminal homicide. *Journal of Criminal Law, Criminology, and Police Science,* 1957, *48,* 1-11.
Wolfgang, M. E., & Weiner, N. (Eds.). *Criminal violence.* Beverly Hills: Sage, 1982.

3
The Measurement of Anger as a Multidimensional Construct

Judith M. Siegel
UCLA School of Public Health

Research on risk factors for cardiovascular diseases has identified a number of behavioral attributes that characterize persons prone to poor cardiovascular health. These attributes include a constellation of behaviors called the Type A behavior pattern, life dissatisfaction, anxiety, self-abasement, status incongruity, and angry feelings. Although the Type A behavior pattern has received the strongest empirical support in terms of its relationship with coronary heart disease (CHD), there is evidence which suggests that anger, a component of the Type A behavior pattern, may be a predictor of a wide range of cardiovascular diseases including hypertension and atherosclerosis. In this paper, the evidence supportive of a relationship between anger[1] and cardiovascular disease will be reviewed, followed by preliminary data relevant to the development of a multidimensional inventory of anger.

Anger has been identified as a potential risk factor for cardiovascular disease via three pathways: (1) its relationship with elevated blood pressure (BP), (2) as a major component of the Type A behavior pattern, and (3) its relationship to coronary atherosclerosis. With regard to the first pathway, in the inaugural issue of *Psychosomatic Medicine,* Alexander (1939) described a tentative hypothesis concerning an association between suppressed anger and elevated BP. According to Alexander, the person with elevated BP is caught in a psychodynamic conflict of passiveness and hostile impulses. When these impulses are repressed, a chronic tension is created. Since acute elevations of BP are the normal reaction to rage, it was assumed that chronic inhibition of rage would lead to chronic elevations of BP.

In the absence of longitudinal data, it is difficult to conclude that anger (suppressed or otherwise) causes permanent elevations in BP. Furthermore, the necessity of hypothesizing a "psychodynamic" conflict is debatable. Nonetheless, there has accumulated an impressive body of cross-sectional data which suggest

---

Funds for this research were in part provided by a UCLA Faculty Career Development Award to the author, and in part by grant 1-R01 HL25005-01A1, "Noise and the Epidemiology of Blood Pressure," awarded to Lewis Kuller, Principal Investigator, Evelyn Talbott, Gerald Redmond, Karen Matthews, Co-Principal Investigators.

[1] The terms anger and hostility will be used interchangeably. While Buss (1961) differentiates between anger, as an emotional response, and hostility, as a behavioral response, other researchers have not systematically made this distinction.

that conflicts with anger are characteristic of the hypertensive. For example, a series of studies by Harris and Kalis (Harris et al., 1953; Kalis et al., 1961; Kalis et al., 1957) showed that prehypertensive college women (pressures at or above 140/90) and adult female essential hypertensives differed from normotensive controls in that they were more self-punishing and exhibited more signs of suppressing anger. During staged interpersonal dramas, rated by multiple observers who were unaware of the participants' BP status the hypertensives were also described as being maladaptively hostile and assertive.

More recently, research by Hokanson (1961a, 1961b; Hokanson & Burgess, 1962) indicates a relationship between anger expression and vascular processes. Taken together, Hokanson's studies show that BP will rise in response to a variety of frustrations, and in males may return to normal levels more quickly if there is an opportunity to aggress against the equal- or low-status perpetrator of the frustration than with no opportunity to aggress, while in females a "friendly" counter-response is more effective than an aggressive one. However, counter-response to a high status perpetrator may actually be "tension" producing in both men and women. Although Holmes (1966) presents results that are directly contrary to Hokanson, that is, those not allowed to aggress reduced their arousal more, these experimental studies can be interpreted as supporting the hypothesis that conflicts over anger are related to vascular processes. These studies do not clearly show, however, that the mode of expression of the anger is the critical element.

Some of the most interesting evidence for the conflict over anger hypothesis comes from community-based studies. The Israeli Ischemic Heart Disease Study (Kahn et al., 1972) showed that self-reports of brooding and restraint of retaliation in response to being hurt by one's superior are related to incidence of hypertension among 10,000 male civil service workers. In the United States, Harburg and colleagues (Harburg, Blakelock, & Roeper, 1979; Harburg et al., 1973) have demonstrated a relationship between resentment and BP among blacks living in high stress areas of Detroit. Esler and colleagues (Esler et al., 1977) used an adaptation of Harburg's anger items and determined that the hostility-BP relationship may be specific to a particular sub-type of hypertensive (e.g., those with high renin levels).

Baer and colleagues (Baer et al., 1979) used a discriminant function analysis to derive a set of statements that could differentiate hypertensives from normotensives. Subsequent analysis revealed that anxiety and hostility were the most potent discriminators. Finally, a school-based study (Siegel & Leitch, 1981) revealed that adolescents who had elevated blood pressures on two occasions (above the 90th percentile for their age and sex) scored higher on the Edwards Personality Inventory "Becomes Angry" scale (Edwards, 1966) than did normotensive adolescents. This association was mediated by body mass, however.

In sum, that data do support a relationship between anger and elevated BP, although the existing studies cannot rule out the possibility that anger may be secondary to hypertension, either as an emotional response to the diagnosis or as a manifestation of changes of physiology, or both. Longitudinal studies of an initially normotensive cohort are needed. (More extensive reviews of the personality correlated of hypertension can be found elsewhere (Cochrane, 1971; Davies, 1971; McGinn et al., 1964; Harrell, 1980; Diamond, 1982).)

The second pathway through which anger has been related to cardiovascular disease is as a component of the Type A behavior pattern. The Type A individual, who is at elevated risk for CHD, is characterized by extremes of competitive-achievement striving, aggressiveness-hostility, and speed-impatience (Rosenman, 1978). Because Type A classification is typically based on a simple preponderance of Type A characteristics, not all Type As will manifest all Type A characteristics. Using the interview method of Type A classification, the overall behavior type assessment (e.g., Type A or Type B) is essentially a clinical judgment which relies on the interviewer's ratings of behavior and speech characteristics manifested during the interview, and, to a lesser extent, on content of response.

Although this global behavior type assessment is most frequently used as the unit of analysis, it is possible to derive component scores of Type A behavior (e.g., hard-driving, hostility) from the interview ratings. Those studies which do use component scores of Pattern A as predictors of cardiovascular disease make evident the importance of hostility. Jenkins (1966), for example, reported data from the Western Collaborative Group Study, the major prospective investigation of Type A behavior and heart disease. Silent myocardial infarction cases were matched with two controls and compared on demographic and behavior variables. Self-reports of frequent hostility were associated with higher levels of cholesterol in both groups. Cases scored higher on potential for hostility than controls, as assessed by interviewers' ratings. The interviewer's rating of potential for hostility is based on voice cues and on facial and postural gestures exhibited during the interview.

Matthews and colleagues (Matthews et al., 1977) further analyzed data from the Western Collaborative Group Study. CHD cases and healthy controls were compared with regard to their responses to the Type A interview. Of the seven interview items that were capable of discriminating cases from controls, four were related to anger/hostility. Two of these four items were respondents' self-reports of anger (endorsing that their anger is frequently directed outward and that they get angry more than once a week), and two of the items were ratings made by the interviewer (explosive voice modulation and potential for hostility).

Another line of evidence that emphasizes the importance of the anger/hostility component of the Type A pattern comes from studies on the cardiovascular reponses of Type As and Bs. While the two types typically do not differ in baseline levels of the traditional risk factors for heart disease (e.g., BP, serum cholesterol), they do differ in the magnitude of BP and catecholamine response to environmental and biochemical challenges (see Matthews, 1982, for a review of this literature). It is hypothesized that this excessive sympathetic response may be the mechanism through which Pattern A exerts its pathogenic effect. Elevations in systolic BP are thought to damage the inner layer of the coronary arteries, thereby increasing the likelihood of atherosclerosis and subsequent coronary heart disease (Herd, 1978).

Several studies have examined the components of Pattern A as predictors of sympathetic response. For example, Demroski and colleagues (1978) showed that hostility, as rated by the interviewer, is the component most highly predictive of increases in systolic BP in response to challenge. A follow-up study (Dembroski et al., 1979) indicated that individuals who are classified as Type A, and who also are rated by the interviewer as hostile and verbally competitive, maintain a high level of physiological arousal regardless of the level of experimental challenge. Low hostility Type As, on the other hand, exhibit marked arousal only in highly challenging situations and resemble Type Bs in the magnitude of their BP response.

A comparison of cardiac cases and controls also supports the importance of the hostility dimension (Dembroski et al., 1979). Using the structured interview for behavior type classification, cases were more likely to be classified as Type A than controls. More importantly, the cases were rated by the interviewer as more hostile than the Type A controls, even when only Type A cases and controls were compared. Subsequent analysis showed that the Type As exhibited a greater BP response to the experimental tasks than did Type Bs, and that hostility manifested during the interview was related to changes in BP within the Type A sample alone. In sum, research on the Type A behavior pattern indicates that hostility discriminates cardiac cases from controls, and furthermore, that hostility is the component of Pattern A that is most highly predictive of the excessive sympathetic response that characterizes Type As.

The final pathway through which anger is associated with cardiovascular disease is the relationship of anger with coronary atherosclerosis. Williams and colleagues (1980) administered the Type A interview and a battery of self-report instruments to their sample of coronary angiography patients. Included among these instruments were the Minnesota Multiphasic Personality Inventory (MMPI), a depression rating scale, an anxiety rating scale, a life change questionnaire, and a social support network questionnaire. Previous research (Cook & Medley, 1954) had identified a subset of the MMPI items as a measure of hostility. Williams and colleagues report that gender, the MMPI hostility score, and behavior type classification (A or B), in that order, were the strongest (and independent) predictors of degree of atherosclerosis. Additional analyses showed that the MMPI items indicative of chronic hate and anger were the most significant discriminators.

Other studies of the behavioral correlates of heart disease also imply a relationship between anger and atherosclerosis, although they do not present angiographic findings. For example, in a prospective investigation of Swedish workers, Theorell and colleagues (Theorell, Lind, & Floderus, 1975) found that self-report of hostility when faced with delay was predictive of all deaths, myocardial infarctions, and ulcers. Data from the Framingham study showed that anger symptoms (reports of tension, headache, weaness, depression, or nervousness when really angry or annoyed) were associated with CHD prevalence in women under 65 (Haynes et al., 1978). Furthermore, anger-in (not discussing or showing anger) was related to CHD in incidence in both men and women, and this association was independent of the association of Type A behavior and CHD incidence (Haynes, Feinleib, & Kannel, 1980).

A recent study of adolescents provides preliminary evidence that anger is associated with elevations of both the physical (blood pressure, smoking, lack of exercise) and psychological (anxiety, life dissatisfaction, accumulation of life events, self-esteem, and Type A behavior pattern) risk factors for CHD (Siegel, 1984). Anger was measured by a self-report index that yielded factors of frequent anger directed outward and anger producing situations. Of these two factors, frequent anger directed outward was most highly predictive of cardiovascular risk status in the young. In sum, the third pathway suggests that anger is related to the atherosclerotic process and to CHD, independently of the association of Type A behavior and CHD.

Despite the accumulation of evidence concerning anger as potential risk factor for cardiovascular disease, relatively little research has directly focused on anger. The operational definitions of anger have varied considerably across studies, resulting in little comparability of what dimension of anger has been measured. For example, in the community-based studies of Harburg and colleagues (Harburg, Blakelock, & Roper, 1979; Harburg et al., 1973) and the laboratory follow-up of Esler and colleagues (1977), attention was focused on the relationship between suppressed hostility and hypertension. Suppressed hostility was operationalized as self-reports, in response to a hypothetical situation, of holding in anger when attacked and feelings of guilt if anger is displayed. The relationships between other dimensions of anger, such as intensity or frequency, and BP were not reported. The most divergent operational definition of anger from that used by Harburg and colleagues is the measure of chronic hate that was used by Williams and colleagues (Williams et al., 1980) in their study of atherosclerosis. In this study, anger (hostility) was operationalized as the number of positive responses to items such as, "I have often met people who were supposed to be experts who were no better than I." No measure of suppressed hostility was taken.

Thus, at this point we can conclude that suppressed hostility appears to be predictive of hypertension, and chronic hate appears to be predictive of degree of atherosclerosis, but we do not know to what extent suppressed hostility would predict atherosclerosis and vice versa. The point is that each study of anger and cardiovascular disease has used a measure of anger that is unique to that particular study and has rarely looked at more than one disease endpoint or cardiovascular disease risk factor. Furthermore, the measures of anger themselves have not been systematically examined to determine if they are unidimensional, or are, in fact, measuring multiple dimensions of anger.

The data presented here were collected as part of an effort to develop a self-report inventory that measures multiple dimensions of anger. The literature presented above suggests that the following dimensions of anger may be relevant for hypertension and CHD: frequency, duration, magnitude, hostile outlook, range of anger producing situations, and mode of expression. An inventory was constructed, the Multidimensional Anger Inventory (MAI), which contained items that were grouped together a priori and hypothesized to measure each of the above dimensions. This inventory was administered to approximately 200 male and female college students and approximately 350 adult male factory workers. The college students also completed three existing anger inventories so that comparisons would be made among the dimensions of the MAI and scores derived from existing inventories. The factory workers were participants in a study on the long range impact of noise on blood pressure. Thus, measurements of resting blood pressure, blood pressure response to stress, hypertensive medication status, and risk factors for CHD, including Type A behavior, have also been taken on these subjects.

The current report describes the preliminary psychometric work that has been completed for the MAI, including factor analysis, determination of reliability, and comparison with other inventories. The associations with indices of cardiovascular function will be examined at a later date. Together, these data will provide us with findings relevant to whether anger can best be described as a unidimensional or multidimensional construct, and, if it is determined to be multidimensional, which dimension or combination of dimensions is most highly predictive of cardiovascular function. These data will also suggest whether different dimensions of anger are predictive of different indices of cardiovascular function, (e.g., anger-in may predict resting blood pressure whereas hostile outlook may be a better predictor of blood pressure response to stress). These efforts can aid in the development of anger management training which may be incorporated into cardiovascular risk reduction and rehabilitation programs.

SCALE DEVELOPMENT

A 38-item self-report inventory, the Multidimensional Anger Inventory (MAI), was designed to measure the dimensions of anger (frequency, duration, magnitude) the range of situations to which an individual responds with anger, the mode of anger expression, and the extent of hostility in the individual's outlook. The newly developed inventory included items from existing instruments, as well as items constructed specifically for this inventory. The inventory instructions, the items, their source, and the anger dimension they were thought to assess are contained in Appendix 1. It should be noted that the word "source" in Appendix 1 can refer to either the item (or a modification of the item) being adapted from another inventory (e.g., Buss & Durkee, 1957) or it can refer to a theoretical or empirical work in which the authors suggest that certain attitudes or situations are relevant for anger (e.g., Friedman & Rosenman, 1974). As can be seen in Appendix 1, the number of items included to assess the dimensions of anger were: frequency, 5 (e.g., I tend to get angry more frequently than most people); duration, 2 (e.g., When I get angry, I stay angry for hours); magnitude, 4 (e.g., People seem to get angrier than I do in similar circumstances—reverse scored); mode of expression, twelve; hostile outlook, 6 (e.g., People talk about me behind my back); and range of anger-eliciting situation, 9 (e.g., I get angry when someone lets me down). The mode of expression dimension was further divided into four non-independent dimensions: anger-in 6 (e.g., I harbor grudges that I don't tell anyone about); anger-out, 5 (e.g., When I am angry with someone, I let that person know); guilt, 2 (e.g., I feel guilty about expressing my anger); brood, 4 (e.g., Even after I have expressed my anger, I have trouble forgetting about it); and anger-discuss, 1 (e.g., I try to talk over problems with people without letting them know I am angry). The order of the MAI items as presented to the population described below, is contained in Appendix 2. Each of the 38 statements were rated in terms of how self-descriptive they were. Responses ranged from 1 (completely undescriptive) to 5 (completely descriptive).

College Student Sample

The MAI was administered to 198 college students (74 males, 124 females) who received credit for their participation. In addition to completing the MAI, these students also completed short versions of the Buss-Durkee Hostility Inventory (BDHI) (Buss & Durkee, 1957), the Harburg Anger-In/Anger-Out Scale (Harburg et al., 1973), and the Novaco Anger Inventory (Novaco, 1975).

Portions of these inventories were thought to measure all of the hypothesized dimensions of anger, with the exception of frequency, and thus could be used, in part, as a test of validity of the MAI.

The BDHI was designed to primarily assess what people do when angry, and it measures the following dimensions of hostility: assault, indirect hostility, irritability, negativism, resentment, suspicion, and verbal hostility. The 8-item resentment scale, the 5-item negativism scale, and the 10-item suspicion scale, all in true-false response format, were selected for use in this study. The sum of these scales was used as a partial test of the validity of the hostile outlook dimension of the MAI.

The method of measuring anger developed by Harburg (Harburg et al., 1973) focused exclusively on the expression dimension. The Harburg scale described hypothetical situations of arbitrary frustration (e.g., being told off by one's boss for no good reason) and asked respondents to indicate whether they would feel angry or mad and would show it, feel annoyed and would show it, feel annoyed but would keep it in, feel angry or mad but would keep it in, or not feel angry or mad. For the present study, three of Harburg's hypothetical situations were used: being yelled at by a policeman for no good reason, being yelled at by a professor or employer, and being yelled at by a close friend. Each of the above situations was followed by the five category question about anger expression, a question about what the respondent would likely do if the situation actually occurred, and a question about how long it would take the individual to feel like him- or herself again if "you and a policeman (professor/employer, friend) had an argument or fight." The response categories for this latter question were: less than 1 hour (coded as 1), a couple of hours, a day, more than a day, or more than a week (coded as 5).

Responses to the Harburg scale were used as a partial validation of the duration, magnitude and expression dimensions of the new inventory. For duration, a correlation was computed between the sum of the duration items on the MAI and the sum of the three items on the Harburg inventory concerning how long it would take the individual to feel like him- or herself again. A magnitude score was created from the Harburg inventory by recoding the responses such that no anger was coded as 0, either of the two annoyed responses was coded as 1. (hold in or show it), and either of the two angry responses was coded as 2. These responses were summed across the three items and a correlation was computed between this sum and the sum of the MAI magnitude items. Finally, anger-in and anger-out indices were created by summing the number of times the respondent kept the anger or annoyance in, and also summing the number of times he or she showed the anger or annoyance. Correlations were computed between the Harburg anger-in and anger-out scores and the MAI anger-in and anger-out scores.

The Novaco Inventory (Novaco, 1975) primarily assessed the antecedents of anger (anger eliciting situations). The inventory contained 90 potentially anger-arousing situations (e.g., professor who refuses to listen to your point of view), and the respondent was asked to "rate the degree to which the incident described by the item would anger or provoke you." The response categories ranged from not at all (scored as 1) to very much (scored as 5). Half of the Novaco items were randomly selected for use in the present study as a partial validation of both the magnitude and range of situation dimensions of the MAI. A correlation was computed between the MAI magnitude items and the total score on the Novaco inventory (summed across 45 items). For range of situation, a correlation was computed between the sum of the MAI range items and the *number* of items on the Novaco Anger Inventory that the subject indicated would cause some anger or provocation (e.g., those scored as 4 or 5). This comparison was appropriate because the MAI assessed how characteristic it is for the respondent to get angry in a given situation, whereas the Novaco inventory assessed how angry the respondent *would be* in a given situation. A summary of the measures used as a partial validation of the MAI are presented in Table 1.

Factory Worker Sample

The men who completed the MAI were participants in a study of the impact of long-term occupational noise exposure on blood pressure. Only the data relevant to the psychometric properties of the MAI will be presented here. Subjects were drawn from two factory settings near Pittsburgh, Pennsylvania: one with a documented high noise level and one with a low noise level. The two criteria for study participation were age of greater than 40 and less than 60 years, and an employment history of at least ten years in the current job setting. Preliminary screening in the two factories showed that 70% (n = 1000) of the noise exposed group met the age criterion, whereas 60% (n = 387) of the non-exposed group met this criterion. Seventy-five percent of each group had been employed in their respective plants for 10-25 years. As part of the study procedure, the men completed a battery of self-report questionnaires, one of which was the MAI. In total, 288 men participated in this phase of the study. For the psychometric analyses of the MAI, the data from the two factory settings were combined. The mean age for the sample was 54.8, with a standard deviation of 4.2.

Table 1 Validation measures for the multidimensional anger inventory (MAI) dimensions

MAI dimension	Description of validation measure
Duration	Sum of three items on the Harburg Anger-in/Anger-out scale which ask how long the subject would feel angry in response to hypothetical situations.
Magnitude	1. Sum of three items on Harburg Anger-in/Anger-out Inventory which ask if the subject would feel no anger, annoyance, or get mad in response to hypothetical situations. 2. Sum of 45 items on Novaco Anger Inventory that ask the subject to rate the degree to which specific incidents would anger or provoke provoke him/her.
Mode of expression Anger-in	Number of times that subject would respond to one of three hypothetical situations described by Harburg with anger-in.
Anger-out	Number of times that subject would respond to one of three hypothetical situations described by Harburg with anger-out.
Ranger of anger-eliciting situations	The number of incidents on the Novaco Anger Inventory (45 incidents) to which the subject would respond with anger.
Hostile outlook	Sum of the Buss-Durkee Hostility Inventory negativism, resentment, and suspicion scales.

RESPONSES TO THE MULTIDIMENSIONAL ANGER INVENTORY (MAI)

Overview

The psychometric analyses of the MAI are presented in two sections: the responses of the college students and the responses of the factory workers. Means and standard deviations for each MAI item in the college sample are shown first, followed by data relevant to the test-retest reliability of the MAI. To determine whether the hypothesized dimensions of anger are supported by factor analyses, two factor solutions of the MAI are discussed: one with orthogonal rotation and one with oblique rotation. Next, the alpha coefficients, or measures of internal consistency, are presented for both the a priori dimensions of anger and the factor-derived dimensions. Male and female students are compared on each of these dimensions. Finally, the validation of the MAI is explored by examining the correlations between the MAI scale and scores derived from other inventories that measure anger or hostility. For the factory sample, means and standard deviations of responses to each item are shown, followed by the two factor analyses, and presentation of the reliability (alpha) coefficients. Where appropriate, the findings from the two samples are compared.

College Students

The means and standard deviations of the 198 college students' responses to each of the MAI items are presented in Appendix 3. A subgroup of the sample, 27 students, completed a second MAI three to four weeks later. During the previous academic year, 33 college students from the same subject pool also had completed the MAI twice across a three to four week interval. The time 1 with time 2 correlation for each item is contained in Appendix 4. The data are presented for the 33 and 27 college students separately, and for the two samples combined. The average test-retest reliability for the entire inventory is 0.73.

To determine whether the proposed dimensions of the MAI are supported by factor analysis, the items were subjected to a principal component factor analysis with varimax rotation. All of the scale items, excluding the mode of expression items, were included in one factor analysis. The mode of expression items were examined in a separate factor analysis because it was hypothesized that mode of expression may itself include several dimensions.

The factor analysis of all scale items (excluding mode of expression) yielded three factors with eigenvalues greater than one. The items and their factor loadings are presented in Table 2. The first factor, accounting for 64% of the variance, contained items reflecting the frequency, duration, and magnitude dimensions of anger, and was tentatively labeled the general anger factor. The second factor, accounting for 24% of the variance, represented anger-eliciting situations. The third factor accounted for 12% of the variance and was best described as hostile outlook. Thus, it appeared that the frequency, duration, and magnitude dimensions of the anger response were not independent in this population, but instead clustered together into a general anger factor.

The factor analyses of the mode of expression items yielded two factors, which are shown in Table 3. These factors have been tentatively labeled anger-in

Table 2 Factor structure of the multidimensional anger inventory (MAI). College sample: All items excluding mode of expression

Factor 1: General anger (63.7% of the variance)	
1. I tend to get angry more frequently than most people.	.74
R2. Other people seem to get angrier than I do in similar circumstances.*	.53
6. It is easy to make me angry.	.73
9. Something makes me angry almost every day.	.54
10. I often feel angrier than I think I should.	.60
14. I am surprised at how often I feel angry.	.68
17. At times, I feel angry for no specific reason.	.44
18. I can make myself angry about something in the past just by thinking about it.	.39
22. When I get angry, I stay angry for hours.	.41
R25. When I get angry, I calm down faster than most people.	.45
26. I get so angry, I feel like I might lose control.	.53

Factor 2: Range of anger-eliciting situations (24%)	
30b. I get angry when people are unfair.	.50
30c. I get angry when something blocks my plans.	.66
30d. I get angry when I am delayed.	.58
30e. I get angry when someone embarrasses me.	.51
30f. I get angry when I have to take orders from someone less capable than I.	.53
30g. I get angry when I have to work with incompetent people.	.43
30h. I get angry when I do something stupid.	.44
30i. I get angry when I am not given credit for something I have done.	.55

Factor 3: Hostile outlook (12.3%)	
13. Some of my friends have habits that annoy and bother me very much.	.33
17. At times, I feel angry for no specific reason.	.30
21. People can bother me just by being around.	.72
22. When I get angry, I stay angry for hours.	.32
30f. I get angry when I have to take orders from someone less capable than I.	.32
30g. I get angry when I have to work with incompetent people.	.33

*Reverse scored.

and anger-out. As can be seen in Table 3, the items describing brooding and guilt loaded on the anger-in factor.

In the initial conceptualization of the dimensions of anger, the possibility was considered that the dimensions would not be orthogonal. It seemed reasonable, for example, that a person who gets very angry (magnitude) would stay angry for a long time (duration). Thus, the MAI items, excluding mode of expression, were also factor analyzed using oblique rotation. A delta value of zero was used, which allowed for a fairly oblique (correlated) factor solution. Similar to the orthogonal rotation, the oblique rotation of all items, exluding mode of expression, yielded three factors with eigenvalues greater than one, with these factors being a general anger factor, anger-eliciting situations, and hostile outlook.

Overall, the oblique and orthogonal solutions were highly similar. In fact, all of the items contained in the first two orthogonal factors were also contained in oblique factors. Additionally, the first oblique factor included three items reflecting hostile outlook, and the second factor contained two items reflecting frequency. The third oblique factor contained two fewer items than the orthogonal factor (those absent were: "At times I feel angry for no specific

Table 3 Factor structure of the multidimensional anger inventory (MAI). College sample: Mode of expression items.

Item		Loading
Factor 1: Anger-out (62.5% of variance)		
7.	When I am angry with someone, I let that person know.	.51
29.	It's difficult for me to let people know I'm angry.	−.79
Factor 2: Anger-in/brood (37.5%)		
3.	I harbor grudges that I don't tell anyone about.	.31
4.	I try to get even when I am angry with someone.	.41
11.	I feel guilty about expressing my anger.	.47
19.	Even after I have expressed my anger, I have trouble forgetting about it.	.65
20.	When I hide my anger from others, I think about it for a long time.	.40
27.	If I let people see the way I feel, I'd be considered a hard person to get along with.	.40

reason;" "When I get angry I stay angry for hours"), and was thus a more pure reflection of hostile outlook. The oblique rotation of the mode of expression items yielded the identical two factors as the orthogonal rotation. Since the oblique and orthogonal rotations produced essentially the same solution, the orthogonal solution was used for further analysis because it contained fewer overlapping items among the factors.

The alpha coefficients, or internal consistencies, of the entire inventory, the a priori scales, and the factor derived scales are presented in Table 4. With the exception of the a priori mode of expression scales, all of the a priori and factor

Table 4 Internal consistency (alpha) coefficients for the MAI scales: College sample (n = 198)

Scale	Number of items	Alpha
A priori scales		
Total	38	.86
Frequency	5	.78
Duration	2	.55
Magnitude	4	.55
Mode of expression	12	.42
Anger-in	6	.21
Anger-out	5	.13
Brood	4	.33
Guilt	2	.46
Hostile outlook	6	.47
Range of anger-eliciting situations	9	.77
Factor derived scales		
General anger	11	.84
Range of anger-eliciting situations	8	.78
Hostile outlook	6	.64
Anger-in/brood	6	.64
Anger-out	2	.64

derived scales showed acceptable levels of reliability. The overall alpha (0.86) indicated that the scale has a high degree of internal consistency.

The responses of male and female college students were compared on their overall MAI score and on each of the scales. Scale scores were computed by reverse scoring items 2, 15, 23, 24, 25 and summing the individual's responses over the specific items. Males scored higher than females overall, however, their higher scores appear to be restricted to the hostile outlook $t(192) = 3.08$, $p < .005$, and anger-in, $t(192) = 2.33$, $p < .02$, dimensions. These data are presented in Table 5.

As a partial test of the validity of the MAI, correlations were computed among the subject's responses to the Harburg (1973), Novaco (1975), and Buss-Durkee (1957) inventories, and both the hypothesized and factor-derived MAI scales. Validation would be provided if two conditions were met. First, significant correlations should be found between the MAI dimensions and the scores derived from the other inventories that were selected to measure a specific dimension. These expected associations were described earlier in this paper and are outlined in Table 1. Second, the correlations between the MAI scales and conceptually non-similar dimensions derived from other inventories should be lower than the correlations with conceptually similar dimensions.

The data relevant to the validity of the MAI are presented below. The correlation among the MAI scales and the selected validity scores are presented in Table 6. As expected, the MAI duration scale is significantly related to the Harburg duration score, $r(136) = .47$, $p < .001$. The MAI magnitude scale is related to both the Novaco magnitude score, $r(125) = .26$, $p < .005$, and the Harburg magnitude score, $r(135) = .31$, $p < .001$. The MAI anger-eliciting situations scale is highly related to the Novaco anger situation score, $r(124) = .59$, $p < .001$. Last, the MAI hostile outlook scale is related to the BDHI hostile outlook score, which is a sum of the negativism, resentment, and suspicion items,

Table 5 Multidimensional anger inventory (MAI) scale scores of male (n = 73) and female (n = 123) college students

Scale	Males	Females	t	p
A priori scales				
Total	110.57	105.11	2.34	.05
Frequency	11.66	10.62	ns	
Duration	5.33	5.01	ns	
Magnitude	10.55	10.04	ns	
Mode of expression				
Anger-in	18.13	17.24	2.11	.05
Anger-out	14.01	13.69	ns	
Brood	13.16	13.00	ns	
Guilt	5.34	5.24	ns	
Hostile outlook	17.17	15.70	.005	
Range of situations	31.18	30.43	ns	
Factor derived scales				
General anger	27.52	25.63	ns	
Range of situations	27.75	26.99	ns	
Hostile outlook	17.71	16.72	ns	
Anger-in/brood	17.14	15.37	3.19	.005
Anger-out	5.82	6.11	ns	

Table 6 Correlations of multidimensional anger inventory (MAI) scales with validation scales.

MAI scale	Validation scale	r	p
A priori scales			
Duration	Harburg duration	.47	.001
Magnitude	Harburg magnitude	.31	.001
	Novaco magnitude	.26	.005
Anger-in	Harburg anger-in	.12	ns
Anger-out	Harburg anger-out	.02	ns
Range of situations	Novaco situations	.59	.001
Hostile outlook	Buss-Durkee hostility inventory	.46	.001
Factor derived scales			
General anger	Harburg duration	.28	.001
	Harburg magnitude	.29	.005
	Novaco magnitude	.36	.001
Range of situations	Novaco situations	.60	.001
Hostile outlook	Buss-Durkee hostility inventory	.45	.001
Anger-in	Harburg anger-in	.13	ns
Anger-out	Harburg anger-out	.10	ns

$r(128) = .46$, $p < .001$. (It should be noted that the items from the Buss-Durkee Hostility Inventory that were also included in the MAI were deleted for these analyses.) Two of the a priori MAI scales, anger-in and anger-out, were not significantly related to the scales selected for validation. The subjects' reports of how they might respond to an arbitrary abuse of power, as assessed by the Harburg anger-in and anger-out scale, were not related to MAI reports of their habitual styles of anger expression, ($p > .05$).

With regard to the factor derived scales (see Table 6), all of the expected associations were significant, again with the exception of the relationships among the derived anger-in and anger-out scales and the Harburg anger-in and anger-out scores ($p > .05$). Specifically, the MAI general anger scale (Factor 1) was related to the Harburg duration score, $r(134) = .28$, $p < .001$, the Novaco magnitude score, $r(125) = .29$, $p < .005$, and the Harburg magnitude score, $r(131) = .36$, $p < .001$. The anger-eliciting situations scale score (Factor 2) was highly correlated with the Novaco anger situations score, $r(124) = .60$, $p < .001$, and the hostile outlook scale score (Factor 3) was related to the sum of the BDHI negativism, resentment, and suspicion items, $r(128) = .45$, $p < .001$.

In sum, both the a priori and factor-derived MAI scales showed the expected pattern of relationships with the validity inventory scores, with the exception of anger-in and anger-out. While these existing inventories share some common variance with the MAI, it is clear that they do not tap the same content as the MAI.

The second step of the validity procedure was to determine if the correlations between the MAI scales and the appropriate validity scales were higher than the correlations with the conceptually non-similar validation scales. The MAI scales of duration, hostile outlook (a priori and factor derived), and range of anger-producing situations (a priori and factor derived) all showed their highest correlations with the validity scale that was selected to measure the same dimensions. For the magnitude dimension, only the BDHI score (hostile outlook) showed a higher correlation with the MAI magnitude scale, $r(128) = 0.47$, $p < .001$, than did the Harburg magnitude score, $r(135) = .31$, $p < .001$. This was also the case for the factor derived general anger scale, which contained items reflecting frequency, duration, and magnitude. The correlation of the general anger scale with the BDHI score was $r(128) = 0.50$, $p < .001$.

As reported above, the MAI measures of anger-in and anger-out were not significantly related to the anger-in and anger-out scores derived from the Harburg inventory. The MAI anger-in scales (a priori and factor derived) showed higher correlations with the Harburg duration score, the Novaco magnitude score, and the BDHI total score than with the Harburg anger-in score. It should be noted, however, that the Harburg anger-in scale was no more highly correlated with any of the other MAI or validity scales than it was with the MAI anger-in score. It appears, then, that the Harburg anger-in scale is tapping a unique dimension of anger that is not measured by any of the other scales included in this study.

With regard to the MAI anger-out scales, the hypothesized scale was more highly related to all of the other validity scales than it was to the Harburg anger-out score. The factor derived anger-out score, however, was more highly related to the Harburg scale than it was to any other validity scale, even though the correlation was not significant. Similar to the Harburg anger-in scale, the Harburg anger-out scale appeared to be tapping a unique dimension of anger as it shared little common variance with any of the anger measures in this study. The highest correlation for the Harburg anger-out scale was with the factor derived MAI anger-arousing situations scale, $r(134) = .16$, $p = .05$, followed by a negative correlation with the factor derived anger-in, scale $p = .24$, and a positive correlation with the factor derived anger our scale, $p = .25$.

In sum, the pattern of correlations scales show that, in general, the highest correlations between the MAI scales and the validity scales are those that were hypothesized to be strong. This holds true even for the nonsignificant relationships with the Harburg anger-in and anger-out scales.

Factory Workers

The means and standard deviations of the MAI responses of the 288 adult men are presented in Table 7. A comparison of the factory sample's responses with the college students' responses (see Table 1) indicates that the college students scored significantly higher on the total scale score, with means of 107.16 and 100.00, respectively, $t(473) = 4.48$, $p < .01$. Scores on the a priori scales were also compared for the two samples. The college students scored higher than the factory workers on magnitude, $t(473) = 2.80$, $p < .01$; range of anger arousing situations, $t(473) = 4.89$, $p < .01$; anger-in, $t(473) = 6.01$, $p < .01$; anger-out, $t(473) = 4.86$, $p < .01$; and brood, $t(473) = 9.14$, $p < .01$. The two groups did not differ on scale scores of frequency, duration, hostile outlook, and guilt.

The item responses of the factory workers were subjected to a principal components factor analysis with varimax rotation. As described in the analysis of the college student data, all of the scale items, excluding the mode of expression were included in one factor analysis, and the mode of expression items were analyzed in a separate factor analysis.

Table 7 Means and standard deviations of multidimensional anger inventory (MAI) response. Factory sample (n = 288).

	Mean	S.D.
1. I tend to get angry more frequently than most people.	2.19	1.01
*R2. Other people seem to get angrier than I do in similar circumstances.	3.43	.93
3. I harbor grudges that I don't tell anyone about.	2.40	1.17
4. I try to get even when I'm angry with someone.	2.08	1.07
5. I am secretly quite critical of others.	2.36	1.03
6. It is easy to make me angry.	2.23	1.01
7. When I am angry with someone, I let that person know.	3.20	1.08
8. I have met many people who are supposed to be experts who are no better than I.	3.39	1.03
9. Something makes me angry almost every day.	2.05	1.03
10. I often feel angrier than I think I should.	2.49	1.11
11. I feel guilty about expressing my anger.	2.75	1.17
12. When I am angry with someone, I take it out on whoever is around.	2.06	1.07
13. Some of my friends have habits that annoy and bother me very much.	2.76	1.02
14. I am surprised at how often I feel angry.	2.22	1.02
R15. Once I let people know I'm angry, I can put it out of my mind.	3.18	1.16
16. People talk about me behind my back.	2.44	1.02
17. At times, I feel angry for no specific reason.	1.96	1.00
18. I can make myself angry about something in the past just by thinking about it.	2.35	1.15
19. Even after I have expressed my anger, I have trouble forgetting about it.	2.42	1.13
20. When I hide my anger from others, I think about it for a long time.	2.51	1.17
21. People can bother me just by being around.	2.30	1.14
22. When I get angry, I stay angry for hours.	2.17	1.12
R23. When I hide my anger from others, I forget about it pretty quickly.	2.93	1.04
R24. I try to talk over problems with people without letting them know I am angry.	3.12	1.04
R25. When I get angry, I calm down faster than most people.	3.29	1.05
26. I get so angry I feel like I might lose control.	2.02	1.03
27. If I let people see the way I feel, I'd be considered a hard person to get along with.	2.45	1.14
28. I am on my guard with people who are friendlier than I expected.	2.54	1.17
29. It's difficult for me to let people know I'm angry.	2.52	1.03
30A. I get angry when someone lets me down.	3.18	.92
30B. I get angry when people are unfair.	3.44	1.08
30C. I get angry when something blocks my plans.	3.04	.98
30D. I get angry when I am delayed.	3.19	.98
30E. I get angry when someone embarrasses me.	3.19	1.07
30F. I get angry when I have to take orders from someone less capable than I.	2.82	1.11
30G. I get angry when I have to work with incompetent people.	2.88	1.17
30H. I get angry when I do something stupid.	3.48	1.07
30I. I get angry when I am not given credit for something that I have done.	2.88	1.48

*Reverse scored.

The factor analysis of all scale items (excluding mode of expression) yielded three factors with eigenvalues greater than 1. The items and their factor loadings are presented in Table 8. Similar to the college student analysis, the first factor (71% of the variance) contained items reflecting the frequency, duration, and magnitude dimensions, and was tentatively labeled the general anger factor. The second factor (18% of the variance) represented the range of anger-producing

Table 8 Factor structure of the multidimensional anger inventory (MAI). Factory sample: All items excluding mode of expression.

Item	Loading
Factor 1: General anger (71.3% of the variance)	
1. I tend to get angry more frequently than most people.	.67
5. I am secretly quite critical of others.	.41
6. It is easy to make me angry.	.60
9. Something makes me angry almost every day.	.43
10. I often feel angrier than I think I should.	.58
14. I am surprised at how often I feel angry.	.63
17. At times, I feel angry for no specific reason.	.55
18. I can make myself angry about something in the past just by thinking about it.	.48
21. People can bother me just by being around.	.45
22. When I get angry, I stay angry for hours.	.58
R25. When I get angry, I calm down faster than most people.*	.38
26. I get so angry I feel like I could lose control.	.53
Factor 2: Range of anger-eliciting situations (17.9%)	
30a. I get angry when someone lets me down.	.44
30b. I get angry when people are unfair.	.50
30c. I get angry when something blocks my plans.	.67
30d. I get angry when I am delayed.	.64
30e. I get angry when someone embarrasses me.	.58
30f. I get angry when I have to take orders from someone less capable than I.	.34
30g. I get angry when I have to work with incompetent people.	.33
30h. I get angry when I do something stupid.	.57
30i. I get angry when I am not given credit for something I have done.	.52
Factor 3: Hostile outlook (10.8%)	
8. I have met many people who are supposed to be experts who are no better than I.	.37
13. Some of my friends have habits that annoy and bother me very much.	.49
18. I can make myself angry about something in the past just by thinking about it.	.32
21. People can bother me just by being around.	.54
28. I am on my guard with people who are friendlier than I expected.	.42
30a. I get angry when someone lets me down.	.36
30b. I get angry when people are unfair.	.35
30f. I get angry when I have to take orders from someone less capable.	.53
30g. I get angry when I have to work with incompetent people.	.50
30i. I get angry when I am not given credit for something I have done.	.33

*Reverse scored.

situations, and the third factor (11% of the variance) contained items reflecting a hostile outlook. A comparison of this factor structure with the three factor solution yielded by the college student data (see Appendix 4) showed that they are highly similar. In fact, 83% of the items on the first factor were shared, 94% of the items on the second factor were shared, and 50% of the items on the third factor were shared. (The percent of common items was computed as: 2 times the number of shared items, divided by the sum of the number of items on the college factor and the number of items on the factory factor.)

Table 9 Factor structure of the multidimensional anger inventory (MAI). Factory sample: Mode of expression items.

Item	Loading
Factor 1: Anger-in/brood (74% of the variance)	
3. I harbor grudges that I don't tell anyone about.	.61
4. I try to get even when I am angry with someone.	.64
11. I feel guilty about expressing my anger.	.39
12. When I am angry, I take it out on whoever is around.	.58
19. Even after I have expressed my anger, I have trouble forgetting about it.	.75
20. When I hide my anger from others, I think about it for a long time.	.72
27. If I let people see the way I feel, I'd be considered a hard person to get along with.	.47
Factor 2: Anger-out/brood (26%)	
*R23. When I hide my anger from others, I forget about it pretty quickly.	.60
R24. I try to talk over problems with people without letting them know I'm angry.	.45
29. It's difficult for me to let people know I'm angry.	−.49

*Reverse scored.

The factor analysis of the mode of expression items yielded two factors which are shown in Table 9. The first factor was tentatively labeled as anger-in; 92% of the items were shared with the first of the two college students factors (see Table 3). The anger-in factor for the factory population contained items related to holding anger in (e.g., "I harbor grudges that I don't tell anyone about"), as well as brooding (e.g., "Even after I have expressed my anger, I have trouble

Table 10 Internal consistency (alpha) coefficients for the MAI scales: Factory sample (n = 288)

Scale	Number of items	Alpha
A priori scales		
Total	38	.90
Frequency	5	.76
Duration	2	.51
Magnitude	4	.49
Mode of expression	12	.65
Anger-in	6	.42
Anger-out	5	.44
Brood	4	.46
Guilt	2	.31
Hostile outlook	6	.63
Range of anger-eliciting situations	9	.83
Factor derived scales		
General anger	12	.85
Range of anger-eliciting situations	9	.83
Hostile outlook	10	.80
Anger-in/brood	7	.79
Anger-out/brood	3	.51

forgetting about it"). The second factor, tentatively labeled anger-out, shared only one item (40%) in common with the college sample ("It's difficult for me to let people know I'm angry"—negative loading). Unlike the college sample, the anger-out factor for the factory workers contained items related to brooding, as well as anger-out.

The oblique rotation of the factory workers responses produced a solution highly similar to the orthogonal rotation. The first and second factors of the oblique rotation contained all of the items on the orthogonal first and second factors, as well as items representing the other dimensions of anger. The third factor of the oblique and orthogonal solutions was identical, as were the two factors yielded by the analysis of the mode of expression items. Since the orthogonal and oblique rotations produced highly similar terminal solutions, the orthogonal factors were used in further analyses because they contained fewer overlapping items.

The alpha coefficients, or internal consistencies, of the entire inventory, the a priori scales, and the factor derived scales are presented in Table 10. With the exception of the a priori guilt scale, all of the scales showed acceptable levels of reliability (range of alpha = .42 to alpha = .84). The overall alpha (0.90) showed that the scale had a high degree of internal consistency.

REFERENCES

Alexander, F. Emotional factors in essential hypertension: Presentation of a tentative hypothesis. *Psychosomatic Medicine*, 1939, *1*, 173-179.
Baer, P. E., Collins, F. H., Bourianoff, G. G., & Ketchel, M. F. Assessing personality factors in essential hypertension with a brief self-report instrument. *Psychosomatic Medicine*, 1979, *4*, 321-330.
Buss, A. H. *The psychology of aggression.* New York: Wiley, 1961.
Buss, A. H., & Durkee, A. An inventory for assessing different kinds of hostility. *Journal of Consulting Psychology*, 1957, *21*, 343-349.
Cochrane, R. High blood pressure as a psychosomatic disorder: A selective review. *British Journal of Social and Clinical Psychology*, 1971, *10*, 61-72.
Cook, W. W., & Medley, D. M. Proposed hostility and pharisaic-virtue scales for the MMPI. *Journal of Applied Psychology*, 1954, *38*, 414-418.
Davies, M. H. Is high blood pressure a psychosomatic disorder? A critical review of the evidence. *Journal of Chronic Diseases*, 1971, *24*, 239-258.
Dembroski, T. M., MacDougall, J. M., Herd, J. A., & Shields, J. L. Effects of level of challenge on pressor and heart response in Type A and B subjects. *Journal of Applied Social Psychology*, 1979, *1*, 209-228.
Dembroski, T. M., MacDougall, J. M., & Lushene, R. Interpersonal interaction and cardiovascular response in Type A subjects and coronary patients. *Journal of Human Stress*, 1979, *5*, 28-36.
Dembroski, T. M., MacDougall, J. M., Shields, J. L., Petitto, J., & Lushene, R. Components of the Type A coronary-prone behavior pattern and cardiovascular responses to psychomotor challenge. *Journal of Behavioral Medicine*, 1978, *1*, 159-176.
Diamond, E. L. The role of anger and hostility in essential hypertension and coronary heart disease. *Psychological Bulletin*, 1982, *92*, 410-433.
Edwards, A. L. *Edwards Personality Inventory.* Chicago: Science Research, 1966.
Esler, M., Julius, S., Zweifler, A., Randall, O., Harburg, E., Gardiner, H., & DeQuattro, V. Mild high-renin essential hypertension: Neurogenic human hypertension? *New England Journal of Medicine*, 1977, *296*, 405-411.
Friedman, M., & Rosenman, R. H. *Type A behavior and your heart.* New York: Knopf, 1974.
Harburg, E., Erfurt, J. C., Hauenstein, L. S., Chape, C., Schull, W. J., & Schork, M. A. Socio-ecological stress, suppressed hostility, skin color, and black-white male blood pressure: Detroit. *Psychosomatic Medicine*, 1973, *35*, 276-296.

Harburg, E., Blakelock, E. H., & Roeper, P. J. Resentful and reflective coping with arbitrary authority and blood pressure: Detroit. *Psychosomatic Medicine,* 1979, *41,* 189-202.
Harrell, J. P. Psychological factors and hypertension: A status report. *Psychological Bulletin,* 1980, *87,* 482-501.
Harris, R. E., Sokolow, M., Carpenter, L. G., Friedman, M., & Hunt, S. P. Response to psychologic stress in persons who are potentially hypertensive. *Circulation,* 1953, *7,* 874-879.
Haynes, S. G., Feinleib, M., Levine, S., Scotch, N., & Kannel, W. B. The relationship of psychosocial factors to coronary heart disease in the Framingham study: II. Prevalence of coronary heart disease. *American Journal of Epidemiology,* 1978, *107,* 384-401.
Haynes, S. G., Feinleib, M., & Kannel, W. B. The relationship of psychosocial factors to coronary heart disease in the Framingham study: III. Eight-year incidence of coronary heart disease. *American Journal of Epidemiology,* 1980, *111,* 37-58.
Herd, J. A. Physiological correlates of coronary-prone behavior. In: Dembroski, T. M., Weiss, S., Shields, J., et al. (Eds.), *Coronary-prone behavior.* New York: Springer-Verlag, 1978.
Hokanson, J. E. The effects of frustration and anxiety on overt aggression. *Journal of Abnormal Psychology,* 1961a, *62,* 346-351.
Hokanson, J. E. Vascular and psychogalvanic effects of experimentally aroused anger. *Journal of Personality,* 1961b, *29,* 30-39.
Hokanson, J. E., & Burgess, M. The effects of status, type of frustration, and aggression on vascular processes. *Journal of Abnormal and Social Psychology,* 1962, *65,* 232-237.
Holmes, D. S. Effects of overt aggression on level of physiological arousal. *Journal of Personality and Social Psychology,* 1966, *4,* 189-194.
Jenkins, C. D. Components of the coronary-prone behavior pattern: Their relation to silent myocardial infarction and blood lipids. *Journal of Chronic Diseases,* 1966, *19,* 599-609.
Kahn, H. A., Medalie, J. H., Neufeld, H. N., Riss, E., & Goldbourt, U. The incidence of hypertension and associated factors: The Israeli ischemic heart disease study. *American Heart Journal,* 1972, *84,* 171-182.
Kalis, B. L., Harris, R. E., Bennett, L. F., & Sokolow, M. Personality and life history factors in persons who are potentially hypertensive. *Journal of Nervous and Mental Diseases,* 1961, *132,* 457-468.
Kalis, B. L., Harris, R. E., Sokolow, M., & Carpenter, L. G. Response to psychological stress in patients with essential hypertension. *American Heart Journal,* 1957, *53,* 572-578.
Matthews, K. A., Glass, D. C., Rosenman, R. H., & Bortner, R. W. Competitive drive, Pattern A, and coronary heart disease: A further analysis of some data from the Western Collaborative Group Study. *Journal of Chronic Diseases,* 1977, *30,* 489-498.
Matthews, K. A. Psychological Perspectives on the Type A behavior pattern. *Psychological Bulletin,* 1982, *42,* 303-313.
McGinn, N. F., Harburg, E., Julius, S., & McLeod, J. M. A review of research on psychological correlates of blood pressure. *Psychological Bulletin,* 1964, *61,* 209-219.
Rosenman, R. The interview method of assessment of the coronary-prone behavior pattern. In: Demroski, T. M., Weiss, S., Shields, J., et al. (Eds.), *Coronary-prone behavior.* New York: Springer-Verlag, 1978.
Siegel, J. M. Anger and cardiovascular risk in adolescents. *Health Psychology,* 1984, *3,* 293-313.
Siegel, J. M., & Leitch, C. J. Behavioral factors and blood pressure in adolescence: The Tacoma study. *American Journal of Epidemiology,* 1981, *113,* 171-181.
Theorell, T., Lind, E., & Floderus, B. The relationship of disturbing life-changes and emotions to the early development of myocardial infarction and other serious illness. *International Journal of Epidemiology,* 1975, *41,* 281-293.
Williams, R. B., Haney, T. L., Lee, K. L., Kong, V., Blumenthal, J. A., & Whalen, R. E. Type A behavior, hostility, and coronary atherosclerosis. *Psychosomatic Medicine,* 1980, *42,* 539-550.

APPENDIX 1:

Instructions, Anger Dimension, and Source for Multidimensional Anger Inventory (MAI) Items.

Instructions

Everybody gets angry from time to time. A number of statements that people have used to describe the times that they get angry are included below. Read each statement and circle the number to the right of the statement that best describes you. There are no right or wrong answers.

If the statement is completely undescriptive of you, circle a 1.
If the statement is mostly undescriptive of you, circle a 2.
If the statement is partly undescriptive and partly descriptive of you, circle a 3.
If the statement is mostly descriptive of you, circle a 4.
If the statement is completely descriptive of you, circle a 5.

Please answer every item.

Item pool

Dimension	Item	Source
Frequency	1. I tend to get angry more frequently than most people.	Edwards (1966)
	6. It is easy to make me angry.	Edwards (1966)
	9. Something makes me angry almost every day.	
	14. I am surprised at how often I feel angry.	
	17. At times, I feel angry for no specific reason.	
Duration	22. When I get angry, I can stay angry for hours.	Baer et al. (1979)
	R25. When I get angry, I calm down faster than most people.**	
Magnitude	R2. Other people seem to get angrier than I do in similar circumstances.	Baer et al. (1979)
	10. I often feel angrier than I think I should.	
	18. I can make myself angry about something in the past just by thinking about it.	
	26. I get so angry, I feel like I might lose control.	Buss & Durkee (1957)
Mode of expression anger-in	3. I harbor grudges that I don't tell anyone about.	Baer et al. (1979)
	20. When I hide my anger from others, I think about it for a long time.	Kahn et al. (1972)
	R23. When I hide my anger from others, I forget about it pretty quickly.	
	R24. I try to talk over problems with people without letting them know I'm angry.	Harburg et al. (1979)
	27. If I let people see the way I feel, I'd be considered a hard person to get along with.	Buss & Durkee (1957)
	29. It's difficult for me to let people know I'm angry.	

MEASUREMENT OF ANGER AS A CONSTRUCT 79

Item pool

Dimension	Item		Source*
Mode of expression (continued) anger-out	4.	I try to get even when I'm angry with someone.	Baer et al. (1979)
	7.	When I am angry with someone, I let that person know.	Harburg et al. (1973)
	12.	When I am angry with someone, I take it out on whoever is around.	
	15.	Once I let people know I'm angry, I can put it out of my mind.	
	19.	Even after I have expressed my anger, I have trouble forgetting about it.	
Guilt	11.	I feel guilty about expressing my anger.	Harburg et al. (1973)
	29.	It's difficult for me to let people know I'm angry.	
Brood	R15.	Once I let people know I'm angry, I can put it out of my mind.	
	19.	Even after I have expressed my anger, I have trouble forgetting about it.	
	20.	When I hide my anger from others, I think about it for a long time.	Kahn et al. (1972)
	R23.	When I hide my anger from others, I forget about it pretty quickly.	
Anger-discuss	24.	I try to talk over problems with people, without letting them know I'm angry.	Harburg et al. (1979)
Hostile outlook	5.	I am secretly quite critical of others.	Baer et al. (1979)
	8.	I have met many people who are supposed to be experts who are no better than I.	Williams et al. (1980)
	13.	Some of my friends have habits that annoy and bother me very much.	
	16.	People talk about me behind my back.	Buss & Durkee (1957)
	21.	People can bother me just by being around.	Buss & Durkee (1957)
	28.	I am on my guard with people who are friendlier than I expected.	Buss & Durkee (1957)
Ranger of anger- eliciting situations	30.	I get angry when:	
	a.	someone lets me down.	
	b.	people are unfair.	
	c.	something blocks my plans.	Edwards (1966)
	d.	I am delayed.	Friedman & Rosenman (1974)
	e.	someone embarrasses me.	Buss & Durkee (1957)
	f.	I have to take orders from someone less capable than I.	Williams et al. (1980)
	g.	I have to work with incompetent people.	Friedman & Rosenman (1974)
	h.	I am not given credit for something I have done.	Novaco (1975)

*In some cases, the source is another inventory and the item is an exact replicate or slightly modified version of the original item. In other cases, the source is a theoretical or empirical work, not another inventory.
**Indicates that the item is reverse scored.

APPENDIX 2

Order of Multidimensional Anger Inventory (MAI) Items.

1.	I tend to get angry more frequently than most people.
*R2.	Other people seem to get angrier than I.
3.	I harbor grudges that I don't tell anyone about.
4.	I try to get even when I'm angry with someone.
5.	I am secretly quite critical of others.
6.	It is easy to make me angry.
7.	When I am angry with someone, I let that person know.
8.	I have met many people who are supposed to be experts who are no better than I.
9.	Something makes me angry almost every day.
10.	I often feel angrier than I think I should.
11.	I feel guilty about expressing my anger.
12.	When I am angry with someone, I take it out on whoever is around.
13.	Some of my friends have habits that annoy and bother me very much.
14.	I am surprised at how often I feel angry.
R15.	Once I let people know I'm angry, I can put it out of my mind.
16.	People talk about me behind my back.
17.	At times, I feel angry for no specific reason.
18.	I can make myself angry about something in the past just by thinking about it.
19.	Even after I have expressed my anger, I have trouble forgetting about it.
20.	When I hide my anger from others, I think about it for a long time.
21.	People can bother me just by being around.
22.	When I get angry, I stay angry for hours.
R23.	When I hide my anger from others, I forget about it pretty quickly.
R24.	I try to talk over problems with people without letting them know I am angry.
R25.	When I get angry, I calm down faster than most people.
26.	I get so angry I feel like I might lose control.
27.	If I let people see the way I feel, I'd be considered a hard person to get along with.
28.	I am on my guard with people who are friendlier than I expected.
29.	It's difficult for me to let people know I'm angry.
30A.	I get angry when someone lets me down.
30B.	I get angry when people are unfair.
30C.	I get angry when something blocks my plans.
30D.	I get angry when I am delayed.
30E.	I get angry when someone embarrasses me.
30F.	I get angry when I have to take orders from someone less capable than I.
30G.	I get angry when I have to work with incompetent people.
30H.	I get angry when I do something stupid.
30I.	I get angry when I am not given credit for something that I have done.

*Reverse scored.

APPENDIX 3

Means and Standard Deviations of Multidimensional Anger Inventory (MAI) Responses: College Students (n = 198).

		Mean	S.D.
1.	I tend to get angry more frequently than most people.	2.26	1.04
*R2.	Other people seem to get angrier than I do in similar circumstances.	2.55	.90
3.	I harbor grudges that I don't tell anyone about.	2.57	1.07

		Mean	S.D.
4.	I try to get even when I'm angry with someone.	2.52	1.18
5.	I am secretly quite critical of others.	2.90	1.02
6.	It is easy to make me angry.	2.27	1.04
7.	When I am angry with someone, I let that person know.	3.30	1.08
8.	I have met many people who are supposed to be experts who are no better than I.	2.74	.93
9.	Something makes me angry almost every day.	2.07	.98
10.	I often feel angrier than I think I should.	2.61	1.15
11.	I feel guilty about expressing my anger.	2.57	1.21
12.	When I am angry with someone, I take it out on whoever is around.	2.18	.94
13.	Some of my friends have habits that annoy and bother me very much.	2.98	1.08
14.	I am surprised at how often I feel angry.	2.09	1.01
R15.	Once I let people know I'm angry, I can put it out of my mind.	3.05	1.15
16.	People talk about me behind my back.	2.34	.90
17.	At times, I feel angry for no specific reason.	2.34	1.14
18.	I can make myself angry about something in the past just by thinking about it.	2.80	1.10
19.	Even after I have expressed my anger, I have trouble forgetting about it.	2.80	1.10
20.	When I hide my anger from others, I think about it for a long time.	3.45	1.08
21.	People can bother me just by being around.	2.77	1.13
22.	When I get angry, I stay angry for hours.	2.38	1.07
R23.	When I hide my anger from others, I forget about it pretty quickly.	3.77	1.00
R24.	I try to talk over problems with people without letting them know I am angry.	2.94	.97
R25.	When I get angry, I calm down faster than most people.	2.76	1.05
26.	I get so angry I feel like I might lose control.	2.10	1.07
27.	If I let people see the way I feel, I'd be considered a hard person to get along with.	2.18	.93
28.	I am on my guard with people who are friendlier than I expected.	2.53	1.13
29.	It's difficult for me to let people know I'm angry.	2.70	1.23
30A.	I get angry when someone lets me down.	3.43	.99
30B.	I get angry when people are unfair.	3.86	.86
30C.	I get angry when something blocks my plans.	3.27	.97
30D.	I get angry when I am delayed.	3.27	.94
30E.	I get angry when someone embarrasses me.	3.25	1.09
30F.	I get angry when I have to take orders from someone less capable than I.	3.38	1.08
30G.	I get angry when I have to work with incompetent people.	3.24	1.05
30H.	I get angry when I do something stupid.	3.57	1.10
30I.	I get angry when I am not given credit for something that I have done.	3.43	.96

*Reverse scored.

APPENDIX 4

Time 1–Time 2 Correlations for the Multidimensional Anger Inventory (MAI). Sample 1 (n = 33), Sample 2 (n = 27), and Combined (N = 60).

		1	2	Combined
1.	I tend to get angry more frequently than most people.	.49	.72	.61
2.	Other people seem to get angrier than I do in similar circumstances.	.63	.54	.59
3.	I harbor grudges that I don't tell anyone about.	.63	.31	.49
4.	I try to get even when I'm angry with someone.	.20	.69	.25
5.	I am secretly quite critical of others.	.32	.29	.32
6.	It is easy to make me angry.	.24	.59	.37
7.	When I am angry with someone, I let that person know.	.59	.68	.63
8.	I have met many people who are supposed to be experts who are no better than I.	.37	.42	.40
9.	Something makes me angry almost every day.	.62	.20	.43
10.	I often feel angrier than I think I should.	.50	.17	.36
11.	I feel guilty about expressing my anger.	.52	.14	.26
12.	When I am angry with someone, I take it out on whoever is around.	.50	.55	.51
13.	Some of my friends have habits that annoy and bother me very much.	.42	.41	.41
14.	I am surprised at how often I feel angry.	.59	.60	.60
15.	Once I let people know I'm angry, I can put it out of my mind.	.36	.23	.28
16.	People talk about me behind my back.	.62	.72	.65
17.	At times, I feel angry for no specific reason.	.46	.03	.27
18.	I can make myself angry about something in the past just by thinking about it.	.24	.52	.37
19.	Even after I have expressed my anger, I have trouble forgetting about it.	.69	.39	.57
20.	When I hide my anger from others, I think about it for a long time.	.60	.42	.51
21.	People can bother me just by being around.	.55	.32	.46
22.	When I get angry, I stay angry for hours.	.73	.35	.61
23.	When I hide my anger from others, I forget about it pretty quickly.	.44	.48	.46
24.	I try to talk over problems with people without letting them know I am angry.	.51	.64	.56
25.	When I get angry, I calm down faster than most people.	.58	.57	.57
26.	I get so angry I feel like I might lose control.	.23	.55	.37
27.	If I let people see the way I feel, I'd be considered a hard person to get along with.	.51	.71	.59
28.	I am on my guard with people who are friendlier than I expected.	.72	.48	.62
29.	It's difficult for me to let people know I'm angry.	.18	.73	.39
30A.	I get angry when someone lets me down.	.39	.35	.37
30B.	I get angry when people are unfair.	.58	.79	.67
30C.	I get angry when something blocks my plans.	.75	.43	.64
30D.	I get angry when I am delayed.	.70	.08	.49
30E.	I get angry when someone embarrasses me.	.70	.74	.72
30F.	I get angry when I have to take orders from someone less capable than I.	.71	.78	.74
30G.	I get angry when I have to work with incompetent people.	.60	.44	.55
30H.	I get angry when I do something stupid.	.73	.36	.62
30I.	I get angry when I am not given credit for something that I have done.	.74	.40	.66

4
A Microsocial Analysis of Anger and Irritable Behavior

G. R. Patterson
Oregon Social Learning Center

The studies by Williams, Haney, Lee, Kong, Blumenthal and Whalen (1980) and by Spielberger and London (1982) make a convincing case for a variable such as anger playing a key role in placing certain individuals at risk for coronary atherosclerosis and related disorders. The present report is thought of as a methodological contribution to the existing formulations about this key variable. The social interactional perspective taken here emphasizes the fact that angry people often live in angry environments. Many of their angry behaviors could be reactions to irritable intrusions by persons in their immediate social environment. The present report is therefore focused on the use of observational data collected in natural settings and the analysis of the conditional relations between socio-environmental events and the reactions of the "target" individual. The social interactional perspective, as illustrated in this report, is supported by data, collected in the home, that describes the interactions of angry mothers and their problem children.

Most contemporary theorists view anger as one of several outcomes of a process that can be initiated by certain classes of external events. For example, Zajonc (1980) has made an interesting case for the possibility that emotions, such as anger, can be elicited by external events prior to cognitive assessment and interpretation. It is also the case that the individual's reconstruction of the external event, particularly his or her attributions about the intention of the other person involved, serve an arousal-eliciting function (Durel & Krantz, Chap. 14; Novaco, 1973, Chap. 11). In support of this formulation, Novaco (1975) alters the cognitive components of the process to reduce anger. Durel and Krantz (Chap. 14) employ chemical blocking agents to directly reduce the arousal. This writer proposes to add a methodological note to this formulation.

This intent is consistent with Lang's (1983) bio-informational formulation of emotion as involving three interrelated action sets: verbal report, overt motor reactions, and physiological reactions. As he points out, investigators often find only low order positive correlations among these reactions to external stimuli. His formulation outlines the conditions under which one might expect an external stimulus to produce any or all of these reactions. The three reactions are

---

An earlier version of the manuscript was presented at the NIMH sponsored conference on "Prevention Research on Assessment and Intervention for Disabling Anger" at SRI, Stanford, January 1983. This report is based on research funded by the National Institute of Mental Health, Section on Crime and Delinquency, MH 32857.

connected by a network of associations, and some external stimuli will elicit all three—verbal, physiological and motor—while others may produce only one or two. The present report addresses itself to the feasibility of using data collected in natural settings for identifying those stimuli that reliably serve as determinants for these three classes of emotional behavior. The studies of phobias reviewed by Lang (1968) and others showed that fearful verbal reports are not necessarily accompanied by either autonomic arousal or escape avoidant reactions. In the present study, the analogous question concerns the covariation between irritable verbal behavior (scolding), angry motor behavior (hitting, grabbing), and negative affect (angry tone of voice, facial expression).

For the purposes of illustration, this report will search for events in the social environment that elicit mothers' irritable motor behaviors. Are there certain child behaviors that reliably elicit, in a probabilistic sense, these maternal reactions? It turns out that mothers in normal families perform irritable verbal behaviors at the rate of about one every two or three minutes, while they hit, push, or spank only once every 200 minutes (Patterson, 1982). It is obvious, then, that the mothers' irritable verbal behavior and their angry motor behaviors cannot covary in each episode. Under what conditions do they covary? An analysis of data collected with a new code system for a normal sample showed that the mothers' facial expressions and voice tones reflected an angry emotion for an average of about three seconds. It is suggested by Lang's (1983) model, that external stimuli often elicit the mothers' irritable verbal behavior, but this is neither accompanied by, nor does it lead to, angry emotion or hitting. What are the determinants in the social environment that elicit these higher rate maternal irritable behaviors? Under what conditions do they lead to anger and to hitting?

The potential methodological contribution lies in the possibility that sequential data (or diaries) collected in the natural environment might identify those events that reliably elicit the irritable verbal behaviors of the client that, in turn, lead to physiologic arousal or angry motor behaviors such as hitting, or both. There is another potentially useful function that could be served by such analyses. It is the case, for example, that some angry individuals live in angry social environments [e.g., a sizeable proportion of child-abusing parents live with extremely irritable, angry children (Reid, Patterson, & Loeber, 1981)]. As shown in the field studies of these families, much of the parents' irritable behavior is in reaction to the abrasive behavior of the poorly socialized child. It would be revealing to look into the action-reaction patterns in these homes.

What proportion of the irritable verbal behaviors of the Type A or coronary-prone adult (see Rosenman, Chap. 5) are in reaction to the abrasive behavior of a poorly socialized child? What is the quality of life that characterizes the interactions of Type A adults with their families or their colleagues at the office? What are the determinants for the escalation from a few, relatively innocous words to physiologic arousal; or for some individuals, is it the other way around? Simple descriptive data, sequential in form, and collected in natural settings are required to answer these questions.

There is a third potential contribution to be made by a microanalytic approach to sequences of interaction collected in natural settings. It has to do with the possibility that some or many of the irritable verbal behaviors and the angry motor and physiological reactions are elicited by external stimuli that are neutral, at least as they would be coded by an outside observer. Programmatic studies by Dodge and his colleagues (Dodge, 1980; Dodge & Frame, 1982) provide a convincing case for the possibilities that aggressors often make misattributions about the behavior of other persons with whom they are interacting. Behavior viewed by others as neutral or ambiguous are perceived by the aggressive child as indicative of a hostile intention, and therefore as setting the occasion for an attack. The problem is further compounded by the fact that the people interacting with aggressive individuals also make such misattributions. Observation data collected in the homes of families of aggressive boys showed that, given the mother was behaving in a neutral or prosocial fashion, the likelihood was .040 that the problem child would initiate a coercive behavior. Given the problem child had been prosocial or neutral, the comparable likelihood for the mother was .047 (Patterson, 1982). Not only do these surprise attacks contribute to the overall uncertainty in these families, but also place each individual at increasing risk for episodes that may escalate into emotional or extended irritable confrontations. Are the angry adults characterized by the Type A personality also likely to make the misattributions that produce attacks and retaliations from the social environment? To what extent do such angry adults and aggressive children program their own social environments?

Within the present context, it is assumed that the conditional probabilities describing irritable or angry reactions to another person have several interesting characteristics. As noted above, they may reflect, in part, an individual's misattributions of the intentions of others. It is also the case that these values may reflect processes that impinge from outside the immediate interpersonal exchange. As shown in one extended baseline study, on those days characterized by a high density of familial hassles, most of the mothers were observed to be more irritable in their interactions with their children while others seemed to become more distant (Patterson, 1983). The effect was replicated in the study by Wahler and Dumas (1983), who showed that days characterized by stressful exchanges with relatives were also characterized by higher observed rates of maternal irritable behaviors in interacting with their children.

To provide the data base necessary to study such questions, it was first necessary to develop a system for describing sequences of social interactions. Three years of field studies led to the development of a 29-category system for recording interactions among family members (Patterson, Ray, Shaw, & Cobb, 1969). The psychometric studies of reliability, observer presence effects, observer bias, and validity are summarized by Reid (1978). This code was, in turn, improved by adding new categories for the study of prosocial interactions, and making provision for continuous recording of affect and setting changes (Reid, Dishion, Patterson, Gabrielson, & Thibodeaux, 1984). In the new code system, the Family Process Code, the behavior of the target subject and the person with whom the subject is interacting is recorded in real time, and each action is also coded for shifts to positive or negative affect. Affect judgments are based on cues from voice tone and facial expressions. The data collected in the field are stored in a recording device and then fed directly into a computer. The analyses of action and reaction patterns are then relatively straightforward. For the type of patterns discussed in the present report, it is generally the case that three to four hours of home observation are required to form a sufficient data base.

A SOCIAL INTERACTION PERSPECTIVE

The general strategy to be used in examining setting events that determine anger arousal and expression in the home might best be described as "social interactional" (Cairns, 1979; Gottman & Bakeman, 1979; Hartup, 1979; Suomi, Lamb, & Stephenson, 1979) with special application to the coercive processes found in families (Patterson, 1982). This strategy emphasizes the analysis of social interaction sequences to understanding the development of such phenomena as relationships, social skills and deviant behavior.

Recent extensions of this approach by Gottman (1982) and Levenson and Gottman (1983) provide for encoding the ongoing content of behavior with the ongoing physiological measures of affective reactions. The assumption in the present context is that arousal or negative affect on the one hand, and irritable content of ongoing behavior on the other, are separate factors in social behavior, but the two are best studied as they interact with each other. Unlike Gottman, we are relying on facial expression and voice tone as the base for assessing emotion. This is in keeping with the point of view developed by Izard (1979).

Our clinical experience in treating hundreds of families of antisocial children and families of child-abusing parents suggests that there are observable and repeated patterns of interaction that constitute a prelude to anger expression. These patterned preludes are often overlooked by parent and clinician alike. Field observation studies suggest that it is probable that during the early stages of the anger elicitation or "coercion" process both members of a dyad (i.e., husband-wife or mother-child) develop predictable (probabilistic) patterns of irritable initiations, reactions and counter-reactions. These observable patterns proliferate and grow in complexity; one can think of it as a probability tree growing in the family kitchen or living room. The use of a probability tree as a metaphor for these changes was explored in a brief series of papers (Patterson, 1973; 1974). In these patterns, or trees, the likelihood shifts over time that one will start up a conflict, and then, in turn, the other will react in such a way as to perpetuate it.

The development of patterns of irritable action and reaction signifies an overall increase in frequency of coercive events for the dyad. This increase in frequency and pattern development is thought to define a first stage of a process that eventually leads to high-amplitude aggression. During the early stages, many of the irritable exchanges seem to be run off almost automatically and with relatively little affect on the part of either member. In fact, most of these exchanges could be thought of as relatively trivial (e.g., teasing, scolding, nagging, and so forth). But one of the important tenets of coercion theory is that these relatively trivial, or even banal, events serve as the base from which anger and physical injury may result.

Recent publications concerning social cognitions make a compelling argument for the possibility that participants in this process may be relatively unaware of such trivial events or their reactions to them (Nisbett & Wilson, 1977). Given our limited channel capacity, it seems reasonable to suppose that we attend only to those events that demand our attention; trivial, well practiced coercive exchanges with family members might well be overlooked because of their nonsalient, almost automatic quality. In fact, it may be true that much of the detail of what it is that makes a person angry may lie outside his awareness, but could be found in the minutiae of everyday experiences.

As the action-reaction patterns increase in frequency, there is a commensurate increase in the frequency and length of coercive chains. These increases characterize a second stage in development. Both members of the dyad develop synchronous patterns of irritable action and reaction. Both members then learn that if they continue to a third or fourth reaction in the sequence, they are more likely to win (i.e., the other person temporarily withdraws from the exchange). Almost all combinations of dyads from the clinical samples (aggressive and stealers) showed a higher likelihood of extended chains than did comparable dyads from normal families (Patterson, 1982).

It is hypothesized that an increasing incidence of high amplitude, motoric behaviors (e.g., hitting, shoving, grabbing, and kicking) define a third stage of development that places one or more of the participants at risk for physical injury. In the context of familial conflict, we seek to track how it is that a mother may move from scolding to yelling to threatening to physical assault. Paradoxically, research indicates that it is the victim who trains the attacker to gradually increase the attack's intensity (Patterson, 1982).

Given that the members of a dyad have roughly equal status as opponents, a situation characterizing most mother-child dyads for problem families, it is very likely that this will extend the length of their coercive exchanges. The mother's inept use of discipline permits these exchanges to lengthen and occur with increasing frequency. It then becomes probable that, during an extended exchange, one or the other will also increase the intensity of his or her aggressive reactions. There is a reasonable likelihood that this increase in intensity will be effective in achieving a desired result (i.e., the other will give in or back off). The victim's surrender to this high intensity attack increases the probability that future attacks will recur. Considering their equal status, dyad members may exchange roles as initiator and recipient, leading to a gradual increase in intensity to the point that one or both may be at risk for physical injury. The details of the escalation hypothesis are presented by Patterson (1982). A programmatic series of laboratory studies with animal subjects provide strong support for the assumption that the victim's reactions to high intensity attacks is a prime determinant for future occurrences of such attacks (Knutson, Fordyce, & Anderson, 1982; Viken & Knutson, 1983).

It is assumed that the mother's emotional expresson of anger is most likely to occur during extended coercive exchanges or hitting. At the simplest level, one would expect, for example, that sessions characterized by high frequencies of maternal irritable (content) behavior would also be characterized by more negative affect. The mean scores for these two variables should covary significantly. Data will be presented that relate to this form of the hypothesis. On an event-by-event basis, it must also be the case that many of the high rate mother irritable behaviors will not be accompanied by the lower rate emotional events. What is the likelihood of negative emotional events accompanying irritable content behaviors? Finally, we will also explore the role of negative affect as an antecedent, attendant, and subsequent event for maternal hitting, grabbing, and pushing. The first question is concerned with the possibility of identifying certain aspects of the social environment that reliably elicit maternal high rate irritable verbal behavior.

MICROSOCIAL ANALYSES: SEARCH FOR A MOTHER-CHILD PATTERN

Microsocial analyses of interaction sequences provide a detailed account of anger elicitation and expression, and demonstrate significant correlations between the behavior of one person and the reaction of the other. Given the observation of adequate samples of interaction for a dyad, it is possible to identify the pattern of these action-reaction structures. Microsocial structures have been identified for infant-mother interactions (Parke, 1978), married spouses in conflict (Gottman, 1982; Margolin, 1977), parent-child interactions in abused children (Reid, 1982), and parent child interactions for families of antisocial boys (Patterson, 1982). These studies demonstrate that in the context of social interaction, the target subjects' next responses are determined by a joint function of their prior behavior and the previous reaction of the others to that behavior. One can think of the reactions of others, then, as eliciting, in a probabilistic sense, a target subject's next response. In these studies, the likelihood of, say, the mother scolding given the child teasing a sibling is compared to the base rate likelihood for the mother scolding.[1]

Earlier studies of family interaction sequences had identified a pattern of sibling behaviors that reliably elicited a class of socially aggressive behaviors for the target child (Patterson, 1973). Given that the sibling teased, the probability that the target child would react by hitting was .060, and for teasing it was .149. There was, in fact, a network of four other sibling behaviors that also elicited target child hitting and teasing. One could think of target child hitting and teasing as being functionally related to each other; they are members of the same response class in that both are reliably triggered by the same network of five sibling behaviors. Further analyses extended the pattern from two steps—sibling initiate, target child react—to two additional steps (Patterson, 1977, 1982). Given that the target child reacted to siblings by hitting and teasing, there was a significant increase in the likelihood that the sibling would then hit, tease, and yell. This could define the first three steps in an extended coercive chain. The fourth step was that the target child was likely to react to sibling hitting, teasing, and yelling by yet further hitting. It should be noted that the further one proceeds into such a coercive chain, the greater the predictability of the

---

[1] The concept of base rate is deceptively simple. In the example above, it would seem that the appropriate base for comparison would be the likelihood of mother scold in general (e.g., divide the number of scolds by the total number of mother behaviors when interacting with the child). Several writers have pointed out, however, that this ignores the thematic effect of her own prior behavior (Martin, Maccoby, Baran, & Jacklin, 1981; Patterson, 1982). It is possible to partial out this intrasubject effect by using multiple regression with the mother's prior behavior at Time 2 as one beta and child behavior at Time 1 as another (Martin, et al., 1981). Another method (and one that the author feels is conceptually "cleaner") is to consider only that subset of events where the mother is initiating a behavior to the child and was not interacting with the child at Time 2 (Patterson, 1982). This baserate value would then be compared to the conditional likelihood of the mother initiating scolding given the child teases, and that she had not previously been interacting with the child at Time 2.

Given that one wished to confirm that the behavior of the child was causally related to the behavior of the mother, then it is necessary to use either regression formats or limit oneself to initiations. In that the present discussion does not require this stronger statement about the nature of the reaction, no effort was made to partial out the intrasubject components for the analyses.

participants. For example, the general likelihood that the target child would initiate an exchange by hitting was only .010, but given sibling teasing, etc., then target child teasing or hitting, then sibling teasing, hitting or yelling, the likelihood was .450 that the target child would then hit.

To what extent do comparable structures or patterns characterize mother-child interactions? Thus far, only two single-subject analyses have been carried out (Patterson, 1974; Patterson & Moore, 1979). The hypothesis was that there are two- and three-step patterns characterizing mother-child interactions in the home. For a sample of mothers and problem children, there will be a sequence in which the child as provocateur elicits a class of irritable verbal behaviors from the mothers. These maternal irritable behaviors, in turn, will elicit yet further coercive behaviors from the child. The resulting three-step sequence helps us understand how it is that mothers slip into extended coercive exchanges with the child, placing both at risk for escalations in amplitude of aggression.

To test these hypotheses, six observations were made in the homes of 36 families of socially aggressive boys. The interactions of these preadolescent boys and their families were described sequentially on an earlier code system, the Family Interaction Coding System (FICS), described in Reid (1978). The details of the sample and the format for the statistical analyses were described in Patterson (1982).

Figure 1 summarizes the data for a three-step sequence in mother-child interaction. There were four maternal reactions (command, command negative, disapproval, and physical negative) that were controlled by a shared preceding network of child behavior. It can be seen that when children failed to comply, engage in physical negative behavior (push, hit, grab), or tease, the probabilities were greatly enhanced that the mothers would engage in any one of three following reactions: command, command negative, or disapproval. Each of the prior child behaviors was found to result in at least a tenfold increase over the baseline values for each of the four mother reactions. In most instances, the magnitude of increase was even higher.

The child behaviors and the maternal reactions to them define the first two steps in the coercion process. One could think of any of the three child behaviors as being functionally or causally related; each of them has a similar impact on the mother. It can also be said that the maternal reactions of command, command negative, and disapproval form a class of behaviors that are all elicited by a shared set of prior child behaviors, and that the three maternal reactions are also functionally related. Not only are they elicited by a shared network of prior events, but in addition, they all have a similar impact in determining the next reaction of the child. It can be seen in Figure 1 that the child is very likely (.323) to comply at the third step. It seems, then, that maternal command, command negative, or disapproval is often effective, and the problem child actually goes along with her requests. One could think of these child reactions at the third step as reinforcing the mother's reactions. The findings support the idea that there is at least one three-step pattern that characterizes mothers and their irritable verbal interactions with problem children.

The next hypothesis is that the dyads from problem families more frequently engage in extended negative exchanges. In the present study, maternal inability to teach the child to control physical aggression and teasing, together with her

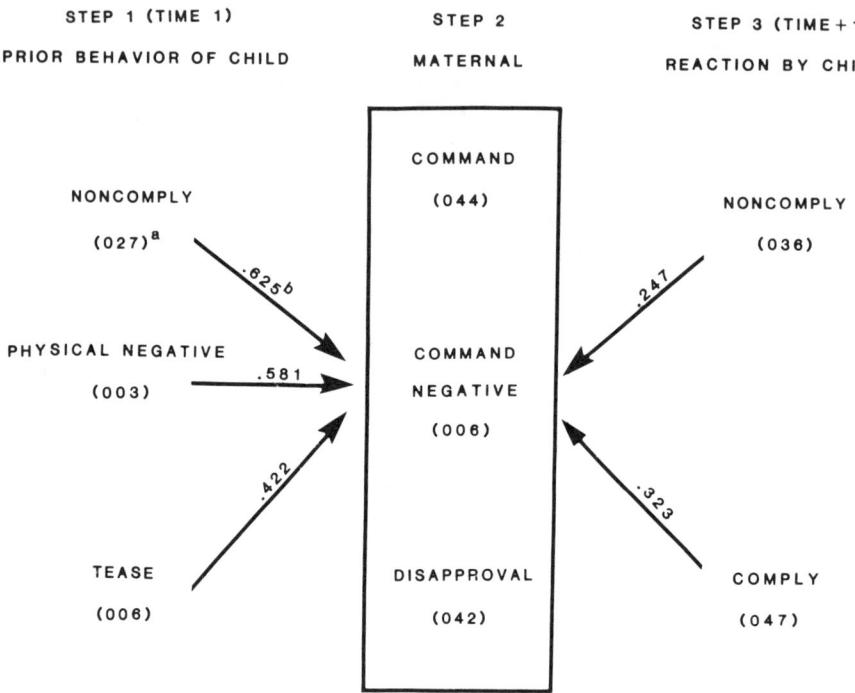

Figure 1 A three-step structure involving a mother's irritable verbal reactions. (*a*) The figures in parentheses refer to the base rate of occurrence for that event (e.g., on the average 2.7% of the children's behavior at Time−1 consisted of noncomply.) (*b*) The conditional likelihood of a mother discipline reaction given the child behavior at Time−1 (e.g., given the child noncomplied, the likelihood of mother command or disapprove was .625).

inability to teach a reasonable degree of compliance, creates a situation where she is constrained to behave in an irritable (command negative and disapproval) fashion. The presence of such extended chains has been demonstrated for families of antisocial and abused children (Patterson, 1982; Reid, 1982; Reid, Taplin, & Lorber, 1981). Observational data analyzed by Reid et al. (1981) showed that from 76% to 83% of coercive events consisted of a *single event.* Someone in the family insults, teases, or scolds another and then stops; no one reacts coercively to it. The whole episode lasts no more than six seconds; about 16% to 21% of the coercive episodes last between 6 and 23 seconds. These are relatively brief three- and four-step sequences. These brief chains are found somewhat less often in normal than in clinical samples, but the differences are not large. What differentiates the samples is that long chains (over 23 seconds) were much more likely to be found in the homes of social aggressors and abused children than in the homes of normals. Given a social aggressive child with an average rate of .8 coercive responses per minute interacting for a 10-hour day, that child could be personally involved in 14 extended chains on any given day.

The findings that extended chains are more likely to occur in the clinical samples is in keeping with the hypothesis. However, the hypothesis stipulated that high intensity maternal behaviors were more likely to occur within extended chains. An analysis by Reid (1982) directly tested this hypotheses. Again, he employed observational data to compare maternal behavior for samples from families of normal, abused, and social aggressor children who are not abused. The findings are summarized in Table 1.

The data suggest that when one considers chains of 23 seconds or longer, there is an increase in the likelihood of high amplitude reactions such as yell, threaten, humiliate, and hit. Within each of the three samples, there seems to be a suggestion of a direct relationship between the likelihood of high amplitude aggression and chain length. The longer the chain, the greater the likelihood of aggression.

Several corollaries follow from this relationship. For example, it should be the case that the more frequently an individual engages in a coercive act, the more likely he or she is to engage in extended chains. This corollary was examined in a study of 33 preadolescent boys referred for treatment of either social aggression or stealing (Patterson, 1979). There was a highly significant correlation between coercive acts and extended chains of coercive behavior for the socially aggressive boys ($r = .76$, $p < .001$). It should also be the case that mothers who engage in high rates of coercive behaviors such as scolding, nagging, and threatening, also tend to engage in high rates of hitting. In a study by Reid et al. (1981), the correlation was .66 ($p < .001$) for one sample of normals, and .36 ($p < .01$) for a sample of nonabused social aggressive boys, and .59 ($p < .05$) for a sample of abused children. The boys in these samples ranged in age from five through 12.

In summary, one of the first steps toward maternal hitting may be characterized by an increase in the rate of coercive behavior by one member of the dyad. This, in turn, would be accompanied by an increase in the occurrence of extended coercive chains, not only with the other dyad member, but perhaps with others in the social milieu. Given the extended chains, it becomes likely that the dyad members, and others as well, will learn to use high amplitude aggressive behaviors. These findings demonstrate the value of direct observation and microsocial analysis of social interactions in determining the causal chains leading to anger and its expression. These analyses also indicate points in the chain at which intervention is most likely to be fruitful in arresting anger escalation. As noted earlier, there is nothing immutable about this sequence. Our experience has shown, for example, that even with extremely disrupted families, an average of 20 hours of therapy produces reductions in the observed rates of irritable behavior for the problem child, the mother, and the siblings (Patterson, Chamberlain, & Reid, 1982; Patterson & Fleischman, 1979). More recent analyses

Table 1 Mean proportions of abusive behaviors by episode length[a]

Length of coercive episode		Antisocial	
	Normal	Nonabusive	Abusive
0 to 11 seconds	.12	.10	.14
12 to 23 seconds	.17	.20	.24
more than 23 seconds	.23	.39	.35

Note. From Reid, 1982.
[a]Threaten, yell, humiliate, or hit.

by Reid (1983) also showed that observed hitting and spanking behaviors for both mothers and fathers of abused children were significantly reduced by such treatment. The innovative interventions described by Novaco in his chapter in this volume are based upon a similar assumption; that is, both parent and Marine Corps drill sergeant can be taught a means of managing their immediate social environment such that their irritable reactions will be reduced.

NEGATIVE ATTRIBUTIONS, AFFECT, AND ANGER

In the preceding section, a general case was made for a process by which both members of a dyad "train" each other to use irritable behaviors; under certain conditions these form predictable, patterned exchanges which, in turn, place both members at risk for engaging in extended chains, including high intensity, aggressive assaults upon each other. What is the role of anger in this process? Certainly, anger is a ubiquitous component reported by everyone, by mothers of problem children as well as by assault-prone police and violent inmates of our prisons (cf. Berkowitz, 1978; Toch, 1969). As we have seen in the preceding section, it is possible to make reliable and informative predictions about aggressive reactions by simply examining the content or type of prior behaviors of the other person. Although not yet tested, it may be assumed that anger would most likely occur during the late segments of extended coercive exchanges. Anger may also serve as a determinant for escalation in the intensity of aggressive behaviors.

The purpose of the following material is to illustrate how a systematic microsocial analysis of the interdependencies in irritable behavior and negative affect might proceed. Because pilot data on mother-child interactions are presented, they are thought to be more illustrative of the approach than confirmatory. The general hypotheses to be explored concern the simultaneous occurrence of irritable content and negative affect, and the possibility that one event precedes or follows the other.

As shown earlier, irritable behaviors on the part of one dyad member elicit irritable reactions in the other member. Might one then conclude that these same behaviors of the one member also elicit anger or negative affect in the other? There are certainly a number of laboratory studies demonstrating that a wide range of aversive stimuli (e.g., heat, noise, insults, frustration) produce reliable increments in autonomic arousal (Bandura, 1973). However, it is also well known that it is the individual's interpretation of the immediate social environment that determines whether the arousal is labelled as anger or anxiety. In social interaction, we have a situation where one or both members may be reacting autonomically to certain behaviors of the other person. We hypothesize that given a past history of conflict, the members of the dyad are more likely to make negative attributions about each other, which increases the likelihood that they would, if asked, label these arousal reactions as anger or frustration. This formulation is in keeping with the programmatic studies of aggressive children by Dodge and his colleagues noted earlier (Dodge, 1980; Dodge & Frame, 1982). Those studies have shown that aggressive children tend to over-attribute hostile intentions to peers, particularly when involved in social exchanges with them.

It is assumed that a history of conflict increases the likelihood that one will view the other person in a negative manner. In fact, it seems likely that irritable content or conflict, arousal, and negative attributions influence each other in a reciprocal fashion; each may function as a positive feedback loop further exacerbating the process. For example, an interesting laboratory analogue study by Kaplan, Burch, and Bloom (1964) showed that dyads who disliked each other were more likely to demonstrate synchronous autonomic reactions during the sessions than were dyads who were positive or neutral about each other. A similar finding has been reported by Levensen and Gottman (1983) for distressed married couples. Is this synchronicity in physiological reactions due to the fact that both members tended to misattribute negative intentions to the other? Or are the attributions a product of the exchange?

The writer assumes that a careful microsocial analysis of angry adults would reveal that many of them live in social environments characterized by frequent attacks by other irritable persons. Understanding and treating such persons should then involve, among other things, training the individuals to carefully monitor their own behavior and the behavior of the other persons triggering the anger. It might also involve a daily diary that describes the negative intentions ascribed to the other person.

How does one assess negative affect in natural settings? Over the last four years, considerable effort has been expended to devise a new observation code for social interaction in the home, one that also makes provision for recording setting changes and changes in affect (Reid et al., 1984). Data were collected using an earlier pilot version of an observational code in roughly a hundred normal families of boys ages 10 through 16. Observer judgment about the neutral shifts to positive or hostile affect is based on changes in facial expression and/or tonal inflections (Patterson & Dishion, 1984). Judgment is made each time the content of an interaction is coded. For each session, the individual's negative affect is described by duration in seconds. Negative affect is a general disposition to react in an angry, irritable fashion to others. Positive affect is a general disposition to react in a warm, friendly fashion. In observational studies of familial interactions, the reliability correlation for affect shift from neutral, across pairs of judges observing the same families on the same occasion, was a modest .58. Our present procedures for recording affect change have been revised, and it is expected that the observer agreement will be considerably improved. Because 28% of the homes were father absent, only the data from mothers were used in the analyses.

The sessions generally lasted about an hour; each family member was observed on three different occasions. Data from the study of these normal families showed that 80% to 90% of the interactions were characterized by neutral affect. Using this instrument, we were curious about how often the average mother might display a positive or negative affect in her interaction with family members. We found, to our surprise, that most of the recorded shifts from neutral affect tended to be positive rather than negative. On the average, the mothers were described as involved in positive affect for a total of 12.6 seconds per session and about three seconds for negative affect. Negative facial expressions and voice changes were relatively brief affairs for mothers of nonproblem families. Those mothers in the sample with problem children engaged in considerably more of the latter.

As a further check on the validity of the instrument as a measure of negative affect, the observers were asked to fill out a questionnaire at the end of each session. They made several global ratings concerning the irritability of the family members. As expected, their global ratings correlated significantly (.46, $p < .001$) with the molecular affect data coded during interactions. The correlation is, of course, not surprising in that both variables were provided by the same observers. However, finding a nonsignificant correlation would raise some doubts about the measure of negative affect. As a second validity check, scores were examined for the mothers on the Hostility subscale (Cook & Medley, 1954) of the Minnesota Multiphasic Personality Inventory. Scores on this scale had been found by Williams et al. (1980) to correlate significantly with the extent of coronary atherosclerosis as determined by angiography. Higher scores on the Hostility subscale mean the individuals describe themselves as suspicious, jealous and hostile in their perceptions of *other* persons. There was a slight but significant trend for high hostility scores to be associated with more negative affect during the home observations. The correlation was a modest $r = .21$ ($p < .05$).

Do the code measures of maternal negative affect correlate with the code measures of maternal irritable reactions to the target child? The correlations are separately summarized in Table 2 for samples of different boys in the fourth, seventh, and tenth grades and for three different irritable reactions. The variable "start up" describes a situation where the target child was behaving in a neutral or even in a positive fashion, and the mother initiated an attack. The first row summarizes the findings; none of these correlations for this variable were significant. This would mean that mothers who were observed to be *most* likely to initiate a fight with the target child were neither more nor less likely to engage in negative affect. It may not be the angry (high negative affect) mother who initiates conflicts.

Notice, however, that the correlations are substantial for the second and third variables, and are moderately consistent across all three grade levels. Mothers coded as higher on negative affect were also coded as more likely to counterattack given a deviant initiation by the child; they were also more likely to persist in being irritable, no matter what the reaction of the child might be. In summary, it seems that maternal negative affect relates not so much to starting conflicts as to extending them once they begin.

Next, mothers were selected who were at the 70th percentile or above for negative affect and at the 70th percentile or above for composite measure of

Table 2 Covariation between negative affect and irritable behavioral content

Mother's irritable reaction to target child (Content)		Correlations for samples			
		Grades			
		Fourth ($N = 25$)	Seventh ($N = 30$)	Tenth ($N = 33$)	All ($N = 88$)
1. Start up conflict	p (M−/Ch+)	.28	.09	.15	.16
2. Counterattack	p (M−/Ch−)	.46*	.58**	.27	.43**
3. Continuance	p (M−/M−)	.31	.56**	.31[a]	.39**

*$p < .05$.
**$p < .001$.

irritable content. Examination of the resulting fourfold table showed that the two classification schemes were significantly correlated. Those mothers at the extreme for negative affect also tended to be at the extreme for irritable content. The contingency coefficient was .43. The findings suggest that mothers who react frequently with an irritable content also tend to react more often with negative affect. Do these events occur as simultaneous events embedded in social interaction or do they occur in sequence, such that one serves as a setting event for the other.

First, the social sequences were analyzed with a six-second "window," whereby the two events were said to co-occur if they both appeared during the same six-second interval. The analysis showed that the likelihood of co-occurrence was .59.

The next issue concerned the likelihood that one event would reliably "trigger" the other (i.e., does negative affect tend to elicit irritable content or the reverse?) The findings showed that if the mother evidenced negative affect, the likelihood that she would display irritable content during the ensuing six seconds was .300. Similarly, if irritable maternal behavior occurred, the likelihood that she would display negative affect in the ensuing six seconds was .280. The observers' judgments thus reflected the fact that negative affect served to elicit negative content about as often as the converse where irritable behavior elicits negative affect. While extremely interesting, the findings should be interpreted with great caution. Both sets of variables were encoded by the same (overworked) observers. In future studies, it will be necessary to use pairs of observers, preferably each independently viewing family interaction; one observer coding affect and the other coding content.

There is another set of data that relates to this general issue. The assumption is that very intense maternal anger is likely to be associated with more extended discipline confrontations; and these confrontations are more likely to occur in clinical than in normal families. A study by Reid (1983) showed that mothers from a sample of distressed families rated their daily discipline confrontations as significantly more angry than did mothers of normal families matched for income and family size. During daily telephone interviews, each mother described the previous day's discipline confrontations, and rated each of them on a seven-point scale, with four being "angry" and seven as "furious." The mean for the mothers from distressed families with abused children was 3.5, significantly greater than the mean of 2.5 for the mothers from normal families. Incidentally, in that same report, Reid showed that after the mothers of the abused children received training in family-management skills, there was a significant reduction in anger during discipline confrontations. In fact, during the post-test, there was no difference in rated anger between mothers of abused and those of normal children. In Reid's programmatic studies of child abusing families, he finds that the mothers *and* fathers are both highly irritable in their exchanges with family members. Because of the high incidence of father-absent homes in these studies, only the data from mothers are cited here.

NEGATIVE AFFECT AND AGGRESSIVE BEHAVIOR

On some occasions, the irritable exchange between mother and child may serve as a kind of interaction trap that gets out of control. What begins as a relatively perfunctory exchange of noncompliance and threats shifts into extended chains that lead to high intensity aggressive behavior. Presumably, the anger, or negative affect, is an accompaniment to (or may even follow) the attack.

To test this hypothesis, data were obtained from a sample of 11 mothers of younger children from Reid's (1983) studies. These mothers were observed to strike, grab, or push their children at relatively high rates during observation sessions. The base rate for high amplitude maternal attacks was .014 (per session). In keeping with these speculations, the likelihood of mother negative affect being coded within the six seconds *following* her attack was .222. In a similar vein, given that she was coded as engaging in negative affect, the likelihood was .034 that she would attack during the same interval. Hitting and negative affect tended to occur together; and the negative emotion also tends to follow her hitting. Both findings are consistent with an entrapment hypothesis.

However, the findings presented earlier also suggested a possibility for yet an additional path, one in which negative affect directly leads to hitting. As Zajonc (1980) points out, it is often the case that a stimulus event elicits an emotional reaction prior to cognitive assessment. It would seem that there might be some stimuli that directly elicit a negative affect, and this, in turn, leads directly to a high intensity attack. This would be roughly analogous to the clinical studies by Toch (1969) and Berkowitz (1978), where both investigators noted a "flash" phenomenon. Following brief interchanges, these violent males reported a flash of intense anger, and then launched a physical attack. The data from the eleven mothers observed to strike their children at high rates were also used to test the "flash" hypothesis. In keeping with the hypothesis, if the mother was coded for negative affect, the likelihood of her hitting within the ensuing six seconds was .035.

The findings are consistent with both the entrapment and the flash hypotheses. Given the small sample size and the modest increment in conditional probability values when compared to the base rate, the findings should be viewed as only illustrative. The findings suggest that there may be several paths to high intensity attack. Some mothers may arrive through the coercion content patterns, escalation route, while others may arrive at the same point by rumination, anger, and explosive rage. It is very likely that the two paths would require different approaches to treatment.

DISCUSSION

The general proposition presented here has been that some of the microanalytic techniques found useful in identifying interactional structure might also be applied to the study of affective reactions. The focus has been on the study of mother-child interactions in natural settings, but the implication is that a similar format might usefully be applied to problems in the area of behavioral medicine as well. What kind of interactional patterns would characterize the exchanges between Type A persons and their colleagues at work or exchanges with their families in the home? Are some of these structures reliably associated with arousal states? If so, then the preventive approach might involve training the patient to track these structures and either alter or avoid them. Our own work with parents involves the assumption that parents can be trained to become more skilled in family-management skills and to more carefully track their social environment. Comparison studies of outcome show significant changes for children and mothers that persist after treatment (Patterson et al., 1982; Patterson & Fleischman, 1979). It remains to be seen whether similar assumptions can be applied to problems within the area of behavioral medicine.

A social interactional perspective in studying mothers of antisocial and abused children has lead us to broaden our view of what the determinants of aggressive behavior might be. Rather than focus only on negative and positive affect toward others, a multilevel assessment forces the investigator to take into account a much wider spectrum of variables. In our own work, it is becoming clear that extrafamilial stressors may severely disrupt the minutiae of microsocial exchanges. For example, mothers severely stressed and without support groups tend to become more irritable when interacting with their children. We believe that these slight altercations can lead to major disruptions in child-rearing processes. We think that disrupted family process generates many products, including maternal anger, depression, and rejection of the child. Are there analagous matrices that should be considered in the study of the Type A person or the hostile individual? Very likely there are, but it will take a broader perspective, including field studies, to determine what the actual situation is.

Microsocial analysis suggests that anger is not just within the individual or within his or her perceptions of the setting. Some of the determinants may actually be in the social environment. Thus, in each person's environment there may be others whose behavior is an important contribution to the triggering negative affect, its associated cardiovascular arousal, and deleterious health consequences. From this perspective, anger and other emotions are the product of a complex process involving subtle interactional patterns that individuals are often not tracking. Nevertheless, they could probably describe these patterns in an interview or in a carefully constructed questionnaire.

It has become part of the conventional wisdom to differentiate between instrumental and hostile aggression (Bandura, 1973; Berkowitz, 1978). The former is presumably determined by reinforcers such as approval, money, or status, while the latter is determined by anger and anticipation of injury to the other person. Findings from our present research program suggests that anger and aggression in the natural environment is more complex. It would seem that both instrumental and hostile aggression may be part of the same complex process, and in many instances one leads to the other. To understand aggression in social interaction such as that occurring in families requires the study of both instrumental and hostile aggression.

In our future research, we propose to further develop strategies to study the structures underlying the experience and expression of anger and aggression. Although our research will continue to develop models based on mother-child interactions, the strategies should apply to the study of anger in other samples and settings. The focus of our research will be on mapping the relationships between attribution, affect, and behavior over time. Specifically, we will study repeated laboratory sessions in which mothers attempt to cope with their preschool children selected for their very high rates of deviant and coercive behavior. Each of the 20 sessions will be coded using the previously described observational rating instrument to describe the interaction structure that characterized each mother-child dyad. A split screen, which includes a closeup of the mothers' facial reactions, will make it possible to more precisely code mothers' positive and negative affective reactions, using detailed systems for coding facial expressions such as that used by Ekman, Friesen, and Ellsworth (1972). The mothers will be asked to view the tapes and give a retrospective account of their feelings and thoughts during the previous session. These accounts will be used to determine the attributional components of the social interaction.

By coding each session for coercive content, negative affect, and negative attribution, we will be in a position to determine the role of these elements in the elicitation, experience, expression, and escalation of interpersonal anger and aggression. First, how do these three elements covary across time? This general design is already being explored for married couples by Gottman and his colleagues.

Is it the case, as hypothesized earlier in this report, that negative attribution is a necessary precursor to negative affect? Is the network of coercive behaviors that elicit irritable responses related to the network that elicits affective and attributional reactions? If a therapist or clinician were successful in having the respondent in a dyad accept a more positive construal of the coercive behavior of the other dyad member, would decreases in negative affect or reductions in irritable and aggressive responses be observed? The formulations by Novaco (see Chap. 11) and others (see Chaps. 12 and 15) would suggest that this would indeed be the case. Microsocial analyses of anger could also be used to examine whether treatment effects will be maintained if the focus of treatment is only on changing the respondent's perceptions and nothing is done to reduce the challenging, coercive behavior of the other member of the dyad. These are the questions for the next generation of social interactional studies. To the extent that anger and aggression increase the risk of disease, then, these future studies of social interaction will be of direct relevance to the field of behavioral medicine.

REFERENCES

Bandura, A. *Aggression: A social learning analysis.* Englewood Cliffs, N.J.: Prentice-Hall, 1973.

Berkowitz, L. Is criminal violence normative behavior? Hostile and instrumental aggression and violent incidents. *Journal of Research in Crime and Delinquency,* 1978, *15,* 148-161.

Cairns, R. B. (Ed.). *The analysis of social interaction: Methods, issues, and illustrations.* Hillsdale, N.J.: Erlbaum, 1979.

Cook, W. W., & Medley, D. M. Proposed hostility and phariasaic-virtue scores for the MMPI. *Journal of Applied Psychology,* 1954, *38,* 414-418.

Dodge, K. A. Social cognition and children's aggressive behavior. *Child Development,* 1980, *51,* 162-170.

Dodge, K. A., & Frame, C. L. Social cognitive biases and deficits in aggressive boys. *Child Development,* 1982, *53,* 626-635.

Ekman, P., Friesen, W. V., & Ellsworth, P. *Emotion in the human face: Guidelines for research and an integration of findings.* New York: Pergamon, 1972.

Gottman, J. Emotional responsiveness in marital conversations. *Journal of Communication,* 1982, *32,* 108-120.

Gottman, J. M., & Bakeman, R. The sequential analysis of observation data. In S. Suomi, M. Lamb, & G. Stephenson (Eds.), *Social interaction analysis: Methodological issues.* Madison: University of Wisconsin Press, 1979.

Hartup, W. W. Levels of analysis in the study of social interaction. An historical perspective. In M. E. Lamb, S. J. Suomi, and G. R. Stephenson (Eds.), *Social interaction analysis: Methodological issues.* Madison: University of Wisconsin Press, 1979.

Izard, C. E. Emotions as motivations: An evolutionary-developmental perspective. In R. Dienstbier (Ed.), *Nebraska Symposium on Motivation, 1978.* Lincoln: University of Nebraska Press, 1979.

Kaplan, H. B., Burch, N. R., & Bloom, S. Physiological covariation and sociometric relationships in small groups. In P. H. Leiderman & D. Shapiro (Eds.), *Psychological approaches to social behavior.* Stanford, Calif.: Stanford University Press, 1964.

Knutson, J., Fordyce, D., & Anderson, D. The escalation of irritable aggression: Control by consequences and antecedents. *Aggressive Behavior,* 1982, *6,* 347–359.

Lang, P. J. Fear reduction and fear behavior: Problems in treating a construct. In J. M. Shlien (Ed.), *Research in psychotherapy* (Vol. 3). Washington, D.C.: American Psychological Association, 1968.

Lang, P. J. Cognition in emotion: Concept and action. In C. Izard, J. Kagan, & R. Zazone (Eds.), *Emotion, cognition, and behavior.* New York: Cambridge University Press, 1983.

Levenson, R. W., & Gottman, J. M. Marital interaction: Physiological linkage and affective exchange. *Journal of Personality and Social Psychology,* 1983, *45*(3), 587–597.

Margolin, G. *A sequential analysis of dyadic communication.* Paper presented at the meeting of the Association for the Advancement of Behavior Therapy, Atlanta, Ga., December, 1977.

Martin, J., Maccoby, E., Baran, K., & Jacklin, C. The sequential analysis of mother-child interaction at 18 months: A comparison of several microanalytic methods. *Developmental Child,* 1981, *17,* 146–157.

Nisbett, R. E., & Wilson, T. D. Telling more than we can know: Verbal reports on mental processes. *Psychological Review,* 1977, *84*(3), 231–259.

Novaco, R. G. *Anger control.* Lexington, Mass.: D. C. Heath, 1975.

Parke, R. D. Perspectives on father-infant interaction. In J. D. Osofsky (Ed.), *Handbook of infancy.* New York: Wiley, 1978.

Patterson, G. R. Changes in status of family members as controlling stimuli: A basis for describing treatment process. In L. A. Hamerlynck, L. C. Handy, & E. J. Mash (Eds.), *Behavior change: Methodology, concepts, and practice.* Champaign, Ill.: Research, 1973.

Patterson, G. R. A basis for identifying stimuli which control behavior in natural settings. *Child Development,* 1974, *45,* 900–911.

Patterson, G. R. Accelerating stimuli for two classes of coercive behaviors. *Journal of Abnormal Child Psychology,* 1977, *5,* 334–350.

Patterson, G. R. A performance theory for coercive family interaction. In R. Cairns (Ed.), *Social interaction: Methods, analysis, and illustrations.* Hillsdale, N.J.: Erlbaum, 1979.

Patterson, G. R. *Coercive family process.* Eugene, Oreg.: Castalia, 1982.

Patterson, G. R. Stress: A change agent for family process. In M. Rutter (Ed.), *Stress, coping, and development in children.* New York: McGraw-Hill, 1983.

Patterson, G. R., Chamberlain, P., & Reid, J. B. A comparative evaluation of a parent-training program. *Behavior Therapy,* 1982, *13,* 638–650.

Patterson, G. R., & Dishion, T. J. *A process model for families of antisocial children,* in preparation.

Patterson, G. R., & Fleischman, M. J. Maintenance of treatment effects: Some considerations concerning family systems and follow-up data. *Behavior Therapy,* 1979, *10,* 168–185.

Patterson, G. R., & Moore, D. Interactive patterns as units of behavior. In S. J. Suomi, M. E. Lamb, and G. R. Stephenson (Eds.), *Social interaction analysis: Methodological issues.* Madison: University of Wisconsin Press, 1979.

Patterson, G. R., Ray, R. S., Shaw, D. A., & Cobb, J. A. *A manual for coding of family interactions* (revised). New York: Microfiche Publications, 1969. (Document 01234, ASIS/NAPS)

Reid, J. B. (Ed.). *A social learning approach to family intervention, Vol. II. Observation in home settings.* Eugene, Ore.: Castalia, 1978.

Reid, J. B. *Social interactional patterns in families of abused and nonabused children: Social and biological origins.* Paper presented at the Society for Research in Child Development Conference on Altruism and Aggression, Washington, D.C., 1982.

Reid, J. B. *Final report: Investigating boys' aggression toward women and girls.* Grant R01 MH25548-83, Oregon Social Learning Center, 1983.

Reid, J. B., Dishion, T., Patterson, G. R., Gabrielson, P., & Thibodeaux, S. *Family interaction code.* Oregon Social Learning Center Technical Report, 1984.

Reid, J. B., Patterson, G. R., & Loeber, R. The abused child: Victim, instigator, or innocent bystander? In D. J. Bernstein (Ed.), *Response structure and organization.* Lincoln: University of Nebraska Press, 1982.

Reid, J. B., Taplin, P. S., & Lorber, R. A social interactional approach to the treatment of abusive families. In R. Stuard (Ed.), *Violent behavior: Social learning approaches to prediction, management, and treatment.* New York: Brunner/Mazel, 1981.

Spielberger, C. D., & London, P. Rage boomerangs. *American Health,* 1982, *1,* 52–56.

Suomi, S., Lamb, M., & Stephenson, G. (Eds.). *Social interaction analysis: Methodological issues.* Madison: University of Wisconsin Press, 1979.

Toch, H. *Violent men:* New York: Aldine, 1969.

Viken, R., & Knutson, J. The effects of reactivity to dorsal stimulation and social role on aggressive behavior in laboratory rats. *Aggressive Behavior,* 1983, *9,* 287–302.

Wahler, R. G., & Dumas, J. E. *Stimulus class determinants of mother-child coercive exchange in multidistressed families: Assessment and intervention.* Paper presented at the Vermont Conference on Primary Prevention of Psychopathology, Bolton Valley, Vermont, June, 1983.

Williams, R. B., Haney, T. L., Lee, K. L., Kong, Y., Blumenthal, J., & Whalen, R. E. Type A behavior, hostility, and coronary atherosclerosis. *Psychosomatic Medicine,* 1980, *42,* 539-549.

Zajonc, R. B. Feeling and thinking: Preferences need no conferences. *American Psychologist,* 1980, *35,* 151-175.

II

HEALTH CONSEQUENCES

It has long been suspected that anger, hostility, and aggression increase risk for cardiovascular disease. The chapters in this section present new evidence documenting this relationship for hypertension and coronary artery disease and indicating the mechanisms that link specific anger dimensions to these disease states.

In "Health Consequences for Anger and Implications for Treatment," Ray Rosenman reviews the evidence relating the sympathetic nervous system to anger and hostility, as well as to hypertension and its coronary heart disease complications. He also presents evidence that anger and hostility are the components of the Type A behavior pattern that largely account for its relationship to heart disease risk. While hostility, aggression, and anger have their origins in the limbic system, Rosenman views these behaviors as the result of social learning. As such, hostility, anger, and aggression are amenable to modification and are appropriate targets for intervention in the treatment of hypertension and prevention of heart disease.

Focusing on hypertension in "Suppressed Anger in Hypertension: Facts and Problems," Stevo Julius and his associates present evidence indicating that some patients with mild hypertension exhibit a unique pattern of interrelated physiological responses and behavioral factors, including unexpressed anger that may play a role in elevating blood pressure in borderline and mild hypertensive individuals. Turning to issues of etiology, Dr. Julius discusses problems that may prevent drawing the popular conclusion that these interrelated factors, including anger, are important in the development of more severe established hypertension.

The prevalence of hypertension is not only twice as great but also is associated with higher mortality rates among black as compared to white Americans. These differences have most often been ascribed to dietary and constitutional or genetic factors. In contrast to these explanations, Doyle Gentry draws upon the literature and his own data to support the hypothesis that certain styles of coping with life strain and hostility are related to blood pressure and may predispose black Americans to hypertension. Like Rosenman, Gentry views these anger-related factors as learned and discusses implications for anger intervention and prevention of hypertension.

In "Behavioral Factors in Hypertension: Cardiovascular Responsivity, Anger, and Social Competence," Stephen Manuck and his associates extend the concept of anger suppression, discussed in the previous chapters, to nonassertiveness. He presents evidence linking these anger-expression factors to stress and cardiovascular reactivity. With regard to the role of reactivity in the development of hypertension, Manuck discusses the literature from the perspective of individual differences and presents recent findings on determinants of hyperreactivity to stressors, including family history of cardiovascular disease.

In "The Health Consequences of Hostility," Redford Williams and his associates show that a psychological characteristic, involving hostility and cynicism, is related cross-sectionally to severity of coronary atherosclerosis, and prospectively to coronary heart disease. Moreover, they report recent findings that indicate increased risk of mortality from all causes among individuals who, when tested, show elevated scores on this psychological dimension. They describe this high-risk psychological characteristic and the questionnaire scale that measures it, presenting data from both psychometric and long-term health outcome studies. The biological pathways whereby hostility and cynicism may be translated into disease processes are speculated upon.

In this volume, the only chapter to focus on the animal model is that by Stephen Manuck and his associates at the Arteriosclerosis Research Center at Bowman Gray School of Medicine. This chapter is included because it presents landmark research documenting causal relationships between hostility and aggression expressed under stressful social conditions and the extent of arteriosclerosis determined by direct assessment of arterial lesions. Such prospective studies linking anger, hostility, and aggression to disease are essential to establish the causal relevance of these characteristics to disease outcomes. In many cases, however, this research cannot be conducted with human subjects; therefore, a comprehensive picture of the health consequences of anger and hostility must rely, at least in part, on animal research. This point is further demonstrated by a study reported by Manuck and his associates on individual differences in animal cardiac reactivity to stress, which constitutes one of only two existing prospective studies connecting cardiovascular reactivity to coronary artery disease.[1] Integrating their animal data into the mosaic of human research on behavioral factors in coronary heart disease, Manuck et al. present a model tracing the mechanisms by which Type A behavior, and particularly hostility, lead to heart disease through enhanced cardiovascular reactivity to stress.

[1] The other study (Keys, A., Taylor, H. L., Blackburn, H., Brozek, J., Anderson, J. T., & Simonson, E. Mortality and coronary heart disease among men studied for 23 years. *Archives of Internal Medicine*, 1971, *128*, 201-214) found diastolic blood pressure response to the Cold Pressor Test to be the most significant variable for CHD prediction in a 23-year prospective study.

5
Health Consequences of Anger and Implications for Treatment

Ray. H. Rosenman
SRI International

This chapter will be concerned with some of the relevant evidence that relates the sympathetic nervous system to hypertension, and hostility/anger dimensions to the pathogenesis of hypertension and its end-organ coronary disease complications. It will be shown that these same dimensions are the probable coronary-prone behaviors that relate Type A behavior pattern to enhanced coronary artery disease and increased incidence of clinical coronary heart disease via enhanced central noradrenergic secretion. Aggression, hostility, and anger dimensions are related to evolutionary gender differences in limbic system anatomy, but evidence will be presented that these are far more learned behaviors that interact with genetic potentials. The role of anger management will be discussed as an appropriate therapeutic intervention in the treatment of hypertension as well as the prevention of coronary heart disease.

Aggression, hostility, and anger are central concepts for theories of personality (Spielberger, Jacobs, Russell, & Crane, 1983). Their maladaptive effects are importantly related not only to psychoneuroses, depression, and schizophrenia, but perhaps equally to hypertension, coronary heart disease (CHD), and CHD complications of hypertension (Diamond, 1982). Although anger is viewed as an emotional reaction (Spielberger et al., 1983; Buss, 1961) and aggression as a behavioral response (Schachter & Singer, 1962), operational distinctions may be difficult since aggressive behavior is often associated with hostility and anger (Spielberger et al., 1983; Diamond, 1982). Some believe that hostile aggression is motivated by anger; others believe that aggression is an inevitable instinctual drive with no necessary causal relationship to hostility (Diamond, 1982).

SOME RELATIONSHIPS OF ANGER DIMENSIONS WITH BLOOD PRESSURE AND CARDIOVASCULAR RESPONSIVENESS

The relationship of anger to hypertension has been studied sporadically for many decades (Brunton, 1909), with much research perhaps too easily dismissed for methodological flaws (Diamond, 1982; Weiner, 1977; Harrell, 1980). However, more recent, carefully performed epidemiological and longitudinal studies have found an association between self-reported ineffective management of anger and either higher resting blood pressure (BP) (Diamond, 1982; Harrell, 1980; Harburg, Blakelock, & Roeper, 1979; Weiner, 1977; Baer, Collins, Bourenoff, & Ketchel, 1979) or sustained hypertension as observed in the 5-year prospective study of Israeli civil servants (Kahn, Medalie, Neufeld, Riss, & Goldbourt, 1972) and in the 20-year prospective study of Harvard undergraduates (McClelland, 1979). Many other studies have found hypertensive subjects to harbor unexpressed hostility and anger (Diamond, 1982) that is associated with exaggerated and more prolonged cardiovascular (CV) responses to a variety of stressful stimuli (Baer et al., 1979; Goldstein, 1981), although generally, if not invariably, shortened (Harburg et al., 1979) when subjects are provided an opportunity to vent their anger (Hokanson, Burgess, & Cohen, 1963).

There is a consensus—if not universal—finding (Goldstein, 1981) that subjects with hypertension tend to exhibit exaggerated CV responses to a variety of stressful stimuli, particularly those of cognitive nature (Brod, Fencl, Hejl, & Jirka, 1959; Shapiro, 1961; Light & Obrist, 1980). Although this does not provide definitive evidence for a causal role in the pathogenesis of hypertension, it is significant that similar responses are observed in normotensive offspring of hypertensive parents and in younger persons with more labile or "borderline" hypertension (Esler, Julius, Zweifler, Randall, Harburg, Gardiner, & DeQuattro, 1977; Esler, Julius, Randall, Ellis, & Kashima, 1975; Falkner, Onesti, Angelakos, Fernandes, & Langman, 1979; Falkner, Onesti, & Angelakos, 1979; Nestel, 1969). The most reactive of such persons are those with high sodium-renin profiles who also exhibit other hemodynamic differences, such as higher baseline cardiac output and heart rate (Esler et al., 1975; Esler et al., 1977), even with normal peripheral vascular resistance (Julius, Quadir, & Gajendragadkar, 1979; Julius & Esler, 1975. Also see Julius, Chap. 6.) It also is significant that adolescents with parental hypertension who progress from "borderline" to sustained hypertension exhibit the greatest CV responses to cognitive stressors (Falkner et al., 1979: Falkner, Onesti, & Hamstra, 1981). Behaviorally induced CV responses tend to reflect stable individual characteristics that usually generalize from the laboratory to naturalistic situations (Manuck, Corse, & Winkelman, 1979; Light, 1981). Chronic stress in certain animals induces sustained hypertension, particularly in association with high plasma renin activity (Henry & Cassel, 1969; Henry & Stephens, 1977; Henry, Stephens, & Santisteban, 1975; Lawler, Barker, Hubbard, & Allen, 1980; Forsyth, 1971).

Lability of both systolic and diastolic blood pressure of sometimes striking degree is physiologically ubiquitous, with predictable variations by time of day, level of anxiety and other emotions, and type of activity. However, using ambulatory monitoring, a recent study finds that the greatest variability correlates with both level of anxiety and level of hostility (Thailer, Friedman, Harshfield, Kleinert, & Pickering, 1982).

RELATIONSHIPS OF STRESSORS TO NEUROHORMONAL RESPONSES AND BLOOD PRESSURE

CV responses to stressful stimuli are associated with neurohormonal changes (Diamond, 1982; Nestel, 1969; Julius & Esler, 1975; Henry & Stephens, 1977; Frankenhaeuser, 1980). However, there appears to be a dissociation between pituitary-adrenal (PA) and sympathetic-adrenal (SA) activity (Frankenhaeuser, Rauste von Wright, Collins, von Wright, Sedvall, & Swahn, 1978). Cannon's oversimplified belief (Cannon, 1932) held that epinephrine (E) is associated with a flight response and norepinephrine (NE) with an active coping or fight response, and these even take different demonstrated limbic pathways (Weiner, 1977; Cannon, 1936; Ax, 1953; Funkenstein, King, & Drolette, 1957; Schachter, 1957). However, it is now preferable to view responses as alpha-adrenergic, which stimulate peripheral vasoconstriction, and beta-adrenergic, which increase heart rate and contraction while inducing vasodilation in the skeletal muscle bed.

PA activation is associated with a conservation-withdrawal type of response, which is often concurrent with negative emotional feelings of distress (Frankenhaeuser, 1980; Frankenhaeuser et al., 1980; Frankenhaeuser, 1982); SA activation occurs more often in response to challenge for control and is associated with positive feelings of alertness and action-proneness (Henry & Stephens, 1977; Lundberg & Frankenhaeuser, 1980). Moreover, PA activation may have a bidirectional response to stressors, either elevating or suppressing secretion of cortisol in association with feelings of high controllability (Frankenhaeuser, 1980). The secretion of E is a basic arousal reaction, which is a sensitive index of response intensity; that of NE is more complex, with less well understood significance (Frankenhaeuser, Mellis, Rissler, Bjorkvall, & Patkai, 1968).

Both the basic E arousal and the NE responses should be considered homeostatic. NE induces a rise of both systolic and diastolic blood pressure and is associated with increased vigilant sensory intake, increased isometric muscle strength, and protection against hemorrhage. It can thus be viewed as preparation for a fight response that is opposite to the vasodilation associated with isotonic exercise. It is not surprising that those responses associated with fear are quite varied and resemble responses during isotonic exercise. Among the various emotions, anger appears to evoke the greatest overall CV responses, and these are antithetical to the responses associated with relaxation. They involve both E and NE in a pattern resembling those associated with isometric exercise, with a rise of both cardiac output and peripheral vascular resistance (Schwartz, Weinberger, & Singer, 1981).

Many emotions induce CV responses whose differences reside in the mix of alpha- and beta-adrenergic secretions. It is primarily the perception of an event that determines the emotional response and hence the psychophysiological consequences (Frankenhaeuser, 1980; Sokolow, Werdegar, Perloff, Cowan, & Brenenstund, 1970). Anger is a cognitive response that is associated with personal appraisal and interpretation (Spielberger et al., 1983; Diamond, 1982; Buss, 1961) and induces an active coping response in the susceptible individual (Frankenhaeuser, 1982; Schwartz et al., 1981). Compared with fear or anxiety, an expressed anger response is associated with relatively smaller rise of heart rate and greater rise of diastolic blood pressure due to peripheral vasoconstriction (Schachter, 1957; Schwartz et al., 1981). The finding that offspring of hypertensive parents, who are at increased risk for sustained hypertension, also exhibit higher baseline systolic blood pressure and higher heart rate response to cognitive stressors (Manuck, Giordani, McQuaid, & Garrity, 1981) may not be a paradox, considering that the special role of anger for hypertension resides in the unique pressor response to unexpressed anger. This response may even play a role in the resetting of baroreceptors, which itself is relevant for hypertension (Schwartz et al., 1981).

Many hypertensive subjects have difficulty expressing aggression, hostility, and anger (Baer et al., 1979; Esler et al., 1977; Alexander, 1939; Steptoe, 1981).

They thereby internalize emotions that may evoke the exaggerated and prolonged CV responses that may be diminished in the laboratory when they are given an opportunity to vent their anger (Hokanson et al., 1963). Assertiveness, viewed as the ability to stand up to one's emotions (Jakubowski & Lange, 1978; Linehan & Egan, 1979), can be operationally defined and objectively assessed (Arkowitz, 1981; Bellack, 1979). Hypertensive subjects often have difficulty with assertiveness (Saslow, Gressel, Shobe, DuBois, & Schroeder, 1950; Wolff & Wolf, 1951; Harris, Sokolow, Carpenter, Freedman, & Hunt, 1953; Kalis, Harris, Sokolow, & Carpenter, 1957) hence ineffective anger management, which has been found capable of classifying persons with higher baseline blood pressure and later higher incidence of hypertension (Kahn et al., 1972; McClelland, 1979; Esler et al., 1977). Such findings have helped to reduce earlier confusion, which resulted from the use of interchangeable psychometric measures that probably in part assessed different dimensions of anger (Spielberger et al., 1983; Diamond, 1982; Stauder, Holroyd, Appel, Gorkin, Uphole, & Saab, 1983). It seems clear that among younger persons of higher risk because of parental hypertension, those who most often progress to sustained hypertension are those who show the most exaggerated catecholamine and CV responses to stressors designed to elicit anger, and the greatest risk occurs among those who are least able to express the anger (Kahn et al., 1972; McClelland, 1979; Falkner et al., 1979). If there actually is a hypertensive personality (Alexander, 1939), it appears to involve an avoidance type of defensiveness that prevents successful adaptation to stressful situations (Shapiro, 1960; Handkins & Munz, 1978; Sapira, Scheib, Moriarty, & Shapiro, 1971; Pilkowsky, Saplding, Shaw, & Korner, 1973). This relationship is relevant to the finding that sustained hypertension is most consistently related to environmental situations that require continuous behavioral adjustments on an individual's part (Gutman & Benson, 1971).

Since anger induced the greatest catecholamine responses (Schwartz et al., 1981) it is relevant that increased plasma levels of the NE transmitter are found in a significant subset of younger subjects with hypertension or with more labile and "borderline" levels of blood pressure (Esler et al., 1977; Nestel, 1969; Julius & Esler, 1975; Steptoe, 1981; Kalis et al., 1957; DeQuattro, Sullivan, Foti, Schoentgen, Bornheimer, Kolloch, Versales, & Levine, 1981; Goldstein, 1981). Although their turnover of NE has not been demonstrated to be abnormal (DeQuattro & Miura, 1974) there may be defective neuronal uptake in some (Esler, Jackson, Bobik, Leonard, Kelleher, Skews, Jennings, & Kornes, 1981). However, plasma dopamine-beta-hydroxylase, the third enzyme in NE biosynthesis, is not different in hypertensive subjects and correlates poorly with SA activity. Moreover, pharmacological agents lower blood pressure in association with depletion of catecholamine, particularly when they deplete NE in peripheral sites (DiPalma, 1961; Weiner, 1977). Nevertheless, there is persuasive evidence that SA activity is increased in a significant subset of hypertensive subjects (Goldstein, 1981; Julius et al., 1979; DeQuattro et al., 1981), that this increase stems from a central origin (DeQuattro et al., 1981; Kawano, Fukiyama, Jakeya, Obo, & Omae, 1982), and that it is in part associated with suppressed hostility (Esler et al., 1977; Sullivan, Schoentgen, DeQuattro, Procci, Levine, & Bornheimer, 1981).

Stressful stimuli that induce active coping are associated with beta-adrenergic CV responses that closely resemble those in "borderline" hypertensive persons

(Esler et al., 1977; Groen, 1982; Julius et al., 1979; Falkner et al., 1981). The catecholamine increase and effects of beta-adrenergic blockade, of course, indicate that the CV responses are SA-mediated.

A relative though not true renal dysfunction is usually believed to be involved in the pathogenesis of sustained hypertension via regulation of electrolytes and blood volume, and over the longer term these may dominate the level at which the BP stabilizes (Guyton, 1980). CV responses to stressful stimuli are enhanced by sodium intake and by potassium depletion (Skrabal, Aubock, & Hortnagl, 1981), and the relatives and offspring of hypertensive subjects often exhibit delayed natriuresis and more rapid contertransport of cellular sodium (Grim, Luft, Miller, Brown, Gannon, & Weinberger, 1979; Canessa, Adragna, Solomon, Connolly, & Tosteson, 1980; Henningsen, Mattsson, Nosslin, Nelson, & Ohlsson, 1979). Renin stimulates release of aldosterone, which in turn stimulates renal sodium reabsorption and potassium excretion, both of which probably sensitize the peripheral vasculature to NE (Parfrey, Vandenburg, Wright, Holly, Goodwin, Evans, & Ledingham, 1981). There is evidence to link aldosterone secretion with dopaminergic-adrenergic systems that are even independent of renin and angiotensin (McKenna, Island, Nicholson, & Liddle, 1979; Whitfield, Sowers, Tuck, & Golub, 1980).

The immediacy and transience of SA-induced CV responses make it difficult to ascribe to them any role beyond initiating increased peripheral vascular resistance, while sustained hypertension probably involves a role of blood volume, cardiac output, and electrolytes (Guyton, 1980). Furthermore, it is plausible that blood-pressure-regulating mechanisms that may trigger initial elevations are different from those that sustain hypertension. A behavioral paradigm of active coping responses is beta-adrenergically mediated. The response to renal nerve stimulation that is beta-adrenergically mediated is one of the three main factors that control release of renin from renal juxtaglomerular cells (Genest, 1977; DeQuattro, Barbour, Campese, Fink, Miand, & Esler, 1977). CV responses to stressful stimuli thus may not be valid indicators of blood pressure dysregulation per se unless they are manifestations of particular control mechanisms.

The complexity of blood pressure regulation indicates that hypertension has multiple causes, as suggested by Page's mosaic model (Page & McCubbin, 1966); but we now accept a sequential pathogenesis for hypertension, and it is clear that beta-adrenergic input can play a culpable role at each of the important stages of this mosaic sequence. It is difficult to avoid suspecting a special role of anger, at least for the level of blood pressure in subjects with hypertension, if not for its pathogenesis (Schachter, 1957). Some cardiologists have long recognized this association. Thus, in 1909 Lauder Brunton discussed the special role of hurry and anger in the etiology of hypertension; he believed that they accelerated atheromatosis. In 1956 Paul Wood noted that hypertension was likely to occur in persons who overreact to certain types of stressful stimuli, a finding that was subsequently emphasized by Nixon (Nixon & Bethel, 1974; Nixon, 1976) and others.

RELATIONSHIPS OF TYPE A HOSTILITY AND ANGER DIMENSIONS TO CHD

It is equally difficult to ignore a special role for anger variables in coronary heart disease (CHD). Type A behavior pattern (TAB) includes a cluster of behavioral dispositions, specific behaviors, and emotional reactions (Rosenman, Friedman, Straus, Wurm, Kositchek, Hahn, & Werthessen, 1964; Rosenman, 1978; Rosenman & Chesney, 1982). Its very conceptualization in the late 1950s delineated specific components, including anger dimensions, that were designed to be assessed and scored in the Structured Interview (SI) (Rosenman et al., 1964; Rosenman, 1978), which was developed initially to assess Type A/B behaviors in the Western Collaborative Group Study (WCGS). Although the reported follow-up analyses were based mainly on global A/B behaviors (Rosenman, Brand, Sholtz, & Friedman, 1976), one prevalence study of the SI responses was done in 25 men who were enrolled in the WCGS but excluded from prospective follow-up because the intake ECG showed that they had suffered a "silent" MI prior to enrollment. This study compared these 25 men with age- and occupation-matched controls and found that the hostility component of the SI was higher in the subjects with prior "silent" MI (Jenkins, 1966). It was therefore decided to examine the components to TAB as determined from the SI in a larger sample of WCGS subjects. In this study Dr. Ray Bortner was asked to do a blind rating of the SI responses of 62 men who subsequently suffered CHD during follow-up, comparing them with the responses of two control subjects who were matched for age and occupation. Other investigators much later have also used the initially conceptualized components (Dembroski, MacDougall, Shields, Petitto, & Lushene, 1978). The untimely death of Dr. Bortner did not permit him to see the fruit of his labors in this initial prospective study of TAB components. The analyses of his ratings of the SI (Matthews, Glass, Rosenman, & Bortner, 1977) showed that, among the specific components of TAB, it was those that related to competitive drive, impatience, and potential for hostility that selectively identified the coronary-prone subjects. A new appraisal of the same data revealed that the anger/hostility dimension is the dominant characteristic among the coronary-prone Type A behaviors (Spielberger, Rosenman, Chesney, & Hecker, to be published), a finding that is fully consonant with the original conception of coronary-prone TAB (Rosenman et al., 1964). Later investigators have not only provided construct validity to the TAB concept (Rosenman & Chesney, 1982) but also have confirmed the relationship of Type A anger dimensions to the incidence of CHD (Haynes, Feinleib, & Kannel, 1980).

Although psychometric measures are able to assess TAB with only limited success (Rosenman & Chesney, 1982), it is significant that hostility/anger items and scales of such measures are found to discriminate A/B behaviors (Rosenman, Rahe, Borhani, & Feinleib, 1976; Chesney, Black, Chadwick, & Rosenman, 1981) as well as to correlate with the enhanced CV responsiveness of Type A subjects (Williams, Lane, Kuhn, Melosh, White, & Schanberg, 1982). It also is significant that psychometric measures of such hostility/anger dimensions are correlated with CHD incidence in other prospectively followed population, such as in the Western Electric Study (Shekelle, Gale, Ostfeld, & Paul, 1983) and in the medical student cohort of the University of North Carolina (Barefoot, Dahlstrom, & Williams, 1983), and are correlated with the severity of basic coronary atherosclerosis in the subjects studied by angiographic methodology (Williams, Haney, Lee, Kong, Blumenthal, & Whalen, 1980; Blumenthal, Williams, Kong, Schanberg, & Thompson, 1978).

The relationship of anger/hostility to CHD is an important one that has led to some confusion. Although TAB has been found (Rosenman et al., 1964) and confirmed (Rosenman & Chesney, 1982) to be a risk factor for CHD, there is considerable evidence that it may be the anger/hostility dimension of TAB that confers coronary-proneness (Matthews et al., 1977: Spielberger et al., to be published; Jenkins, 1966). This emotional characteristic also was found to relate significantly to the incidence of CHD in the Framingham Study (Haynes et al., 1980), but only spuriously apart from TAB since the Framingham Type A Scale was directed primarily at the impatience and accelerated pace of activities of TAB and a separate scale was used to assess the anger/hostility dimension. The same problem appears to arise with the studies that used scales derived from the MMPI (Cook & Medley, 1954; Hathaway & McKinley, 1967) to measure hostility and found predictive correlations with the incidence of CHD (Shekelle et al., 1983; Barefoot et al., 1983) as well as with the severity of coronary atherosclerosis (Williams et al., 1980; Blumenthal et al., 1978). The finding of a relationship of "hostility" to the severity of coronary atherosclerosis in the studies of Shekelle and Barefoot led them to infer that this behavior was independent of TAB. Unfortunately, these authors had failed in their studies to administer the SI to assess either the TAB of their subjects or its hostility/anger dimensions, thus leading to a somewhat spurious conclusion that such behaviors are independent of TAB, when they may in fact be dominant Type A behaviors that relate TAB to CHD (Mathews et al., 1977; Spielberger et al., in press).

One relevant problem is whether these MMPI scales (Cook & Medley, 1954; Hathaway & McKinley, 1967) actually are appropriate for assessment of hostility/anger dimensions. Although there appears to be some correlation with these traits (Spielberger et al., 1983), the reader is referred to the paper by Megargee included in this book. He points out that these MMPI scales have not been validated by studies which provide construct validity to the belief that they measure hostility/anger and aggression, and that perhaps they provide evidence to the contrary. It has been pointed out (Shekelle et al., 1983; Barefoot et al., 1983) that these psychometric measures probably assess the quality and quantity of social supports (Berkman & Syme, 1979) rather than hostility/anger characteristics. The validity of these as measures of anger dimensions must be further questioned in view of the finding that, in the cited prospective studies, the scales were found to be related not only to incidence of CHD but also to mortality from cancer and from all causes (Shekelle et al., 1983; Barefoot et al., 1983).

TAB is a characteristic coping style that is considered by some to be a response to environmental threats to a Type As control (Glass, 1977; Glass & Contrada, 1982). This interpretation may be oversimplified since it is probably an enhanced sense of competitiveness at a cognitive level that provides the substrate for most Type A behaviors, including aggressive drive, accelerated pace of activities, and anger/hostility. Possibly to avoid anxiety from threat of failure (Glass, 1977) Type As usually have an achievement orientation that seeks an aggressive approach and accelerated pace of activities (Frankenhaeuser, 1980; Rosenman et al., 1964; Rosenman & Chesney, 1982; Ray & Bozek, 1980). They appear to be predisposed to enhanced response to hostile interaction, even when the latter is inappropriately perceived (Frankenhaeuser, 1980; Frankenhaeuser et al., 1980). Type As exhibit enhanced catecholamine release during competitive laboratory stressors (Friedman, Byers, Diamant, & Rosenman, 1960) and, in dyad competition, it is not surprising that Type A subjects exhibit an increased hostility when paired with other Type As who exhibit similar behaviors (Frankenhaeuser et al., 1980; Dembroski et al., 1978). One has only to audit the challenge-type SIs of severe Type As to understand how such behaviors are readily induced in the susceptible individual (Rosenman, 1978).

The mix of neurohormonal secretion in response to stressful stimuli can be variable (Frankenhaeuser et al., 1980; Dembroski et al., 1978; Williams et al., 1982; Glass & Contrada, 1982). However, male Type As are generally found to respond to overstimulation with higher E response (Glass, Drakoff, Contrada, Hilton, Kehoe, Mannucci, Collins, Snow, & Elting, 1980) and to competitive physical activity and cognitive tasks with higher NE response, compared to Type Bs. Augmented cortisol secretion may occur in response to situations requiring vigilance, but not in those requiring rapid information processing. An increase of cortisol secretion appears to occur with low controllability (Frankenhaeuser, 1980; Glass et al., 1980). However, since the pituitary-adrenal system tends to be deactivated in response to controllability, a decrease of cortisol secretion is exhibited by Type As in situations where they anticipate high controllability (Frankenhaeuser et al., 1980; Frankenhaeuser, 1982). It is clear that the degree of perceived control is an important modulating influence which tends to reduce negative feelings and to enhance positive feelings of arousal (Frankenhaeuser, 1980). For example, Type As may exhibit no increase of catecholamines on a self-paced reaction time task (Frankenhaeuser et al., 1980). There are important sex differences in the responses to stressful stimuli, however (Frankenhaeuser, 1980).

Aggressive, hostile individuals are found to excrete more norepinephrine compared with more passive or anxious subjects (Friedman et al., 1960). It is thus not surprising that the greatest Type A/B differences are found in CV response to stressful stimuli that elicit hostility/anger (Frankenhaeuser, 1980; Dembroski et al., 1978 and 1979; Glass et al., 1980). The relatively greater response of systolic blood pressure (Manuck & Garland, 1979; Manuck, Craft, & Gold, 1978) confirms a beta-adrenergically mediated mechanism (Nestel, 1969).

The above-described evidence supports the belief that CV responsiveness is a marker for CHD. It also supports the role of Type A hostility/anger dimension that has been found to correlate with greater severity of coronary atherosclerosis (Blumenthal et al., 1978) and higher incidence of CHD in Type A subjects of both sexes (Rosenman et al., 1976; Matthews et al., 1977; Haynes et al., 1980; Jenkins, 1966).

It should be recalled that stressful stimuli that evoke cardiodynamic patterns observed in "borderline" hypertensive subjects and in offspring of hypertensive parents (Falkner et al., 1979; Julius & Esler, 1975) are those that involve beta-adrenergically mediated active coping responses (Falkner et al., 1979; Light, 1981). Many consider CV responsiveness to be a marker for hypertension as well as for CHD. However, although Type As have been found to exhibit greater variability of blood pressure than Type Bs (see Siegel, Chap. 3; Scherwitz, Berton, & Leventhal, 1978; Siegel, Matthews, & Leitch, 1983; Manuck et al., 1979), there do not appear to be significant A/B differences in the prevalence or incidence of sustained hypertension (Rosenman et al., 1964; Shekelle, Schoenberger, & Stamler, 1976). This finding might be considered evidence against a role of vascular hyperresponsiveness in the pathogenesis of hypertension. This seeming paradox might in part be reconciled by the fact that TAB is associated with rapid expression and overt manifestations of aggression, hostility, and anger (Rosenman et al., 1964; Rosenman & Chesney, 1982) that are antithetical to those of many subjects with hypertension. In our current review of the psychological variables associated with CHD in the WCGS, it will be of interest to determine whether Type As who suppressed hostility and anger exhibited higher rates of hypertension, with a converse finding for Type Bs who were able to express such emotions. Glass (1977) has offered another explanation by finding that when Type As perceive a failure of efforts to control stressful stimuli and events, they cease their enhanced active coping responses, thereby diminishing sympathetic-adrenal activity and perhaps even increasing parasympathetic activity. Nevertheless, the hypothesis that CV responsiveness provides a marker for hypertension must be questioned for many reasons, among which is the fact that the enhanced responsiveness of males compared with females is not related to differential rates of hypertension.

It is probably more productive to consider that CV responsiveness provides a marker for CHD complications of hypertension rather than for hypertension itself. Enhanced CV responsiveness characterizes subjects with manifest CHD as well as with sustained hypertension. It is similarly found in their respective offspring, as well as in Type A compared with Type B children (Siegel et al., 1983; Matthews & Jennings, 1984; Lundberg, 1983; Matthews, 1982), a relevant finding in considering the observed familial similarity of A/B behavior patterns (Bortner, Rosenman, & Friedman, 1970). What remains unclear is whether the differences in responsiveness are variably due to a genetic predisposition for CV responsiveness, a psychological predisposition to experience anger, or experientially conditioned SA overreactivity.

GENETIC, EVOLUTIONARY, AND ENVIRONMENTAL FACTORS IN HOSTILITY AND ANGER DIMENSIONS

The studies of anthropologists can provide insight into certain aspects of the problem of aggression and hostility/anger. For the present purposes, I am indebted to the lucid writings of Ashley Montagu (Montagu, 1976; Turnbull, 1978) and have attempted to summarize relevant material. A major belief holds that humans are genetically and instinctively aggressive by reason of evolutionary heritage. The limbic system, which is associated with aggression, has a three-fold evolutionary development in which the amygdala is identified with aggression. However, the amygdala's existence does not necessarily mean that the brain is programmed instinctually for aggression. Thus, its stimulation in animals does not elicit aggressive behaviors unless these were previously learned. Moreover, its stimulation in human subjects variously causes anxiety, depression, anger, fright, and horror, but not an attack behavior. The Type A male child is found to be achievement-oriented, but often also comes from a home that is similarly oriented (Frankenhaeuser, 1980). Thus, a child, at least in part, learns aggression by approval, enhanced status, and rewards for such behavior. It is likely that behaviors arise out of an interaction of genetic potentials and environmental factors, but personality traits, behaviors, and attitudes are probably far more the result of environmental than inherited variables (Montagu, 1976).

The drive for preservation of species and self leads to the type of aggression that is biologically adaptive, life-serving, and phylogenetically programmed. This type is common to both animals and humans; most other forms of aggression are not. The latter, which can be biologically maladaptive, probably arise out of the human experience since they are almost exclusively found in human beings. Indeed, the principal factor operating in animal evolution is identified as cooperation rather than conflict (Montagu, 1976; Turnbull, 1978). Almost all aggressive behavior in animals is directed at acquisition and retention of food and at establishment of a dominance relationship, rather than at inflicting injury. Life or death fights other than for food and survival are quite rare in animals; their conflicts consist mainly of the baring of teeth and butting of horns, which are relatively harmless trials of strength and mutual appraisal for hierarchical dominance and social order, and in fact serve to keep divisiveness, aggression, and fighting to a minimum (Montagu, 1976). An animal usually kills for food or defense, but only rarely for aggressive purposes. Even in primates, as in lower animals, most fighting is a ritualized process which preserves the species and is very different from innate aggression that has killing as the goal. Thus, man does not fight wars merely because animals are territorial or because they have aggressive goals for domination which, however, do not involve destruction. There is no innate aggressiveness in chimpanzees; they do not fight among themselves, nor do males strike females. They prevent fighting among their offspring merely by a stylized type of stare (Pfeiffer, 1981).

The belief of Ardrey that man became man when he became aggressive and learned to hunt has been largely discarded by anthropologists such as Johanson, Leakey, and Montagu, who have observed that the key to man's evolution is cooperative culture (Montagu, 1976; Turnbull, 1978). The evolution of *Homo sapiens* appears to stem from an ability to live in effective groups, compared with other protohominids such as the Australopithecines, who failed in this regard.

In *The Brothers Karamazov,* Dostoevsky, in his discussion of cruelty to children, has Ivan paint a Nietzschean picture of human aggression, but resents reference to man as sometimes being bestial, pointing out that only humans, not animals, exhibit such behaviors. In *Notes from the Underground,* he observes that it is civilization rather than evolution that has increased instrumental aggression in humans. Montagu (1976) points out that drive is different from instinct, which is a phylogenetically programmed and fixed action pattern designed to react to a specific stimulus in an organized and biologically adaptive manner that is characteristic for any given species. Aggressive behavior is not necessarily instinctive in humans since it in fact is not stereotyped or inevitable, and does not appear in vacuo. By analogy, sexual drive may be instinctively fueled by hormonal actions on the brain. However, although born with a capacity for sexual activity, humans must learn how to perform. Montagu questions whether we are correct to describe Neanderthals as bestial when they were the first to bury their dead on a bed of flowers, surrounded by objects placed there for their final journey. In many primitive societies today the key behavior is cooperation (Turnbull, 1978).

Cultures do not differ by reason of genetic factors but from variable experience. A genetic contribution probably lies behind most human behaviors, but it may be the socialization, conditioning, and learning from infancy on that far more determine much behavior, probably including many Type A behaviors as well as the behaviors observed in subjects with hypertension. There is doubtless genetic influence on the limbic system's neuronal and receptor distributions, which are variably influenced in the interaction with cognitive appraisals and somatic feedbacks. Morphology, biochemistry, neuroanatomy, and behavior are inextricably intertwined in evolutionary development, but there is increasing evidence for a major effect of behavioral changes on the other parameters (Judson, 1983). Darwinian tradition, carried forward by followers such as E. Mayr and E. O. Wilson, is increasingly being challenged by evidence that evolution is not fully responsible for shaping human traits, which may not be merely transmitted by genes but influenced by cultural factors in many of their important characteristics. For example, Tanner (1981) hypothesizes that progressive reduction of the size of canine teeth may have resulted from preferential female selection of males with smaller canines, which are associated with less aggressive behavior, a cultural behavior influence that accordingly could be held responsible for shaping the development of a physical trait. Tanner (1981) also hypothesizes that more social, less aggressive, and less disruptive males may have been more often selected as sexual partners during human evolution, and the change in mating patterns may therefore have increased sociability, not only between males and females but even between males themselves.

There is no brain center that compels us to become aggressive; therefore, aggression is not inevitable. We are born with a potential for aggression, but the behavior must be learned. After all, Darwin taught that there is a competition for existence but never stated that this involved aggression rather than cooperation. He did not confuse aggressive drive with instinct (Montagu, 1976).

Some relevant effects of the environment were recently reviewed in a symposium held at Johns Hopkins Medical School and elsewhere (Konner, 1982; Mandell, 1982). These reviews point out how parental abuse and neglect are associated with alcoholism in youth, and parental crime and abuse with increased aggression in children. Observing hostile aggression on the sporting fields increases aggressive behavior among many spectators who identify with the players (Pfeiffer, 1981). It is the culture that encourages bone-jarring football tackles and the rituals of ice hockey duels, as well as the unregulated competition of the industrial world and the concept that the strongest is the most fit. An anthropologist at the University of Pennsylvania, Peggy Reaves Sanday, compared scores of cultures and found that rape neither is universal nor stems from a biological drive, but is instead a conditioned response to the way certain kinds of societies are organized (Benderly, 1982). She found certain behaviors to be common to rape-prone societies, including a tolerance for violence and the encouragement of males at all ages to be aggressive, tough, and competitive. The typical rapist is not sexually deprived but is a hostile and aggressive male who enjoys violence toward females (Olmert, 1982). Rape is not inherent in the sex relationship and remains unknown in many simpler African societies whose people live in harmonious groups that place high value on the nurturance and fertility of the female. Rape-free societies do not have exclusively male clubs or special political and religious groups that exclude females, and they do not have machos, which in Spanish means "male of animal species." This absence of male aggression and violence may be due to the fact that such societies also have no lack of land and resources as well as no need for competitive survival like that which, for example, characterized the trigger-happy American frontiersman, the

Southern planter outnumbered by restive slaves, the Israelis who approached Canaan, or the Azande conquerors of neighboring African tribes (Montagu, 1976).

SEX DIFFERENCES IN AGGRESSIVENESS, ANGER DIMENSIONS, AND CARDIOVASCULAR RESPONSIVENESS

It is accepted that there is a difference between sexes in aggressiveness, hostility, and anger (Waldron, 1976). These "masculine" behaviors not only comprise the major components of coronary-prone TAB (Rosenman & Chesney, 1982), but may underlie in general the higher rates of CHD that occur in males. Differences in various abilities, such as male visual-spatial skills and female verbal and fine-coordination skills, can be correlated with evolutionary differences of brain structure (Konner, 1982). Sex hormones in the brain structure, which doubtless have certain evolutionary influences, are found in the hypothalamus, which controls hormone production and is genetically primed for differential development. Sex hormones acting on the brain at critical periods determine gender roles and associated behaviors (Gelman, 1981). Although biological inheritance of such factors is thereby determined by hormones, the genetic basis is reinforced by cultural institutions (Waldron, 1976).

Aggression is closely linked with testosterone (Scaramella & Brown, 1978). Male behaviors in female offspring are increased when testosterone is given to pregnant animals; female children whose mothers accidentally received it during pregnancy ("Sexual Behavior," 1979) show similar behaviors. There are sex differences in hypothalamic nuclei density and synaptic neuronal connections that can be masculinized by administration of testosterone. This fact, of course, suggests that the basic mammalian plan is female and remains so unless "told" otherwise by testosterone (Konner, 1982). The superiority of the female for survival was recognized by both Montagu (1976) and Mark Twain (Murphy, 1982) who humorously stated that the Bible was written by men who understood and feared the obviously greater sexual competence of the female. Males have adopted many practices to impose restrictions on females via social convention (Murphy, 1982). A similar male apprehension probably underlies abominable practices (Bernardez-Bonesatti, 1982; Symons, 1979) such as clitoral excision in certain African tribes (Favazza, 1983). Montagu (1976) understood the potential for the superior female constitution, noting that male dominance is more "noise than substance" and that male initiative may primarily be a defense of relative sexual weakness. He correctly pointed out that some cultural practices are a reversal of natural orders and a biological denial that has transcended nature by turning it upside down.

Humans undergo a psychosexual differentiation before birth that affects both brain and behaviors. This belief was confirmed (Konner, 1982) in the famed Dominican Republic families that produced 38 offspring from 23 interrelated families, after many generations of intermarriage in three villages. Among them were 19 females at birth who failed to develop secondary sex characteristics at prepuberty but later underwent complete physical and psychological masculinization. They were found to exhibit a genetic male chromosome pattern which lacked the enzyme involved in male sex hormone synthesis that changes testosterone into dihydrotestosterone (DHT). The lack of DHT induced the female appearance at birth and prepuberty, while the presence of testosterone engendered normal male puberty. It is significant that these individuals required no special training for adoption of male behaviors, indicating that gender differences in aggressive behaviors are associated with brain differences ("Sexual Behaviors," 1979).

However, humans are probably becoming less captive to their hormones. In the studies by Frankenhaeuser and associates (Collins & Frankenhaeuser, 1978), it has been observed, for example, that the sexes have grown more similar as females develop in a more "masculine" direction. It remains to be seen whether females are in fact less aggressive and competitive as they move into new occupations and combative sports (Waldron, 1976; Gelman, 1981; Murphy, 1982; "Women," 1980; Bernardez-Bonesatti, 1982). The explosive growth of such sports activities has been found to be making females more assertive, independent, ambitious, and confident ("Women," 1980). It may be that young females never had adequate opportunity to become more aggressive and competitive ("Women," 1980). Thus, although gender roles are genetically related, they are not unalterably determined by biology and are partly a cultural product (Konner, 1982). Puberty may store muscle and fat differently between the sexes, but this is not the total story. The presence or absence of testosterone does not prevent individuals from learning behaviors that are shaped by social and environmental conditions. The male winner of a gold medal in the 1964 Olympic 400-meter freestyle swim would have placed fifth among the more competitive females who swam the same race in the 1980 Olympic match (Gelman, 1981). It will be of future interest to observe whether changes of sex hormone ratios occur as females adopt a more competitive role in society.

Testosterone correlates with aggressive behaviors (Scaramella & Brown, 1978). In prison inmates, males with the highest levels have the earliest age at first arrest (Konner, 1982). However, its level is subject to environmental influence. For example, when a monkey is introduced into a cage with established dominance, the newcomer exhibits a rapid drop of plasma testosterone, but when placed in a cage of females in heat, testosterone rises sharply. Some years ago, Zumoff and associates (Zumoff, Rosenfeld, Friedman, Sanford, Byers, Rosenman, & Hellman, 1978) made a "blind" analysis of plasma and urinary steroids which were obtained for them from groups of classic Type A and B males subjects. Two significant A/B differences were found. The Type As showed higher daytime excretion of testosterone glucuronide, probably because of increased rate of its production, while the Type Bs showed higher plasma DHT levels. This difference is significant because in females the DHT/testosterone ratio is much higher than in males. These findings become more significant with the confirmation by Williams et al. (1982) of an increased testosterone response to certain stressful stimuli in Type A subjects. In view of sex differences in CHD incidence, it is relevant that testosterone increases and estradiol decreases arterial wall hypertrophy in experimental hypertension and that testosterone increases the frequency of arterial thrombosis after intimal injury is induced.

It also is relevant to examine sex differences of SA responses. In general, there appear to be no differences of baseline plasma catecholamines or cortisol (Frankenhaeuser et al., 1980). There are significant differences in response to stressors, as well as in coping (Frankenhaeuser, 1982). Males exhibit greater overall catecholamine responses to stressful stimuli and to challenges that are reflected in different coping patterns on the emotional level. However, the lower catecholamine responses by females to acutely stressful situations are not accompanied by less efficient coping or achievement. Frankenhaeuser and associates (1980) have pursued this subject in a series of elegant studies which consistently find that psychological factors are determinants of different neuroendocrine responses to stressful stimuli. They observed that females cope more economically than males in achievement situations, being more vulnerable only in areas where they are traditionally expected to show greater competence than males. In view of the sex differential in CHD incidence and the relevance of psychophysiological responsiveness, it is thus particularly significant that the consistently observed lower female response to stressful stimuli is not associated with either less efficient coping or lower achievement.

SOME RELATIONSHIPS OF EMOTIONS TO CNS RECEPTORS

The above discussion is concerned mainly with several aspects of the role of anger dimensions for hypertension, Type A behavior pattern, and CHD. In view of their biobehavioral nature, it is not entirely presumptuous for a cardiologist to look briefly at some aspects of related psychological factors. The rapidly developing science of neurochemical pathology has shown a chemistry of emotions that can be manipulated by opening or closing brain receptor binding sites. This field was particularly stimulated by the finding that Parkinson's disease is associated with a deficiency of the dopamine transmitter, while an increased number of brain dopamine receptors has been found to be present in schizophrenia (Marsden, 1982; Snyder, 1982; Knight, 1982; Thal, 1983). Fundamental abnormalities may reside either in the dopamine system or in one linked to dopamine neurons (Knight, 1982; Thal, 1983). It may be relevant to hypertension that norepinephrine plays a supportive role in the motor actions of dopamine, with a link between dopaminergic-adrenergic systems that affect aldosterone secretion independent of renin and angiotensin (McKenna et al., 1979; Whitfield et al., 1980). Neuroleptic drugs block norepinephrine as well as dopamine receptors (Snyder, 1982), and clonidine, the alpha-agonist that is so useful for treatment of hypertension by decreasing hypothalamic adrenergic secretion, appears to be an effective neuroleptic agent for treatment of certain schizophrenic symptoms (Snyder, 1982) and panic syndromes (Hoehn-SAric, Merchant, Keyser, & Smith, 1981). There is evidence of catecholamine hypofunction in endogenous depression (van Pragg, 1982), while brain neurotransmitters that are involved in anxiety states include dopamine and norepinephrine (Braestrup, 1982).

At the University of Utah, Reimherr and Wood have observed that central nervous system stimulants can favorably affect personality problems associated with adult hyperactivity, including motor hyperactivity, attention deficits, moodiness, and explosive tempers (*Research Resources Reporter,* 1982), some of which resemble certain Type A behaviors (Chesney, Black, Chadwick et al., 1980; Rosenman & Chesney, 1982). In such hyperactive subjects, the stimulants induce easier concentration, less attention wandering, less talkativeness, slowed thinking, and increased listening to spouses—the latter, incidentally, being a major complaint of the spouses of many Type A males. These benefits are similar to those observed in hyperactive children treated with amphetamines, and are quite different from the exhilaration, loquaciousness, restlessness, and excitement that these same agents may induce in normal adults. One inference is that patients who are responsive to central nervous system (CNS) stimulants may be hyperactive because of a persistent biological abnormality that may be inherited, with certain childhood manifestations being forerunners of difficulties in adult life (*Research Resources Reporter,* 1982).

Hyperactivity is associated with a deficiency of dopamine, one neurotransmitter that controls emotional responses and complex movements (Thal, 1983). CNS stimulants are far more effective than tricyclic antidepressants in controlling both hyperactive children and adults. They increase dopaminergic activity, in contrast to antidepressants, which increase noradrenergic and serotonergic neurotransmitter brain activities.

A major brain dysfunction has never been found for anxiety, and perhaps one should not be looked for in considering anxiety as a prerequisite for a well-functioning person and in view of its important role in evolution and species survival (Braestrup, 1982). However, it is possible to consider pathological anxiety as a marginal type of overreaction in otherwise normal neuronal circuits (Braestrup, 1982).

On the other hand, anxiety may have an underlying chemical basis, considering that benzodiazepines appear to act directly against anxiety by attaching to binding receptor sites in the brain of many species, including humans. Moreover, there appears to be an evolutionary development of such receptors since they are absent in sharks and species below their level of development. Finally, the severe form of spontaneous anxiety found in the panicogenic syndrome, which is often associated with mitral valve prolapse, is also associated with excessive secretion of epinephrine and is responsive to such neuroleptic drugs as clonidine, benzodiazepines, and alprazolam, all of which inhibit the locus ceruleus (Hoehn-Saric et al., 1981). Further examination of this new field of neurochemistry is beyond the scope of this writer. However, it may be useful to speculate that certain coronary-prone behaviors similarly may be marginal overreactions associated with biological dysfunctions that involve one or more brain neurotransmitters, but without measurable deviations from normal.

IMPLICATIONS FOR THERAPEUTIC APPROACHES

It also is beyond the present purpose to point out more than briefly some implications for therapeutic approaches based on the above discussion. In a recent report from the National Academy of Sciences' Medical Institute (Hamburg, Elliott, & Parron, 1982), it was stated that medical research should be redirected to focus on motivating persons to change their lifestyles as the most important step in preventing disease. It was pointed out that the first step is to identify those behaviors which are risk factors for disease and then to determine whether their change would serve the purpose of prevention. The present volume is directed at only one such behavior, and other chapters will address the issue of modifying such anger behaviors. Coping emerges as one of the most important constructs in stress theory (Glass, 1979; Mills, 1976) with a growing consensus that it is a major determinant of adverse psychophysiological responses

(Roskies & Lazarus, 1980; Vickers, Hervig, Rahe, & Rosenman, 1981). It therefore becomes advisable to view treatment measures not only in the context of the stressors and their psychophysiological responses but also with a view to individual coping resources (Frankenhaeuser, 1980; Roskies & Lazarus, 1980). It should be important to match various therapeutic measures according to the differences in such responses. For example, relaxation methodologies might prove to be of greatest benefit for subjects with anxiety, and cognitive approaches for those with anger responses that particularly involve beta-adrenergically mediated mechanisms. Thus, behavioral therapy directed at anxiety appears to be more appropriate for fear responses, while assertiveness training and modification of maladaptive anger are probably more appropriate for hypertension and CHD (Schwartz et al., 1981). Our increasing knowledge of the variable individual responses that involve the PA and SA systems makes it possible to assess the roles of these responses in psychological abnormalities as well as in hypertension and CHD. This knowledge should permit more specifically aimed behavioral as well as pharmacological therapy (Rosenman & Friedman, 1977; Rosenman, 1978; Rosenman, 1983).

It appears unlikely that the scientific approach will reduce the impact of environmental stressors, which are probably increasing at an ever accelerating rate. It may be possible to reduce their impact in some by paying greater attention to proper fit between behavior pattern and occupation (Chesney, Sevelius, Black, Swan, & Rosenman, 1981). For example, Type As suffer much less distress (Chesney et al., 1981) when they work at their appropriate accelerated pace and with an adequate arousal level, which however, may be inappropriate for Type B individuals (Frankenhaeuser & Johansson, 1981).

Exercise provides many psychological and somatic benefits and may be a useful adjunct for therapy (Sjoberg, 1980; Elliot & Zeiner, 1979). When properly pursued, it is accompanied by physiologically normal homeostatic responses, but its CV risks (Friedman, Manwaring, Rosenman, Donlon, Ortega, & Grube, 1973) may be increased when it is performed in an angry compared with a relaxed mood.

Another approach might consider altering traditional stereotypic male behaviors. Studies by Frankenhaeuser et al. (Frankenhaeuser, 1978; Collins & Frankenhaeuser, 1978; Frankenhaeuser et al., 1980) suggest that increased Type A behavior in females may not necessarily be associated with increased risk of either hypertension or CHD.

Antihypertensive pharmacological approaches must consider that hypertension is not a disease state but only a state of elevated blood pressure, as long emphasized by G. Pickering (1968), who also pointed out that treatment should be directed at prevention of its end-organ complications rather than only at lowering of the blood pressure level. It must now be recognized that the so-called step-care approach is aimed primarily at lowering of the blood pressure, and that this has failed in clinical trials to reduce the CHD complications of hypertension (Freis, 1982), perhaps even increasing it by excessive emphasis on diuretic medications ("Multiple risk factor intervention trial," 1982) that stimulate norepinephrine secretion (Lake, Ziegler, Coleman, & Kopin, 1979). The regulation of the blood pressure, whether normal or elevated, involves two major systems; and, regardless of which is more involved in the etiology of an individual's hypertension, it is not possible to reduce the influence of either system without respectively stimulating the other's input. Diuretics, for example, stimulate adrenergic activity, and it appears only logical that their administration should invariably be accompanied by medication directed at either reducing or blocking excess noradrenergic secretion, with adequate replacement of potassium chloride to diminish arteriolar responsiveness induced by its depletion (Skrabal et al., 1981; Parfrey et al., 1981).

The future probably holds great promise for the development of new pharmacological agents that will have ever more precise ability to act at the desired receptor sites, providing a new method for "behavioral therapy." In any event, whether in the present world or the future, even more complex world, the helathy individual will probably be one who avoids habitually disturbing homeostatic mechanisms (Nixon & Bethel, 1974; Nixon, 1976; Ketterer, 1982). Although it is necessary for those who deal in the science of stress to pontificate about complex systems of CV and other responses to the environment, it is remarkable how many senior scientists have reached the conclusion that an element of humor to replace anger is advisable for adequate coping with ones milieu (Selye, 1976).

REFERENCES

Alexander, F. Emotional factors in essential hypertension: Presentation of a tentative hypothesis. *Psychosomatic Medicine*, 1939, *1*, 173-179.
Arkowitz, H. The assessment of social skills. In M. Hersen & A. S. Bellack (Eds.), *Behavioral assessment: A Practical Handbook* (Second Edition). New York: Pergamon, 1981.
Ax, A. F. The physiological differentiation between fear and anger in humans. *Psychosomatic Medicine*, 1953, *5*, 443-442.
Baer, P. E., Collins, F. H., Bourenoff, G. C., & Ketchel, M. F. Assessing personality factors in essential hypertension with a brief self-report instrument. *Psychosomatic Medicine*, 1979, *16*, 321-330.
Barefoot, J. C., Dahlstrom, W. G., & Williams, R. B. Hostility, CHD incidence and total mortality: A 25-year follow-up study of 255 physicians. *Psychosomatic Medicine*, 1983, *45*, 59-63.
Bellack, A. S. A critical appraisal of strategies for assessing social skill. *Behavioral Assessment*, 1979, *1*, 157-176.
Benderly, B. L. Rape-free or rape-prone societies. *The Sciences*, 1982, *22*, 40-43.
Berkman, L. F., & Syme, S. L. Social networks, host resistance, and mortality: A nine-year follow-up study of Alameda County residents. *American Journal of Epidemiology*, 1979, *109*, 186-204.
Bernardez-Bonesatti, T. Women and anger. *The Sciences*, 1982, *22*, 21-33.
Blumenthal, J. A., Williams, R., Kong, Y., Schanberg, S. M., & Thompson, L. W. Type A behavior and angiographically documented coronary disease. *Circulation*, 1978, *58*, 634-639.
Bortner, R. W., Rosenman, R. H., & Friedman, M. Familial similarity in Pattern A behavior: Fathers and sons. *Journal of Chronic Diseases*, 1970, *23*, 39-43.
Braestrup, C. Neurotransmitters and CNS disease: Anxiety. *Lancet*, 1982, *2*, 1030-1034.
Brod, J., Fencl, V., Hejl, Z., & Jirka, J. Circulatory changes underlying blood pressure elevation during acute emotional stress (mental arithmetic) in normotensive and hypertensive subjects. *Clinical Science*, 1959, *18*, 269-279.
Brunton, L. An address on blood pressure in man: Its estimation and indication for treatment. *British Medical Journal*, 1909, *2*, 64-67.
Buss, A. H. *The psychology of aggression*. New York: Wiley, 1961.
Canessa, M., Adragna, N., Solomon, J. S., Connolly, T. M., & Tosteson, D. C. Increased sodium-lithium countertransport in red cells of patients with essential hypertension. *New England Journal of Medicine*, 1980, *302*, 772-776.
Cannon, W. B. *The wisdom of the body*. New York: Norton, 1932.

Cannon, W. B. *Bodily changes in pain, hunger, fear, and rage.* New York: Appleton-Century-Crofts, 1936.
Chesney, M. A., Black, G. W., Chadwick, J. H., & Rosenman, R. H. Psychological correlates of the coronary-prone behavior pattern. *Journal of Behavioral Medicine,* 1981, *4,* 217-230.
Chesney, M. A., Sevelius, G. G., Black, G. W., Swan, G. E., & Rosenman, R. H. Work environment, Type A behavior, and coronary disease risk factors. *Journal of Occupational Medicine,* 1981, *23,* 551-555.
Cook, W. W., & Medley, D. M. Proposed hostility and pharisaic-virtue scales for the MMPI. *The Journal of Applied Psychology,* 1954, *38,* 414-418.
Collins, A., & Frankenhaeuser, M. Stress responses in male and female engineering students. *Journal of Human Stress,* 1978, *4,* 43-48.
Dembroski, T. M., MacDougall, J. M., Herd, J. A., & Shields, J. L. Effects of level of challenge on pressor and heart responses in Type A and B subjects. *Journal of Applied Social Psychology,* 1979, *9,* 209-228.
Dembroski, T. M., MacDougall, J. M., Shields, J. L., Petitto, J., & Lushene, R. Components of Type A coronary-prone behavior pattern and cardiovascular responses to psychomotor challenge. *Journal of Behavioral Medicine,* 1978, *1,* 159-176.
DeQuattro, V., Barbour, B. H., Campese, V., Fink, E. J., Miand, L., & Esler, M. Sympathetic nervous hyperactivity in high-renin hypertension. *Mayo Clinic Proceedings,* 1977, *52,* 369-373.
DeQuattro, V., & Miura, Y. In J. Laragh (Ed.), *Hypertension Manual.* New York: Dun-Donnelley, 1974.
DeQuattro, V., Sullivan, P., Foti, A., Schoentgen, S., Bornheimer, J., Kolloch, R., Versales, G., & Levine, D. Central noradrenergic mechanisms in hypertension and in postural hypotension. In J. Laragh, F. Buhler, & D. Seldin (Eds.), *Frontiers in hypertension research.* New York: Springer-Verlag, 1981.
Diamond, E. L. The role of anger and hostility in essential hypertension and coronary heart disease. *Psychological Bulletin,* 1982, *92,* 410-433.
DiPalma, J. R. In A. N. Brest & J. H. Moyer (Eds.), *Hypertension-recent advances: The second Hahnemann Symposium on hypertensive disease.* Philadelphia: Lea and Febiger, 1961.
Elliot, S. K., & Zeiner, A. R. Effects of physical fitness training on resting and reactive blood pressures of normotensive and hypertensive firemen. *Psychophysiology,* 1979, *16,* 200. (Abstract)
Esler, M., Jackson, G., Bobik, A., Leonard, P., Kelleher, D., Skews, H., Jennings, G., & Kornes, P. Norepinephrine kinetics in essential hypertension: Defective neural uptake of norepinephrine in some patients. *Hypertension,* 1981, *3,* 149-156.
Esler, M., Julius, S., Randall, O. S., Ellis, C. N., & Kashima, T. Relation of renin status to neurogenic vascular resistance in borderline hypertension. *American Journal of Cardiology,* 1975, *36,* 708-715.
Esler, M., Julius, S., Zweiffer, A., Randall, O., Harburg, E., Gardiner, H., & DeQuattro, V. Mild high-renin essential hypertension: Neurogenic human hypertension? *New England Journal of Medicine,* 1977, *296,* 405-411.
Falkner, B., Onesti, G., & Angelakos, E. T., Fernandes, M., & Langman, C. Cardiovascular response to mental stress in normal adolescents with hypertensive parents. *Hypertension,* 1979, *1,* 23-30.
Falkner, B., Onesti, G., & Hamstra, B. Stress response characteristics of adolescents with high genetic risk for essential hypertension: A five-year follow-up. *Clinical and Experimental Hypertension,* 1981, *3,* 583-591.
Favazza, A. R. The greatest flavor of mankind and other abominations. *MD,* 1983, 213-216.
Forsyth, R. P. Regional blood flow changes during 72-hour avoidance schedules in the monkey. *Science,* 1971, *173,* 546-548.
Frankenhaeuser, M. *Psychoneuroendocrine sex differences in adaptation to the psychosocial environment.* New York: Academic, 1978.
Frankenhaeuser, M. Psychobiological aspects of life stress. *Coping and Health.* New York: Plenum, 1980.
Frankenhaeuser, M. The sympathetic-adrenal and pituitary-adrenal response to challenge: Comparison between the sexes. In T. M. Dembroski, T. H. Schmidt, & G. Blumchen (Eds.), *Biobehavioral bases of coronary heart disease.* Basel, N.Y.: Karger, 1982.

Frankenhaeuser, M., & Johansson, G. On the psychophysiological consequences of understimulation and overstimulation. In L. Levi (Ed.), *Society, stress and disease, Vol. IV: Working life.* New York: Oxford University Press, 1981.
Frankenhaeuser, M., Lundberg, U., & Forsam, L. Dissociation between sympathetic-adrenal and pituitary-adrenal responses to an achievement situation characterized by high controllability: Comparison between Type A and Type B males and females. *Biological Psychology,* 1980, *10,* 79-91.
Frankenhaeuser, M., Mellis, I., Rissler, A., Bjorkvall, C., & Patkai, P. Catecholamine excretion as related to cognitive and emotional reaction patterns. *Psychosomatic Medicine,* 1968, *30,* 109-120.
Frankenhaeuser, M., Rauste von Wright, M., Collins, A., von Wright, J., Sedvall, G., & Swahn, G. Sex differences in psychoneuroendocrine reactions to examination stress. *Psychosomatic Medicine,* 1978, *40,* 334-343.
Friedman, M., Byers, S. O., Diamant, J., & Rosenman, R. H. Plasma catecholamine response of coronary-prone subjects (Type A) to a specific challenge. *Metabolism,* 1975, *4,* 205-210.
Friedman, M., Manwaring, J. H., Rosenman, R. H., Donlon, G., Ortega, P., & Grube, S. M. Instantaneous and sudden death: Clinical and pathological differentiation in coronary artery disease. *Journal of the American Medical Association,* 1973, *225,* 1319-1328.
Friedman, M., St. George, S., Byers, S. O., & Rosenman, R. H. Excretion of catecholamines, 17-ketosteroids, 17-hydroxy-coricoids, and 5-hydroxyindole in men exhibiting a particular behavior pattern (A) associated with high incidence of clinical coronary artery disease. *Journal of Clinical Investigation,* 1960, *39,* 758-764.
Freis, E. P. Should mild hypertension be treated? *New England Medical Journal,* 1982, *307,* 306-309.
Funkenstein, D. H., King, S. H., & Drolette, M. *Mastery of stress.* Cambridge, Mass.: Harvard University Press, 1957.
Gelman, E. Lions vs. Tigers. *Newsweek,* May 1981, p. 75.
Genest, J. *Hypertension.* New York: McGraw-Hill, 1977.
Glass, D. C. *Behavior patterns, stress, and coronary disease.* Hillsdale, N.J.: Erlbaum, 1977.
Glass, D. C. Behavior patterns, stress, and catecholamines. In *Yearbook of Science and the Future.* Chicago: Encyclopaedia Britannica, 1979.
Glass, D. C., & Contrada, R. J. Type A behavior and catecholamines: A critical review. In C. Raymond Lake & Michael Ziegler (Eds.), *Norepinephrine: Clinical aspects.* Baltimore: Williams & Wilkins, 1982.
Glass, D. C., Krakoff, L. R., Contrada, R., Hilton, W. F., Kehoe, K., Mannucci, E. G., Collins, C., Snow, B., & Elting, E. Effect of harrassment and competition upon cardiovascular and plasma catecholamine responses in Type A and Type B individuals. *Psychophysiology,* 1980, *17,* 453-463.
Goldstein, I. B. Assessment of hypertension. In C. K. Prokop & L. A. Bradley (Eds.), *Medical psychology: Contributions to behavioral medicine.* New York: Academic, 1981.
Grim, C. E., Luft, F. C., Miller, J. Z., Brown, P. L., Gannon, M. A., & Weinberger, M. H. Effects of volume expansion and contraction in normotensive first-degree relatives of essential hypertensives. *Journal of Laboratory and Clinical Medicine,* 1979, *94,* 764-771.
Groen, J. J. Stress has same response in hypertensives and normotensives. *Journal of Psychosomatic Medicine,* 1982, *26,* 141-154.
Gutmann, M. C., & Benson, H. Interaction of environmental factors and systemic arterial blood pressure: A review. *Medicine,* 1971, *50,* 543-553.
Guyton, A. C. *Circulatory physiology III: Arterial pressure and hypertension.* Philadelphia: Saunders, 1980.
Hamburg, D. A., Elliott, G. R., & Parron, D. L. (Eds.),. *health and behavior, frontiers of research in the biobehavioral sciences.* Washington, D.C.: National Academy, 1982.
Handkins, R. E., & Munz, D. C. Essential hypertension and self-disclosure. *Journal of Clinical Psychology,* 1978, *34,* 870-875.
Harburg, E., Blakelock, E. H., & Roeper, P. J. Resentful and reflective coping with arbitrary authority and blood pressure: Detroit. *Psychosomatic Medicine,* 1979, *41,* 189-202.
Harrell, J. P. Psychological factors and hypertension: A status report. *Psychological Bulletin,* 1980, *87,* 482-501.
Harris, R. E., Sokolow, M., Carpenter, L. G., Jr., Freedman, M., & Hunt, S. P. Responses to

psychologic stress in persons who are potentially hypertensive. *Circulation,* 1953, *7,* 874-879.
Hathaway, S. R., & McKinley, J. C. *Minnesota multiphasic personality inventory manual* (revised edition). New York: Psychological Corp., 1967.
Haynes, S. G., Feinleib, M., & Kannel, W. B. The relationship of psychosocial factors to coronary heart disease in the Framingham study. Part III: Eight-year incidence of CHD. *American Journal of Epidemiology,* 1980, *3,* 37-58.
Henningsen, N. C., Mattson, S., Nosslin, B., Nelson, D., & Ohlsson, O. Abnormal whole-body and cellular (erythrocyte) turnover of 22Na in normotensive relatives of probands with established essential hypertension. *Clinical Science,* 1979, *57,* 3215-3245.
Henry, J. P., & Cassel, J. C. Psychosocial factors in essential hypertensive: Recent epidemiologic and animal experimental evidence. *American Journal of Epidemiology,* 1969, *90,* 171-200.
Henry, J. P., & Stephens, P. M. The social environment and essential hypertension in mice: Possible role of the innervation of the adrenal cortex. In *Stress, Health and Social Environment.* New York: Springer-Verlag, 1977.
Henry, J. P., Stephens, P. M., & Santisteban, G. A. A model of hypertension showing reversibility and progression of cardiovascular complications. *Circulation Research,* 1975, *36,* 156-164.
Hoehn-Saric, R., Merchant, A. F., Heyser, M. L., & Smith, F. K. Effects of clonidine on anxiety disorders. *Archives of General Psychiatry,* 1981, *39,* 1278-1282.
Hokanson, J. E., Burgess, M., & Cohen, M. F. Effects of displaced aggression on systolic blood pressure. *Journal of Abnormal and Social Psychology,* 1963, *67,* 214-218.
Hyperactivity problems identified in adults. *Research Resources Reporter,* November 1982, pp. 10-11.
Jakubowski, P., & Lange, A. J. *The assertive option: Your rights and responsibilities.* Champaign, IL: Research, 1978.
Jenkins, C. D. Components of the coronary-prone behavior pattern: Their relation to silent myocardial infarction and blood lipids. *Journal of Chronic Diseases,* 1966, *19,* 599-609.
Judson, H. F. An empirical presence. *The Sciences,* May 1983, 20-23.
Julius, S., & Esler, M. Autonomic nervous cardiovascular regulation in borderline hypertension. *The American Journal of Cardiology,* 1975, *36,* 685-696.
Julius, S., Quadir, H., & Gajendragadkar, S. Hyperkinetic state: A precursor of hypertension? A longitudinal study of borderline hypertension. *Mild Hypertension: Natural History and Management.* Chicago: Pitman, 1979.
Kahn, H. A., Medalie, J. H., Neufeld, H. N., Riss, E., & Goldbourt, U. The incidence of hypertension and associated factors: The Israeli ischemic heart disease study. *American Heart Journal,* 1972, *84,* 171-182.
Kalis, B. L., Harris, R. E., & Sokolow, M., & Carpenter, L. G. Response to psychological stress in patients with essential hypertension. *American Heart Journal,* 1957, *53,* 572-578.
Kawano, Y., Fukiyama, K., Jakeya, Y., Obo, T., & Omae, T. Elevated plasma catecholamines without alteration in cardiovascular responsiveness in growing men with borderline hypertension. *American Heart Journal,* 1982, *104,* 1351-1356.
Ketterer, M. W. Lateralized representation of affect, affect cognizance, and the coronary-prone personality. *Biological Psychology,* 1982, *15,* 171-189.
Knight, J. G. Neurotransmitters and CNS disease: Dopamine-receptor stimulating autoantibodies: A possible cause of schizophrenia. *Lancet,* 1982, *2,* 1073-1075.
Konner, M. *The tangled wing.* New York: Holt, 1982.
Lake, C. R., Ziegler, M. G., Coleman, M. D., & Kopin, I. J. Hydrochlorothiazide-induced sympathetic hyperactivity in hypertensive patients. *Clinical Pharmacology Therapy,* 1979, *26,* 428-432.
Lawler, J. E., Barker, G. G., Hubbard, J. W., & Allen, M. T. The effects of conflict on tonic levels of blood pressure in the genetically borderline hypertensive rat. *Psychophysiology,* 1980, *17,* 363-370.
Light, K. C. Cardiovascular responses to effortful active coping: Implications for the role of stress in hypertension development. *Psychophysiology,* 1981, *18,* 216-225.
Light, K. C., & Obrist, P. A. Cardiovascular reactivity to behavioral stress in young males with and without marginally elevated causal systolic pressures: A comparison of clinic, home and laboratory measures. *Hypertension,* 1980, *2,* 802-808.

Linehan, M. M., & Egan, K. J. Assertion training for women. In A. S. Bellack & M. Hersen (Eds.), *Research and practice in social skills training.* New York: Plenum, 1979.
Lundberg, U. Note on Type A children and cardiovascular responses to challenge in 3-6 year old children. *Journal of Psychosomatic Research,* 1983, *23,* 281-288.
Lundberg, U., & Frankenhaeuser, M. Pituitary-adrenal and sympathetic-adrenal correlates of distress and effort. *Journal of Psychosomatic Research,* 1980, *24,* 125-130.
Mandell, W. *Medical World News,* October 11, 1982, p. 40.
Manuck, S. B., Corse, C. D., & Winkelman, P. A. Behavioral correlates of individual differences in blood pressure reactivity. *Journal of Psychosomatic Research,* 1979, *23,* 281-288.
Manuck, S. B. Craft, S., & Gold, K. J. Coronary-prone behavior pattern and cardiovascular response. *Psychophysiology,* 1978, *15,* 403-411.
Manuck, S. B., & Garland, F. N. Coronary-prone behavior pattern, task incentive and cardiovascular response. *Psychophysiology,* 1979, *16,* 136-142.
Manuck, S. B., Giordani, B., McQuaid, K. J., & Garrity, S. J. Behaviorally-induced cardiovascular reactivity among sons of reported hypertensive and normotensive parents. *Journal of Psychosomatic Research,* 1981, *25,* 261-269.
Marsden, C. D. Neurotransmitters and CNS disease: Basal ganglia disease. *Lancet,* 1982, *2,* 1141-1146.
Matthews, K. A. Psychological perspectives on the Type A behavior pattern. *Psychological Bulletin,* 1982, 293-323.
Matthews, K. A., Glass, D. C., Rosenman, R. H., & Bortner, R. W. Competitive drive, Pattern A, and coronary heart disease: A further analysis of some data from the Western Collaborative Group Study. *Journal of Chronic Diseases,* 1977, *30,* 489-498.
Matthews, K. A., & Jennings, J. R. Cardiovascular responses of boys exhibiting the Type A behavior pattern. *Psychosomatic Medicine,* 1984, *46,* 484-497.
McClelland, D. C. Inhibited power motivation and high blood pressure in men. *Journal of Abnormal Psychology,* 1979, *88,* 182-190.
McKenna, T. J., Island, D. P., Nicholson, W. E., & Liddle, G. N. Dopamine inhibits angiotensive stimulated aldosterone synthesis in bovine adrenal cells. *Journal of Clinical Investigation,* 1979, *64,* 287-291.
Mills, I. H. The disease of failure of coping. *The Practitioner,* October 1976, 529-538.
Montagu, A. *The nature of human aggression.* Oxford: Oxford University Press, 1976.
Multiple risk factor intervention trial: Risk factor changes and mortality results. *Journal of the American Medical Association,* 1982, *248,* 1465-1477.
Murphy, R. F. Man's culture and woman's nature. *Annals of the New York Academy of Science,* 1982, 15-24.
Nestel, P. J. Blood pressure and catecholamine excretion after mental stress in labile hypertension. *Lancet,* 1969, *1,* 694-696.
Nixon, P. B. F., & Bethel, J. N. Preinfarction ill health. *American Journal of Cardiology,* 1974, *33,* 446-449.
Nixon, P. G. F. The human function curve. *The Practitioner,* 1976, *217,* 765-771 and 935-944.
Olmert, O. Medieval mayhem. *Smithsonian,* 1982, 34-36.
Page, T. H., & McCubbin, J. W. Section 2. In W. F. Hamilton & P. Dow (Eds.), *Handbook of physiology: Circulation* Vol. 1. Washington, D.C.: American Physiological Society, 1966.
Parfrey, P. S., Vandenburg, M. J., Wright, P., Holly, J. M. R., Goodwin, F. J., Evans, E., & Ledingham, J. M. Blood pressure and hormonal changes following alterations in dietary sodium and potassium in mild essential hypertension. *Lancet,* 1981, *i,* 59-63.
Pfeiffer, J. E. The apish origins of human tension: The case of the amiable chimps and the nervous baboons. *Harvard Magazine,* 1981, 55-60.
Pickering, G. *High blood pressure.* New York: Grune & Stratton, 1968.
Pilkowsky, I., Spalding, D., Shaw, J., & Korner, P. I. Hypertension and personality. *Psychosomatic Medicine,* 1973, *35,* 50-56.
Ray, J. J., & Bozek, R. Dissecting the A-B personality type. *British Journal of Medical Psychology,* 1980, *53,* 181-186.
Rosenman, R. H. The interview method of assessment of the coronary-prone behavior pattern. In T. M. Dembroski, S. M. Weiss, J. L. Shields, S. G. Haynes, & M. Feinleib (Eds.), *Coronary-prone behavior.* New York: Springer-Verlag, 1978.
Rosenman, R. H. The role of Type A behavior pattern in ischemic heart disease:

Modification of its effects by beta-blocking agents. *British Journal of Clinical Practice,* 1978, *32*(1), 58-66.

Rosenman, R. H. Coronary-prone behavior pattern and coronary heart disease: Implications for the use of beta-blockers in primary prevention. In R. H. Rosenman (Ed.), *Psychosomatic risk factors and coronary heart. Indications for specific preventive therapy.* Bern: Huber, 1983.

Rosenman, R. H., Brand, R. J., Sholtz, R. I., & Friedman, M. Multivariate prediction of coronary heart disease during 8.5 year follow-up in the Western Collaborative Group Study. *American Journal of Cardiology,* 1976, *37,* 903-910.

Rosenman, R. H., & Chesney, M. A. Stress, Type A behavior and coronary disease. In L. Goldberger & S. Breznitz (Eds.) *The handbook of stress: Theoretical and clinical aspects.* New York: MacMillan, 1982.

Rosenman, R. H., & Friedman, M. Modifying Type A behavior pattern. *Journal of Psychosomatic Research,* 1977, *21,* 323-331.

Rosenman, R. H., Friedman, M., Straus, R., Wurm, M., Kositchek, R., Hahn, W., & Wethessen, N. T. A predictive study of coronary heart disease: The Western Collaborative Group Study. *Journal of the American Medical Association,* 1964, *189,* 15-22.

Rosenman, R. H., Rahe, R. H., Borhani, N. O., & Feinlab, M. Heritability of personality and behavior. *Acta Geneticae Medicae et Gemellologiae,* 1976, *25,* 221-224.

Roskies, E., & Lazarus, R. S. Coping theory and the teaching of coping skills. In P. O. Davidson & S. M. Davidson (Eds.), *Behavioral medicine: Changing health life styles.* New York: Brunner/Mazel, 1980.

Sapira, J. D., Scheib, E. T., Moriarty, R., & Shapiro, A. P. Differences in perception between hypertensive and normotensive populations. *Psychosomatic Medicine,* 1971, *33,* 239-250.

Saslow, G., Gressel, G. C., Shobe, F. O., DuBois, P. H., & Schroeder, H. A. Possible etiological relevance of personality factors in arterial hypertension. *Psychosomatic Medicine,* 1950, *12,* 292-302.

Scaramella, T. H., & Brown, W. A. Serum testosterone and aggressiveness in hockey players. *Psychosomatic Medicine,* 1978, *40,* 262-267.

Schachter, J. Pain, fear, and anger in hypertensives and normotensives: A psychophysiologic study. *Psychosomatic Medicine,* 1957, *19,* 17-29.

Schachter, S., & Singer, J. E. Cognitive, social, and physiological determinants of emotional state. *Psychological Review,* 1962, *69,* 379-399.

Scherwitz, L., Berton, K., & Leventhal, H. Type A behavior, self-involvement and cardiovascular response. *Psychosomatic Medicine,* 1978, *40,* 593-609.

Schwartz, G. E. Weinberger, D. A., & Singer, J. A. Cardiovascular differentiation of happiness, sadness, anger and fear following imagery and exercise. *Psychosomatic Medicine,* 1981, *43,* 343-364.

Selye, H. *Stress in health and disease.* New York: Butterworth, 1976.

Sexual behavior and the sex hormones. Editorial, *Lancet,* 1979, *2,* 17-18.

Shapiro, A. P. Psychophysiological mechanisms in hypertensive vascular disease. *Annals of Internal Medicine,* 1960, *53,* 64-83.

Shapiro, A. P. An experimental study of comparative responses of blood pressure to different noxious stimuli. *Journal of Chronic Diseases,* 1961, *13,* 293-311.

Shekelle, R. B., Gale, M., Ostfeld, A. M., & Paul, O. Hostility, risk of CHD, and mortality. *Psychosomatic Medicine,* 1983, *45,* 109-114.

Shekelle, R. B., Schoenberger, J. A., & Stamler, J. Correlates of the JAS Type A behavior score. *Journal of Chronic Diseases,* 1976, *29,* 381-394.

Siegel, J. M., Matthews, K. A., & Leitch, C. J. Blood pressure variability and the Type A behavior pattern in adolescents. *Journal of Psychosomatic Medicine,* 1983, *27,* 265-272.

Sjoberg, H. Physical fitness and mental performance during and after work. *Ergonomics,* 1980, *23,* 977-985.

Skrabal, F., Aubock, J., & Hortnagl, M. Low sodium-high potassium diet for prevention of hypertension: Probable mechanisms of action. *Lancet,* 1981, *2,* 895-900.

Snyder, S. H. Neurotransmitters and CNS disease: Schizophrenia. *Lancet,* 1982, *2,* 970-973.

Sokolow, M., Werdegar, D., Perloff, D. B., Cowan, R. M., & Brenenstund, H. Prelminary studies relating portably recorded blood pressure to daily life events in patients with essential hypertension. In M. Koster, H. Musaph, & P. Visser (Eds.), *Psychosomatics in essential hypertension.* Basel, N.Y.: Karger, 1970, (Biblioteca Psychiatrica, No. 44)).

Spielberger, C. D., Jacobs, G. A., Russell, S., & Crane, R. S. Assessment of anger: The State-Trait Anger Scale. In J. N. Butcher & C. D. Spielberger (Eds.), *Advances in personality assessment*, Vol. 2 Hillsdale, N.J.: Erlbaum, 1983.

Spielberger, C. D., Rosenman, R. H. *A reanalysis of coronary-prone Type A behavior in the Western Collaborative Group Study*, to be published.

Stauder, L. J., Holroyd, K. A., Appel, M. A., Gorkin, L., Uphole, V. K., & Saab, P. G. *Anger and essential hypertension: A factor analysis of measures used in recent research.* Presented at the Society of Behavioral Medicine, Baltimore, March 2-5, 1983.

Steptoe, A. *Psychological factors in cardiovascular disorders.* New York: Academic, 1981.

Sullivan, P., Schoentgen, S., DeQuattro, V., Procci, W., Levine, D., & Bornheimer, J. Anxiety and neurogenic tone—at rest and in stress, in primary hypertension. *Hypertension*, 1981, *3*, 125-130.

Symons, D. *The evolution of human sexuality.* Oxford: Oxford University Press, 1979.

Tanner, N. M. *On becoming human.* Cambridge, Mass.: Harvard University Press, 1981.

Thailer, S. A., Friedman, R., Harshfield, G. A., Kleinert, H. D., & Pickering, T. G. *Analysis of behavioral interactions in blood pressure variability.* Presented at Association for Advancement of Behavior Therapy, Los Angeles, November 19-21, 1982.

Thal, C. D. Neurotransmitters in neurologic diseases. *Medical Times*, 1983, *3*, 29-33.

Turnbull, C. M. The politics of non-aggression. In A. Montagu (Ed.), *Learning non-aggression: The experience of non-literate societies.* Oxford: Oxford University Press, 1978.

van Pragg, H. N. Neurotransmitters and CNS diseases: Depression. *Lancet*, 1982, *2*, 1259-1263.

Vickers, R. R., Harvig, L. K., Rahe, R., & Rosenman, R. H. Type A behavior pattern and coping and defense. *Psychosomatic Medicine*, 1981, *43*, 381-396.

Waldron, I. Why do women live longer than men? *Journal of Human Stress*, 1976, *2*, 2-13.

Weiner, H. *Psychobiology and human disease.* New York: Elsevier, 1977.

Whitfield, L., Sowers, J. R., Tuch, M. L., & Golub, M. S. Dopamine control of plasma catecholamine and aldosterone response to acute stimuli in normal men. *Journal of Clinical Endocrinology and Metabolism*, 1980, *51*, 724-729.

Williams, Jr., R. B., Haney, T. L., Lee, K. I., Kong, Y., Blumenthal, J. A., & Whalen, R. E. Type A behavior, hostility, and coronary atherosclerosis. *Psuchosomatic Medicine*, 1980, *42*, 539-549.

Williams, Jr., R. B., Lane, J. D., Kuhn, C. M., Melosh, W., White, A. D., & Schanberg, S. M. Type A behavior and elevated physiological and neuroendocrine responses to cognitive tasks. *Science*, 1982, *218*, 483-485.

Wolff, H. S., & Wolf, S. A summary of experimental evidence relating life stress to the pathogenesis of essential hypertension in man. In E. T. Bell (Ed.), *Hypertension: A symposium.* Minneapolis: University of Minnesota Press, 1951.

Women. The new wave in sports. *MD*, December 1980.

Wood, P. *Disease of the heart and circulation.* London: Eyre & Spottiswoode, 1956.

Zumoff, B., Rosenfeld, R. S., Friedman, M., Byers, S. O., Rosenman, R. H., & Hellman, L. *Comparison of plasma and urinary steroids in men with Type A and Type B behavior patterns.* Conference proceedings No. 231, pp. A12-1-A12-8, Prospective medicine opportunities in aerospace medicine. Advisory Group for Aerospace Research and Development, North Atlantic Treaty Organization, 1978.

6

Suppressed Anger in Hypertension: Facts and Problems

Stevo Julius, Robert Schneider, and Brent Egan
University of Michigan Medical School

If psychobehavioral factors do play a role in the development of hypertension, the pathophysiologic mechanism of these behavioral influences must be through some change in the neurohumoral control of the circulation. Furthermore, if behavioral changes are the cause and not the consequence of the high blood pressure, alterations in the neurohormonal control of the circulation must be present already in early phases of hypertension.

Hemodynamic studies in borderline and mild hypertension (for definition see (1)) have convinced us that a substantial proportion of patients with borderline and mild hypertension has a strong neurogenic component in the maintenance of their elevated blood pressure. Also, through psychometric assessment we have found certain characteristic behavioral patterns in these individuals. An unproven implication of our research is that this association between behavioral patterns and autonomic dysfunction in borderline and mild hypertension may be etiologic, that is, that the abnormal behavior causes abnormal autonomic function. It must be said, however, that our studies are cross-sectional, and we have no evidence of behavioral factors preceding and later leading to hypertension. There are also other disturbing questions that caution against presuming from our, and other investigators', findings a sequence of (a) behavioral changes, and (b) excessive blood pressure responsiveness that lead to (c) permanent state of hypertension.

In this paper we will present the existing data favoring a role for anger and other behavioral factors in the development of hypertension, but will also point out the problems and deficiencies in the field. The ultimate purpose is to suggest research agenda for the future. Much more work is needed before we can comfortably conclude that behavioral factors play a role in the genesis of human essential hypertension.

HEMODYNAMIC AND PHARMACOLOGIC EVIDENCE

As stated earlier, if psychosomatic factors are important in the development of hypertension, some abnormality in the autonomic nervous control of the circulation ought to be found in the early phases of hypertension. For many years it has been known that the hemodynamic pattern of borderline hypertension is different from established, more severe, hypertension. Whereas in established hypertension the blood pressure elevation is invariably associated with a high vascular resistance, among patients with borderline hypertension many have an elevation of the cardiac output (2, 3). There are a few factors that can cause an elevation of the cardiac output: increased blood volume, reduced oxygen content of the blood (i.e., anoxemia), increased metabolic rate, and central nervous influence. There is no evidence for anoxemia in borderline hypertension and the blood volume is, in fact, decreased (4). On the other hand, the metabolic rate in borderline hypertension is increased (5-7). This increase, then, could be responsible for the high cardiac output but the hemodynamic picture in borderline hypertension is quite different from other elevated metabolic states, such as hyperthyroidism or physical exercise. In these states there is a substantial decrease of vascular resistance. Consequently, the systolic blood pressure is elevated but the diastolic reading is usually decreased so that the mean blood pressure remains unchanged.

In borderline hypertension, the mean blood pressure is significantly increased. A detailed analysis of the hemodynamics of borderline hypertension shows that the vascular resistance, though numerically normal, is in fact elevated if the high levels of cardiac output are taken into account. When we plotted vascular resistance at similar levels of cardiac output, patients with borderline hypertension consistently had higher values than normotensive control subjects (7). Furthermore, with appropriate tests (tilt, exercise, volume expansion, autonomic blockade) it was clear that, although blood pressure responses in borderline hypertensives are similar to the control subjects', at these increased blood pressure levels the vascular resistance of borderline hypertensives is always significantly elevated (8, 9). Reasonably, an enhanced sympathetic drive could account for all the observed phenomena in borderline hypertension, cardiac output and metabolic rate reflecting an excessive beta-adrenergic drive, and abnormal resistance reflecting an enhanced alpha-adrenergc drive.

We first tested whether the cardiac output elevation may be neurogenic (10) by using large intravenous doses of both propranolol (to block the beta-adrenergic drive) and atropine (to block the parasympathetic inhibition of the heart). The cardiac output elevation in patients with hyperkinetic borderline hypertension was fully normalized by this pharmacologic blockade of the autonomic influences on the heart. The higher cardiac output was due to a higher stroke volume and a faster heart rate, which were both corrected after autonomic blockade, and the values became similar to those in normotensive control subjects. We could, therefore, confidently conclude that the cardiac output elevation in hyperkinetic borderline hypertension is mediated through autonomic nervous influences.

A detailed analysis of these experiments provided further interesting insights. As can be seen from Figure 1, blocking the sympathetic drive to the heart was not sufficient to normalize the cardiac output. After large doses of propranolol, the cardiac output was still higher than in normotensive controls. In addition, we had to block the parasympathetic influence on the heart with atropine in order to normalize the cardiac output. Because the sympathetic and parasympathetic control of the heart were both involved in this abnormality of the cardiac output, it was very likely that the abnormality came from the central nervous

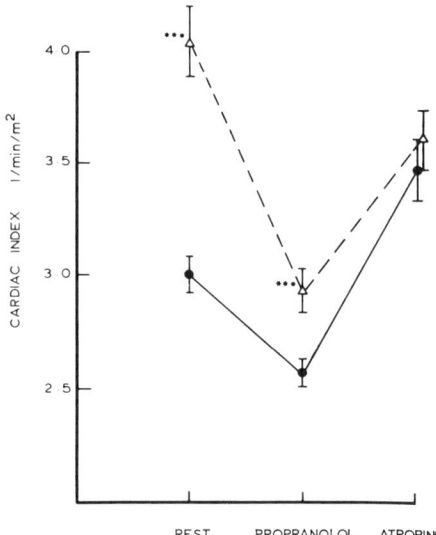

Figure 1 Influence of the stepwise blockade of the autonomic system on cardiac index. First, propranolol 0.2 mg/kg i.v. was given and the measurement taken seven minutes after completion of the injection. Another measurement was taken seven minutes after atropine 0.04 mg/kg i.v. Patients were selected from an elevated cardiac index (one S.D. above the mean of the control.) There were 25 such patients (triangles) and 29 (circles) control subjects. ***$p < 0.001$.

system. This was important because Frohlich, et al. found that some normotensive and some mildly hypertensive subjects had an increased sensitivity of beta-adrenergic receptors, which was responsible for their hyperkinetic circulation (11). There was no evidence that our patients had a peripheral beta-receptor hypersensitivity. In fact, we (12) and others (13) found a decreased beta-adrenergic responsiveness in such patients.

Figure 1 further suggests that the autonomic abnormality in borderline hypertension is central, rather than being related to abnormal peripheral receptors. Size of the change in cardiac output after beta-blockade represents the amount of sympathetic drive to the heart, whereas the degree of change after atropine reflects the amount of parasympathetic inhibition of the heart. When presented in this light, Figure 1 clearly suggests that the sympathetic drive to the heart is increased and the parasympathetic inhibition is decreased in hyperkinetic borderline hypertension (10).

Such a reciprocal relationship in the sympathetic and parasympathetic control of the heart is characteristic of the functional organization in the cardiovascular centers in the medulla oblongata. Whenever the cardiovascular centers receive a signal calling for a change in the autonomic outflow, the response is always integrated—increased sympathetic combined with a decreased parasympathetic discharge and vice-versa. Thus the abnormality in borderline hypertension seems to occur in the integrative areas of central nervous cardiovascular control.

The next step in our investigation of the autonomic involvement in borderline hypertension was to induce a complete receptor blockade of the heart (as before) and also of the peripheral alpha-adrenergic receptors. This was necessary because normalization of the elevated cardiac output did not result in blood pressure returning to the normal range (10). After cardiac blockade, hyperkinetic patients responded with an elevation of the vascular resistance and continued to maintain their blood pressure elevation. We speculated that this elevation of vascular resistance may be neurogenic and should be readily abolished with alpha-adrenergic blockade with phentolamine.

In the next two series (14, 15), however, there were only a few patients with hyperkinetic circulation (defined as a cardiac output 2 S.D. above the control mean). Total autonomic blockade fully normalized the blood pressure elevation in only about 30% of patients with borderline hypertension (14) and mild established hypertension (15). These 30%, whose blood pressure normalized after autonomic blockade could justifiably be termed as having a "neurogenic" hypertension. The major characteristics of these neurogenic hypertensives were an elevated plasma norepinephrine, elevated plasma renin, and signs of enhanced cardiac sympathetic drive (larger changes in heart rate and pre-ejection period after propranolol, increased resting heart rate).

The extensive increase of the sympathetic drive in high-renin neurogenic hypertension (to the heart and arterioles and presumably to the juxtaglomerular cells in the kidneys) further complemented our initial observation, that the abnormal autonomic control of the circulation in borderline hypertension originates in the central nervous system. As indicated earlier, we have evidence that the abnormality involves reciprocal changes in sympathetic and parasympathetic outflow, and therefore points toward an abnormal integration of the autonomic control of the circulation (16).

What could disrupt the integration of the autonomic control in borderline hypertension? Alteration in afferent baroreceptor input may cause similar effects; however, in our tests the baroreceptor sensitivity in borderline hypertension is normal (17), though others find the sensitivity to be decreased (18). The decreased sensitivity observed in borderline hypertension is probably secondary and not a primary phenomenon. In Eckberg's work, the baroreceptor sensitivity mirrored the degree of blood pressure elevation, even in the borderline hypertension range; those with mildest blood pressure elevation had a normal baroreceptor function (19).

If the abnormality is not caused by an erroneous afferent input from arterial baroreceptors, it could be caused by descending pathways converging on the cardiovascular centers. For example, psychosomatic influences descend upon the cardiovascular centers and can elicit substantial changes in the integration of autonomic tone (20). Consequently, it was appropriate to investigate whether certain behaviors or personality traits are more prominent in borderline hypertension and, if they are, how they relate to the autonomic abnormality.

PSYCHOBEHAVIORAL EVIDENCE

In our first study (21) we used Cattel's 16 personality factor questionnaire to test the subjects' perceptions of their usual behavior; hemodynamics or hormonal profiling were not included in these studies. Subjects were selected for their initially high (>140) or low (<110) systolic blood pressure. Initial systolic blood pressure correlated significantly and positively with submissiveness, sensitivity, sociability and suspiciousness. When subjects were classified according to their repeated blood pressure readings, those who maintained consistently high readings had significantly higher scores on submissiveness, sensitivity and sociability. Anxiety correlated with the initial blood pressure levels, but when classified by blood pressure category, those with consistently high readings had normal anxiety scores.

In this study, we tested 12 pairs of "high" and "low" blood pressure individuals in a paradigm of experimental yielding. This involved assessing individuals' attitudes to certain selected topics of interest, such as capital punishment, juvenile delinquency, and other controversial topics. Later, the subjects were matched with a partner who had different blood pressure classification and held an opposing opinion. Subjects were requested to arrive, through discussion, at a compromise opinion. Subjects with high blood pressure reported liking more intensely their low blood pressure partners. They anticipated that they would not yield but, in fact, did yield during the discussion. They also stated after the interaction that they truly and privately changed their opinion. This behavioral experiment fully confirmed the self-described submissiveness found with the 16-PF questionnaire.

The 16-PFQ test measurements were repeated on a group of medical students in Yugoslavia. The original work was published in Serbo-Croatian (22), but the essential results have subsequently been published in English (23). Two of the factors found to be characteristic for high blood pressure individuals in our study in Ann Arbor were again found in Zagreb. Thus, Yugoslav students living in an entirely different environment were more sociable and more submissive if their blood pressure tended to be high. The high blood pressure students in Zagreb were also described as enthusiastic and less shy. It is truly fascinating to find that in two different cultures subjects with borderline hypertension describe themselves as being outward oriented but submissive to other people. We privately speculated that such a constellation of behavior may lead to difficulties in expressing anger.

Many years later, and after Dr. Harburg independently confirmed his intuitive feeling that "ability to express anger" may relate to blood pressure elevation (24), we were able to test the relationship between the variables and the autonomic nervous abnormalities in mild hypertension (15). By that time, much more was known about the autonomic abnormality in borderline hypertension and our conceptual understanding of behavioral factors had progressed. From a previous publication (14), it was known that patients with high-renin are those with the clearest neurogenic hypertension. It was also shown that the autonomic abnormality originates in the central integrative areas of cardiovascular control (16).

We were interested to learn whether patients with mild but established hypertension and high-renin values have characteristics similar to patients with borderline hypertension (15). It was shown that patients with more advanced hypertension still have signs of extensive autonomic hyperactivity and that their hypertension can be abolished with autonomic blockade. These patients were ideal candidates to evaluate the question of association between behavior and autonomic nervous dysfunction. The behavior-oriented questionnaires included IPAT anxiety scale, Buss-Durkey personality inventory, Cattel's 16-personality factors questionnaire and Harburg's "anger-in/anger-out" scale. In this study, again, the high-renin neurogenic hypertensives were proven to be submissive on the 16-PFQ test. This, then, was the third time that submissiveness was found. The steady appearance of this factor in three different populations over a ten-year span is impressive indeed. In the 1977 study, patients with neurogenic hypertension also had higher scores on "super ego." On the Buss-Durkey scale, the neurogenic (high-renin) hypertensives showed significantly less verbal aggressive action and permitted less overt irritability; thus, a submissive, highly controlled and less aggressive personality was described by these tests. However, these overtly less aggressive and more complacent subjects clearly demonstrated more suppressed hostility by the Harburg scale. As Harburg had anticipated, these individuals were prone to hold anger in, and were incapable of expressing it.

DOES ABNORMAL BEHAVIOR LEAD TO NEUROGENIC HYPERTENSION?

In spite of the association described earlier, there are serious problems and large gaps in our knowledge that speak against a quick generalization from our data to a strong role of behavioral factors in the development of human hypertension. These problems will now be briefly described; a detailed discussion would exceed the purpose of this presentation.

1. Do neurogenic, hyperkinetic patients with borderline hypertension develop sustained hypertension?

Although a larger than normal proportion of patients with borderline hypertension develop future established essential hypertension, the absolute number of those developing hypertension is not overwhelming. In fact, more than four-fifths of all patients with borderline hypertension will never develop hypertension (1). Obviously only some of the patients have a special tendency toward hypertension, and the others harbor a clinically insignificant condition. Are the neurogenic borderline hypertensives therefore at a higher risk, or is the neurogenic borderline hypertension an innocuous and transient condition?

As indicated earlier, the hyperkinetic state in borderline hypertension is clearly neurogenic. The hallmark of this condition, tachycardia, has been shown to be an independent risk factor predicting future hypertension (25, 26). The predictive strength of tachycardia is low, which must mean that only a few patients with hypertension are recruited from the pool of patients with neurogenic stigma. However, the proportion of hypertensives [borderline (27) or established (28)] who underwent a neurogenic borderline phase seems to be sufficiently high to enable investigators to find a substantial number of patients with fast heart rates, in the presence of normal cardiac output and elevated vascular resistance. In the case of more advanced hypertension, one must be cautious, for some of the tachycardia may be secondary to the blood pressure elevation, in that it reflects a subclinical sign of a failing heart.

Catecholamines tend to be elevated in neurogenic borderline hypertension. If one believes that a large number of patients with essential hypertension previously underwent a neurogenic hyperkinetic phase, then one would expect a substantial proportion of patients with essential hypertension to have elevated plasma norepinephrine. This, however, is not the case. As Goldstein has shown in his review (29), norepinephrine is elevated only in young patients with hypertension. This lack of evidence for neurogenic established hypertension is quite disconcerting. It either means that only a few of the hyperkinetic-neurogenic patients enter the large pool of patients with essential hypertension, or that a yet unexplained resetting of the central nervous drive occurs in the course of hypertension. Although it has frequently been suggested that the mechanisms in the course of hypertension may change, and that in later phases the blood pressure is maintained by secondary humoral and anatomic changes, the mechanism whereby the nervous system would be reset to function normally has never been elucidated.

2. What is the mechanism of transition from hyperkinetic to normokinetic hypertension?

Because patients with neurogenic borderline hypertension have a high cardiac output, while patients with established hypertension have normal cardiac output, one must explain how the cardiac output would become normal and how vascular resistance would increase in the course of hypertension. This is conceptually an easier task than explaining the disappearance of the elevated norepinephrine in the course of hypertension.

We postulated that with advancing hypertension the responsiveness of heart rate and contractility to excessive stimulation would decrease (30). This phenomenon of decreased end-organ responsiveness to prolonged increases of sympathetic tone has been observed frequently. In the heart, it may not only be due to receptor down-regulation but also to complex biochemical and structural changes in the course of myocardial hypertrophy (31). We have shown evidence for decreased sympathetic responsiveness in "normokinetic" borderline hypertension (27) and also that the heart actually receives more sympathetic drive. But this drive is needed just to maintain the cardiac output at a normal level. The argument that the normokinetic state may have evolved from a previously hyperkinetic heart is supported by the observation that patients with normal cardiac output, like the high cardiac output patients, still show signs of decreased inhibition of the vagus nerve (28).

An alternative hypothesis for the normalization of the elevated cardiac output was also proposed. It assumes that the elevated output may become normal through the mechanism of autoregulation (32). When the total body flow (cardiac output) exceeds the metabolic needs of the tissues, a total body *non-neurogenic* autoregulation occurs; the vascular resistance is increased, and the cardiac output returns to normal. Although this mechanism occurs in volume-expanded animals and anephric humans (i.e., without functional kidneys) (33), it probably does not occur in hyperkinetic borderline hypertension. We (7) and others (5, 6) have shown that the oxygen consumption in borderline hypertension is increased and the cardiac output is appropriately adjusted to this increase. Thus, the stimulus to autoregulate is absent; there are no signs of a "luxurious perfusion" exceeding the metabolic needs of the body to trigger autoregulation. The autoregulatory theory, however, does have one advantage. It not only explains the normalization of the cardiac output but also the increase of vascular resistance in the hypothetical transition from the high-output to high-resistance hypertension.

Our hypothesis of decreased sympathetic responsiveness as a factor in the normalization of the output also requires an explanation as to why the vascular resistance increases. This can be explained by structural changes in the arterioles, including the media hypertrophy that encroaches upon the vessel lumen. As Folkow proposed (34) and Sivertsson demonstrated in humans (35), such hypertrophic vessels become over-responsive to normal vasoconstricting stimuli. Over-responding of hypertensive patients to alpha-adrenergic blockade has been described by Buehler and co-workers (36), but their claim of a *specific* hypersensitivity of alpha-receptors cannot be substantiated. As reported in their study, the possible effect of hypertension in increasing vascular hypertrophy have not been entirely ruled out.

In summary, we postulate, but have no proof, that if changing from high-output to high-resistance occurs in the natural history of hypertension, this is done by decreased cardiac responsiveness to sympathetic stimuli and by a hypertrophy-induced hyperresponsiveness of arterioles.

3. How are personality, blood pressure hyperresponsiveness, and blood pressure variability related to the development of hypertension?

Several investigators found increased blood pressure responsiveness to mental stress in borderline hypertensives (37-39). However, blood pressure responses to stimuli such as dynamic exercise (5-7), isometric exercise (40) and volume expansion (6, 7) have been normal. The blood pressure response to upright posture is debatable, as some have found excessive increases (41, 42) in diastolic blood pressure while others have not (9). Thus, there is some laboratory evidence that blood pressure variability is increased in borderline hypertensives. Because this is particularly true with regard to certain types of mental stress, it suggests involvement of psychobehavioral characteristics.

Another group that displays cardiovascular hyperresponsiveness in the laboratory is that exhibiting the Type A coronary-prone behavior pattern. These subjects show greater increases of blood pressure (and heart rate and catecholamines) when challenged with mental stressors than do Type B controls (42). However, the resting baseline blood pressure of Type As are not elevated. The Type A subjects differ from neurogenic hypertensives in their personality and behavioral characteristics. The Type A behavior pattern is typified by hostility, competitiveness and aggressiveness, as well as time urgency (43, 44). Compared with the anger-in characterization (15) of neurogenic hypertensives, these individuals direct anger out. Thus, blood pressure hyperresponsiveness to mental stress may be associated with different personality characteristics than those known to be associated with an increase of the average blood pressure.

Despite the laboratory evidence for blood pressure hyperresponsiveness in borderline hypertensives, the majority of investigators have not found increased variability in this group of patients during ambulatory blood pressure monitoring (45, 46). Responsiveness to mental stress is only one of the factors that influences blood pressure variability. As indicated earlier, with the exception of mental stress, patients with borderline hypertension respond normally to other pressor stimuli. It appears that in the natural setting during ambulatory blood pressure monitoring, normal regulation of blood pressure responsiveness to various stimuli prevails, and the hyperresponsiveness to mental stress is not sufficient to materially influence the overall blood pressure variability.

Perhaps of greater clinical significance, blood pressure variability is not an independent predictor of hypertensive complications (47). This observation makes it even less likely that blood pressure variability is involved in the development of hypertension. In other words, if variability led to hypertension, then variability should carry a poorer prognosis. Furthermore, the reproducibility of increased blood pressure variability is essentially nonexistent in individuals examined biennially, while the level of the blood pressure is reasonably reproducible (48).

Although evidence indicates behavioral traits are involved in the pathogenesis of hypertension, increased blood pressure variability is not likely to be the mechanism. Evidence implicating other mechanisms has been reported by Hollenberg, who found increased renal vascular resistance responses to mental stress in borderline hypertensives (49). However, no differences in blood pressure responses were noted in this study. Interestingly, Light et al. found that greater sodium retention was associated with a larger heart rate response during mental stress in a subgroup of patients with either borderline hypertension or a positive family history of hypertension (50).

In summary, there is evidence for both specific behavioral traits and increased pressor response to mental stresses in the laboratory in borderline hypertensives. However, blood pressure variability does not appear excessive under free-living conditions. Furthermore, increased variability was not reproducible in the Framingham study and was not an independent predictor of morbidity or mortality. Thus, in studies investigating the relationship between behavioral characteristics and hypertension it would be prudent to concentrate on other factors than the blood pressure variability.

REFERENCES

1. Julius, S., & Schork, M. A. Borderline hypertension—A critical review. *Journal of Chronic Diseases,* 1971, *23,* 723-754.
2. Widimsky, J., Fejfarova, M. H., & Fejfar, Z. Changes of cardiac output in hypertensive disease. *Cardiologia,* 1957, *31,* 381-389.
3. Eich, R. H., Peters, R. J., Cuddy, R. P., & Smulyan, H. The hemodyamics in labile hypertension. *American Heart Journal,* 1962, *63,* 188-195.
4. Julius, S., Pascual A. V., Reilly, K., & London, R. Abnormalities of plasma volume in borderline hypertension. *Archives of Internal Medicine,* 1971, *127,* 116-119.
5. Lund-Johansen, P. Hemodynamics in early essential hypertension. *Acta Medica Scandinavica, Supplement,* 1967, *482,* 1-105.
6. Sannerstedt, R. Hemodynamic response to exercise in patients with arterial hypertension. *Acta Medica Scandinavica, Supplement,* 1966, *458,* 1-83.
7. Julius, S., & Conway, J. Hemodynamic studies in patients with borderline blood pressure elevation. *Circulation,* 1968, *38,* 282-288.
8. Julius, S., Pascual, A. V., Sannerstedt, R., & Mitchell, C. Relationship between cardiac output and peripheral resistance in borderline hypertension. *Circulation,* 1971, *43,* 382-390.
9. Sannerstedt, R., Julius, S., & Conway, J. Hemodynamic response to tilt and beta-adrenergic blockade in young patients with borderline hypertension. *Circulation,* 1970, *42,* 1057-1064.
10. Julius, S., Pascual, A. V., & London, R. Role of parasympathetic inhibition in the hyperkinetic type of borderline hypertension. *Circulation,* 1971, *44,* 413-418.
11. Frohlich, E. D., Tarazi, R. C., & Dustan, H. P. Hyperdynamic beta-adrenergic circulatory state: Increased beta-receptor responsiveness. *Archives of Internal Medicine,* 1969, *123,* 1-7.
12. Julius, S. Neurogenic component in borderline hypertension. In S. Julius & M. Esler (Eds.), *The nervous system in arterial hypertension,* Springfield, Ill.: Thomas, 1976.
13. Bertel, O., Buhler, F. R., Kowski, W., & Lutold, B. E. Decreased beta-adrenoreceptor

responsiveness as related to age, blood pressure, and plasma catecholamines in patients with essential hypertension. *Hypertension,* 1980, *2,* 130–138.
14. Esler, M. D., Julius, S., Randall, O. S., Ellis, C. N., & Kashima, T. Relation of renin status to neurogenic vascular resistance in borderline hypertension. *American Journal of Cardiology,* 1975, *36,* 708–715.
15. Esler, M., Julius, S., Zweifler, A., Randall, O., Harburg, E., Gardiner, H., & DeQuattro, V. Mild high-renin essential hypertension. Neurogenic human hypertension? *New England Journal of Medicine,* 1977, *296,* 405–411.
16. Julius, S., & Esler, M. Autonomic nervous cardiovascular regulation in borderline hypertension. *American Journal of Cardiology,* 1975, *36,* 685–696.
17. Julius, S., & Hansson, L. Hemodynamics of prehypertension and hypertension. *Verhandlungen der Deutschen Gesellschaft für Innere Medizin,* 1974, *80,* 49–58.
18. Takeshita, A., Tanaka, S., Kuroiwa, A., & Nakamura, M. Reduced baroreceptor sensitivity in borderline hypertension. *Circulation,* 1975, *51,* 738–742.
19. Eckberg, D. L. Carotid baroreflex function in young men with borderline blood pressure elevation. *Circulation,* 1979, *59,* 632–636.
20. Hilton, S. M. Inhibition of baroreceptor reflexes on hypothalamic stimulation. *Journal of Physiology (London),* 1963, *165,* 56–57.
21. Harburg, E., Julius, S., McGinn, N. F., McLeod, J., & Hoobler, S. W. Personality traits and behavioral patterns associated with systolic blood pressure levels in college males. *Journal of Chronic Diseases,* 1964, *17,* 405–414.
22. Julius, S. Psihosomatske znacajke studenata a povisenim sistolickim tlakom. Unpublished thesis for Sc.D. Degree, University of Zagreb, 1964.
23. Julius, S. The psychophysiology of borderline hypertension. In *Brain, Behavior, and Bodily Disease.* H. Weiner, M. A. Hofer, & A. J. Stunkard (Eds.), New York: Raven, 1981.
24. Harburg, E., Erfurt, J. C., Hauenstein, L. S., Chape, C., Schull, W. J., & Schork, M. A. Socio-ecological stress, suppressed hostility, skin color, and black-white male blood pressure: Detroit. *Psychosomatic Medicine,* 1973, *35,* 276–296.
25. Levy, R. L., White, P. D., Stroud, W. D., & Hillman, C. C. Transient tachycardia: Prognostic significance alone and in association with transient hypertension. *Journal of the American Medical Association,* 1945, *129,* 585–588.
26. Paffenbarger, R. S., Jr., Thorne, M. C., & Wing, A. L. Chronic disease in former college students–VIII. Characteristics in youth predisposing to hypertension in later years. *American Journal of Epidemiology,* 1968, *88,* 25–32.
27. Julius, S., Randall, O. S., Esler, M. D., Kashima, T., Ellis, C. N., & Bennett, J. Altered cardiac responsiveness and regulation in the normal cardiac output type of borderline hypertension. *Circulation Research,* (Supplement I), 1975, *36–37,* I199–I207.
28. Korner, P. I., Shaw, J., Uther, J. B., West, M. J., McRitchie, R. J., & Richards, J. G. Autonomic and non-autonomic circulatory components in essential hypertension in man. *Circulation,* 1973, *48,* 107–117.
29. Goldstein, D. S. Plasma norepinephrine in essential hypertension. A study of the studies. *Hypertension,* 1981, *3,* 48–52.
30. Julius, S. Psychophysiologic evidence for the role of the nervous system in hypertension. In A. Amery, (Ed.), *Hypertension cardiovascular disease: Pathophysiology and treatment.* Belgium: Nijhoff, 1982.
31. Trimarco, B., Volpe, M., Ricciardelli, B., Picotti, F. B., Galva, M. D., Petracca, R., & Condorelli, M. Studies of the mechanisms underlying impairment of beta-adrenoceptor-mediated effects in human hypertension. *Hypertension,* 1983, *5,* 584–590.
32. Cowley, A. W., Jr. The concept of autoregulation of total blood flow and its role in hypertension. *American Journal of Medicine,* 1980, *68,* 906–916.
33. Coleman, T. G., Bower, J. D., Langford, H. G., & Guyton, A. C. Regulation of arterial pressure in the anephric state. *Circulation,* 1970, *42,* 509–514.
34. Folkow, B. Role of vascular factor in hypertension. *Contrib Nephrol,* 1977, *8,* 81–94.
35. Silvertsson, R. The hemodynamic importance of structural vascular changes in essential hypertension. *Acta Physiologica Scandinavica Supplementum* 343, 1970, *79,* 3–56.
36. Amann, F. W., Bolli, P., Kiowski, W., & Buhler, F. R. Enhanced alpha-adrenoreceptor-mediated vasoconstriction in essential hypertension. *Hypertension,* (Supplement I), 1981, *3,* I119–1123.

37. Nestel, P. J. Blood pressure and catecholamine excretion after mental stress in labile hypertension. *Lancet,* 1969, *1,* 692-694.
38. Falkner, B., Onesti, G., Angelakos, E. T., Fernandes, M., & Langman, C. Cardiovascular response to mental stress in normal adolescents with hypertensive parents. Hemodynamics and mental stress in adolescents. *Hypertension,* 1979, *1,* 23-30.
39. Light, K. C., & Obrist, P. A. Cardiovascular reactivity to behavioral stress in young males with and without marginally elevated casual systolic pressures. Comparison of clinic, home, and laboratory measures. *Hypertension,* 1980, *2,* 802-808.
40. Sannerstedt, R., & Julius, S. Systemic haemodynamics in borderline arterial hypertension: Response to exercise before and under the influence of propranolol. *Cardiovascular Research,* 1972, *6,* 398-403.
41. Frohlich, E. D., Tarazi, R. C., Ulrych, M., Dustan, H. P., & Page, I. H. Tilt test for investigating a neural component in hypertension. Its correlation with clinical characteristics. *Circulation,* 1967, *36,* 387-393.
42. Hull, D. H., Wolthuis, R. A., Cortese, T., Longo, M. R., Jr., & Triebwasser, J. H. Borderline hypertension versus normotension: Differential response to orthostatic stress. *American Heart Journal,* 1977, *94,* 414-420.
43. Matthews, K. A. Psychological perspectives on the Type A behavior pattern. *Psychological Bulletin,* 1982, *91,* 293-323.
44. Chesney, M. A., Black, G. W., Chadwich, J. H., & Rosenman, R. H. Psychological correlates of the Type A behavior pattern. *Journal of Behavioral Medicine,* 1981, *4,* 217-229.
45. Horan, M. J., Kennedy, H. L., & Padgett, N. E. Do borderline hypertensive patients have labile blood pressure? *Annals of Internal Medicine,* 1981, *94(Part I),* 466-468.
46. Floras, J. S., Hassan, M. O., Sever, P. S., Jones, J. V., Osikowska, B., & Sleight, P. Cuff and ambulatory blood pressure in subjects with essential hypertension. *Lancet* 1981, *2,* 107-109.
47. Sokolow, M., Wedegar, D., Kain, H. K., & Hinman, A. T. Relationship between level of blood pressure measured casually and by portable recorder, and severity of complications in essential hypertension. *Circulation,* 1966, *34,* 279-298.
48. Kannel, W. B., Sorlie, P., & Gordon, T. Labile hypertension: A faulty concept? The Framingham study. *Circulation,* 1980, *61,* 1183-1187.
49. Hollenberg, H. K., Williams, G. H., & Adams, D. F. Essential hypertension: Abnormal renal vascular and endocrine responses to a mild psychological stimulus. *Hypertension,* 1981, *3,* 11-17.
50. Light, K. C., Koepke, J. P., Obrist, P. A., & Willis, P. W., IV. Psychological stress induces sodium and fluid retention in men at high risk for hypertension. *Science,* 1983, *220,* 429-431.

7
Relationship of Anger-Coping Styles and Blood Pressure among Black Americans

W. Doyle Gentry
University of Virginia

Benign essential hypertension is epidemic in the United States. Approximately one in every five adult Americans is thought to have hypertension, that is, blood pressure above 160 mm Hg systolic and/or 95 mm Hg diastolic (Moss & Scott, 1976). Hypertension accounts for at least 60,000 American deaths annually and is a major contributing (risk) factor in the 1.5 million heart attacks and strokes occurring each year in this country (Kannel, 1974; NHBPEP, 1976). It also ranks as the fourth most common diagnosis at physician office visits, accounting for 3.5% of all such visits each year (Madden, Turner & Eckenfels, 1982).

Hypertension, however, does not affect all segments of American society equally. It is noticeably greater among American blacks, increases with age in all persons, is higher for males than females, and is greater for persons who reside in high socioecological stress areas (Fries, 1973; James & Kleinbaum, 1976; Roberts & Maurer, 1976).

In this chapter, we are especially concerned with the disparity in hypertension rates characterizing black compared to white Americans. The prevalence of hypertension is twice as high among black Americans as compared to whites, and it is estimated that blacks have between six and fifteen times higher mortality due to hypertension and/or hypertension-related diseases (Thompson, 1980).

To date, research investigating the causes underlying black-white blood pressure differences has tended to focus on differences in genetic makeup (Schull, Harburg, Schork, Weener & Chape, 1977) and diet. Less often, if at all, has research centered on possible psychosocial differences between these two race groups. In this chapter, we will offer empirical evidence which suggests that such factors (e.g., anger-coping styles) do, in fact, operate to influence human blood pressure and thereby increase one's chances of developing hypertensive disease, and that these factors distinguish between black and white Americans.

SUPPRESSED ANGER AND HYPERTENSION

Over 40 years ago, Franz Alexander (1939) offered the tentative hypothesis that "chronic inhibited rage may lead to a chronic elevation of the blood pressure." He observed that hypertensives belong to a group of persons caught in an "emotional paralysis," unable to fully express anger in the form of aggressive behavior (toward the provocative agent) because of competing tendencies toward passive, dependent, and anxious behavior.

Research since that time has kept this hypothesis alive (Weiner, 1977). For example, in a recent 5-year prospective study of 10,000 Israeli male civil service employees, Kahn, Medalie, Neufeld, Riss, and Goldbourt (1972) found that those individuals who reported a tendency to "brood when hurt by a supervisor," "restrain retaliation when hurt by a supervisor," "keep conflict with wife to self," and/or "brood when hurt by co-workers" had a much higher incidence of hypertension (rate = 81/1,000) as compared to individuals not so characterized (rate = 35/1,000). Only nine out of ninety biomedical and behavioral variables studied predicted theincidence of hypertension in this population at a level significantly above chance ($p = .01$), and two of these nine dealt with the respondents' tendency to suppress work-related anger.

Similarly, Baer, Collins, Bourianoff, and Ketchel (1979) noted that the most discriminating item on their brief 16-item psychosocial screening questionnaire designed to differentiate between hypertensives and normotensives was, "I tend to harbor grudges that I don't tell anybody about." Thirty-seven percent of their screened hypertensives responded in the affirmative to this item, as compared to twenty-seven percent of the screened normotensives.

Finally, our own recent research on this topic (Gentry, Chesney, Gary, Hall & Harburg, 1982; Gentry, Harburg & Hauenstein, 1973; Harburg, Erfurt, Hauenstein, Chape, Schull, & Schork, 1973; Harburg, Blakelock & Roeper, 1979) suggests that persons who habitually express anger in some form when provoked by others have lower systolic and diastolic pressure than persons who habitually inhibit (suppress) such feelings, the average magnitude of difference being approximately ± 3-4 mm Hg. The observed differential risk for hypertension is these same individuals is 1.636 to 1 (Table 1). About one out of five "anger-in" respondents were diagnosed hypertensive, as compared to one out of eight "anger-out" respondents.

Anger suppression combines with other behavioral risk factors (Gentry et al., 1982), such as race, sex, and socioecological stress area, to create group differences in "at risk" status for hypertension that range from less than 7% (for white females who reside in low stress areas and who express their anger openly) to 39% (for black males, residing in high stress areas, who suppress anger). Table

Table 1 Odds of being classified hypertensive and odds ratios between behavioral factors

Factors		Odds	Odds ratio[a]
Race	Black	0.2043	1.642
	White	0.1244	
Sex	Male	0.1952	1.498
	Female	0.1303	
Socioecological stress area	High	0.1924	1.456
	Low	0.1321	
Anger expression	Low	0.2039	1.636
	High	0.1247	

[a]Odds ratios describe the relative risk for hypertension associated with being black vs. white, male vs. female, and so forth.

Table 2 Differential risk (odds) of being
classified hypertensive
associated with presence of
behavioral factors

Risk factors present	Odds
4	0.3860
3	0.2481
2	0.1594
1	0.1025
0	0.0658

Note. 4 = black, male, high stress area, low anger expression; 0 = white, female, low stress area, high anger expression.

2 illustrates the differential risk (odds) of being classified hypertensive associated with the presence or absence of these various behavioral factors.

SUPPRESSED ANGER AMONG BLACK AMERICANS

Given the long-standing link between suppressed anger and hypertension noted above, it seems logical to explain at least part of the observed differences in black-white blood pressure in terms of anger-coping styles. In a recently published study (Gentry, Chesney, Kennedy, Hall, Gary & Harburg, 1983), we noted that black and white adult Americans differed somewhat in their habitual propensity for expressing versus suppressing anger across a wide range of anger-provoking interpersonal situations (Table 3). In this study of 1,006 residents of Detroit, we found that black males were significantly more likely to hold anger in than were other race-sex groups (Table 4), as were individuals residing in high verus low socioecological stress areas.

Elsewhere (Gentry, 1972), we had previously noted a similar tendency of black males to fail to express anger openly when provoked in an experimental situation, as compared to black females. That is, whereas male and female black college students reported increased anger, elevated blood pressure, and heightened verbal aggressivity upon being insulted by a white student examiner, only the black females registered their overt (aggressive) dislike and disapproval of the person delivering the insult.

Other researchers in the past have found blacks and whites to differ in their respective tendencies toward suppressed anger. Crain and Weisman (1972), for example, found that blacks and poorly educated persons were much less likely to

Table 3 Hypothetical anger situation and multiple-choice response
categories: "If your boss got angry and blew up at you for
no good reason, how would you feel?"

Anger-out	Anger-in
Angry or mad and show it.	Annoyed, but would keep it in.
Annoyed and would show it.	Angry or mad, but would keep it in.
	Wouldn't get angry, mad, or annoyed.

Table 4 Distribution of anger-coping tendencies as a function of race-sex interaction

Tendencies	Black		White	
	Male	Female	Male	Female
Anger-in	58 (23%)	46 (18%)	33 (14%)	48 (19%)
Anger-out	195	212	209	205

recall angry feelings in the past than were their white and/or highly educated counterparts. Yarrow (1958) observed that black children, when faced with provocation, tended to limit expression of emotionality to covert (fear, withdrawal) rather than overt (fighting, obscene language) behaviors. Forbes and Mitchell (1971), in related fashion, reported that, even though adult black females attributed more blame to a white-frustrating-a-black than a black-frustrating-a-white, they did not demonstrate anticipated feelings of anger or outwardly directed aggression.

Other writers such as Grier and Cobbs (1968) and Baughman (1971) support this notion: that is, that black Americans by-and-large suppress expression of anger, particularly black males. Grier and Cobbs, in fact, suggest that black males grow up with male models characterized as weak, powerless, inferior, and totally dependent on whites who in turn fascinate and attack them, as well as in a mother-son relationship, the primary goal of which is the blunting of masculine assertiveness and aggressivity. The likelihood of the latter, maternal influence, appears high even today given the fact that over 40% of all black American families are headed by females (Madden, Turner & Eckenfels, 1982). Baughman (1971) adds that blacks have for-the-most-part tended to avoid dealing with anger, especially that provoked by whites, by resorting to behaviors such as (1) displacement of aggression into other blacks; (2) attempts to "remain unaffected by" such feelings (denial); (3) wit and humor; and (4) identification with the oppressor (whites). In no case, however, do such attempts lead to a full, complete acknowledgement and/or open expression of the angry emotion. This unresolved anger may also account for much of the observed hostility (attitude) characterizing blacks as compared to whites (Mussen, 1953).

SUPPRESSED ANGER AND HYPERTENSION IN BLACK AMERICANS

In two as yet unpublished studies, we are beginning to understand the dynamics of suppressed anger-hypertension risk in black Americans. In the first study (Kennedy, Chesney, Gentry, Gary, & Harburg, Note 1), using data from the Detroit sample, we examined the combined effects of anger-coping styles and self-reported hostility toward whites on diastolic blood pressure in 489 adult black men and women. As in our previous studies, subjects represented both high and low socioecological stress areas, the latter defined in terms of both social instability (e.g., crime and divorce rates) and socioeconomic status (e.g., median income and education). Blood pressure was measured directly by trained nurse-observers of the same race in the respondents' homes prior to their completing a lengthy public health questionnaire. The latter contained multiple questions about anger expression tendencies (Table 3) and hostile attitudes toward whites. The type of questions used to define respondent's level of inter-racial hostility (high versus low) included the following: "Sometimes I hate white people," "When I'm in a place where all of the people are white, I often feel I'm in enemy territory," and, "I am most at ease when I am with blacks and there are no whites present."

As Figure 1 shows, results of this study revealed that anger-coping style mediates the relationship between self-reported hostility and diastolic pressure. That is, blacks who are high in hostility *and* tend to keep anger suppressed have without question the highest mean diastolic pressures. All other combinations of these two variables resulted in significantly lower pressures. Presumably, the hostility carried around by blacks high in this behavioral (attitudinal) trait triggers anger (emotion), which when suppressed leads to elevated blood pressure, the latter at a level (in this particular instance) comparable to that seen in hypertensives. This observation held true for both black men and women.

In our second study (Chesney, Gentry, Gary, Kennedy, & Harburg, Note 2), we also noted that anger-coping style could mediate the otherwise pathologic relationship between *life strain* and elevated diastolic blood pressure in both blacks and whites. These data are presented in Figures 2 and 3. *Job strain* here refers to self-reported failure to have a (1) chance to earn more money, (2) chance to work with friendly people, (3) chance to learn new skills or use one's present skills, (4) chance for job security, and (5) chance to advance at work. *Family strain* similarly refers to self-acknowledged failure to (1) spend time with spouse, (2) make decisions with spouse, (3) have good sex with spouse, (4) receive appreciation from spouse, and (5) spend time with children and be a good parent. Blacks and whites who are high in either type of life strain *and* who also suppress anger in day-to-day life situations (including those involving spouse and children, as well as boss) run the risk of significantly elevated diastolic pressure, compared to those persons who do not experience strain and/or express their anger (in some form) as they experience it.

The importance of such relationships for better understanding the differential risk for hypertension between the two race groups rests in the fact that we already have data which indicates that blacks, at least black males, are more

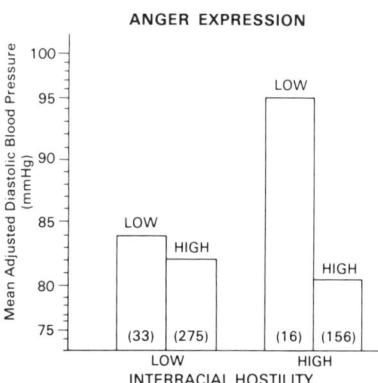

Figure 1 Combined effects of interracial hostility and anger-coping style on diastolic blood pressure. (Numbers in parentheses refer to group size.)

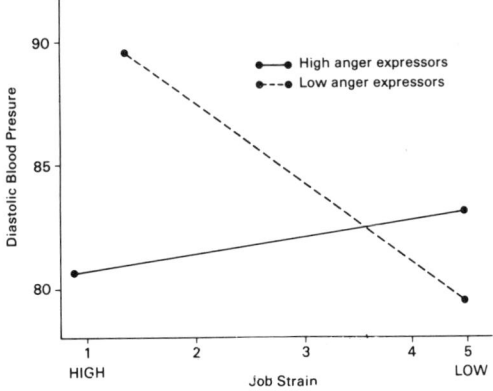

Figure 2 Mediating effect of anger-coping style on the relationship between job strain and blood pressure.

likely to suppress anger (Gentry et al., 1983) and our general observation/belief that black Americans on the whole are more likely to experience life strain in the form of unrealized expectations, failure, and frustration at work and home.

It would seem that it is the combination of hostility and anger suppression, rather than either variable alone, that offers the greatest "risk" for hypertension: what Harburg et al. (1979) have labeled "chronic resentment."

FUTURE RESEARCH ISSUES

Clearly, our understanding of the potential role of psychosocial or behavioral factors influencing black-white blood pressure differences is at best limited. We have tried here to argue that anger-coping styles, particularly in combination with hostility, play a key role in predisposing black Americans to this dread disease. But what about other biomedical and/or behavioral factors (e.g., family history of hypertension) that may also play either an additive or interactive role in

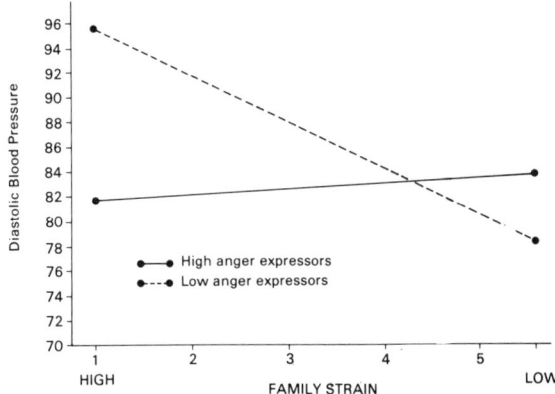

Figure 3 Mediating effect of anger-coping style on the relationship between family strain and blood pressure.

defining risk? Pairing up anger-in tendencies and self-reported levels of hostility with other known etiologic contributors seems like a reasonable first step. Also, it would seem important to begin researching the developmental history of anger suppression in different race groups. Is it, as Baughman (1971) suggests, primarily a function of fear of counter-aggression in blacks versus guilt in whites that serves as a barrier to free, adaptive expression of anger?

Some of our earlier research (Gentry et al., 1973), as well as still unpublished data, would support such a thesis, elevated blood pressure appears related to guilt over anger expression in whites, but not blacks, and whites are about twice as likely to admit to feeling guilty after expressing anger than are blacks. Alexander (1939) earlier speculated that anger suppression in blacks may represent overlearned self-control of such impulses (emotion) which was adaptive early on in adjusting to a new (slave) culture, yet persists to some degree today with maladaptive consequences.

Elsewhere (Gentry, Chesney, Gary, Hall, Harburg & Kennedy, 1983), we have reported preliminary data which suggests that anger-coping styles are learned and may, in fact, be reflected in the behavior of blacks and whites during childhood years, for example, in terms of their reaction to parental punishment. We found a greater percentage of persons who admitted in retrospect that they "resisted" parental punishment, rather than "gave in," among anger-out (79%) compared to anger-in (21%) respondents. Also, we found that certain psychological traits or attributes of one's dominant parent (i.e., one who generally got their way in parental disputes), involving both affective and disciplinary styles, were to some extent related to the development of adult anger-coping styles. That is, anger-in respondents, black or white, were more likely to remember their parents as loving, warm, close, easy-going, and relaxed individuals, in contrast to anger-out respondents who recalled their parents as being cold, distant, strict, tense, and excitable.

Finally, it would seem that we now have sufficient data outlining the relative risk of hypertension associated with anger-in tendencies to embark on some intervention research. We have some clues already as to where and to whom such intervention efforts should be targeted: that is, blacks, black males, persons poorly educated, and those residing in high socioecological stress areas. We have some data to suggest that these maladaptive styles are most likely learned early on in life and thus will have to be *un*learned, requiring some type of psychotherapeutic intervention strategy (e.g., assertive training). And, referring to Table 2, we can even begin to estimate the ultimate therapeutic pay-off in terms of reducing this one component of risk that is, estimating risk for hypertension if three risk factors are present instead of four, two instead of three, one instead of two, and so forth. As far as we are aware, no efforts have been made thus far to package, much less to try out, intervention programs specifically addressing the issue of anger-coping style(s) and/or hostility. The work of Bach and Goldberg (1972) and Burns (1980) among others would serve as a starting point in this regard.

REFERENCES

Alexander, F. Emotional factors in essential hypertension. *Psychosomatic Medicine*, 1939, *1*, 173-179.

Bach, G. R., & Goldberg, H. *Creative aggression.* New York: Doubleday, 1974.
Baer, P. E., Collins, F. H., Bourianoff, G. G., & Ketchel, M. F. Assessing personality factors in essential hypertension with a brief self-report instrument. *Psychosomatic Medicine,* 1979, *41,* 321-330.
Baughman, E. E. *Black Americans.* New York: Academic, 1971.
Burns, D. D. *Feeling good.* New York: Morrow, 1980.
Crain, R. L., & Weisman, C. S. *Discrimination, personality, and achievement: A survey of northern blacks.* New York: Seminar, 1972.
Forbes, G. B., & Mitchell, S. Attribution of blame, feelings of anger, and direction of aggression in response to interracial frustration among poverty-level female negro adults. *Journal of Social Psychology,* 1971, *83,* 73-78.
Fries, E. D. Age, race, sex, and other indices of risk in hypertension. *American Journal of Medicine,* 1973, *55,* 275-280.
Gentry, W. D. Biracial aggression: I. Effect of verbal attack and sex of victim. *Journal of Social Psychology,* 1972, *88,* 75-82.
Gentry, W. D., Chesney, A. P., Gary, H. E., Hall, R. P., & Harburg, E. Habitual anger-coping styles: I. Effect on mean blood pressure and risk for essential hypertension. *Psychosomatic Medicine,* 1982, *44,* 195-202.
Gentry, W. D., Chesney, A. P., Kennedy, C. D., Hall, R. P., Gary, H. E., & Harburg, E. The relation of demographic attributes and habitual anger-coping styles. *Journal of Social Psychology,* 1983, *121,* 45-50.
Gentry, W. D., Harburg, E., & Hauenstein, L. Effects of anger expression/inhibition and guilt on elevated diastolic blood pressure in high/low stress and black/white females. *Proceedings of American Psychological Association,* 1973, 115-116.
Grier, W. H., & Cobbs, P. M. *Black rage.* New York: Basic, 1968.
Harburg, E., Blakelock, E. H., & Roeper, P. J. Resentful and reflective coping with arbitrary authority and blood pressure: Detroit. *Psychosomatic Medicine,* 1979, *41,* 189-202.
Harburg, E., Erfurt, J. C., Hauenstein, L. S., Chape, C., Schull, W. J., & Schork, M. A. Socio-ecological stress, suppressed hostility, skin color, and black-white male blood pressure: Detroit. *Psychosomatic Medicine,* 1973, *35,* 276-296.
James, S. A., & Kleinbaum, D. G. Socioecologic stress and hypertension related mortality rates in North Carolina. *American Journal of Public Health,* 1976, *66,* 354-358.
Kahn, H. A., Medalie, J. H., Neufeld, H. N., Riss, E., & Goldbourt, U. The incidence of hypertension and associated factors: The Israel ischemic heart disease study. *American Heart Journal,* 1972, *84,* 171-182.
Kannel, W. B. Role of blood pressure in cardiovascular morbidity and mortality. *Progress in Cardiovascular Disease,* 1974, *17,* 5-24.
Madden, T. A., Turner, I. R., & Eckenfels, E. J. *The health almanac.* New York: Raven, 1982.
Moss, A., & Scott, G. Hypertension: United States, 1974. *Advance Data,* USDHEW, HRA, November, 1976.
Mussen, P. H. Differences between the TAT responses of Negro and white boys. *Journal of Consulting Psychology,* 1953, *17,* 373-376.
NHBPEP. *Guidelines for the education and management of the hypertensive patient.* DHEW Publication (NIH), 1976, 76-744.
Roberts, J., & Maurer, K. Blood pressure of persons 6-74 years of age in the United States. *Advance Data,* USDHEW, HRA, October 18, 1976.
Schull, W. J., Harburg, E., Schork, M. A., Weener, J., & Cape, C. Heredity, stress and blood pressure, a family set method—II. Family aggregation of hypertension. *Journal of Chronic Diseases,* 1977, *30,* 659-669.
Thompson, G. E. Hypertension: Implications of comparisons among blacks and whites. *Urban Health,* May 1980, 31-33.
Weiner, H. *Psychobiology and human disease.* New York: Elsevier, 1977.
Yarrow, M. R. Interpersonal dynamics in a desegregation process. *Journal of Social Issues,* 1958, *14,* Whole No. 1.

REFERENCE NOTES

1. Kennedy, C. D., Chesney, A. P., Gentry, W. D., Gary, H. E., & Harburg, E. *Anger-coping style as a mediator in the relationship between hostility and blood pressure.* Unpublished manuscript, 1984.
2. Chesney, A. P., Gentry, W. D., Gary, H. E., Kennedy, C., & Harburg, E. *Anger-coping style as a mediator in the relationship between life strain and blood pressure.* Unpublished manuscript, 1984.

8
Behavioral Factors in Hypertension: Cardiovascular Responsivity, Anger, and Social Competence

Stephen B. Manuck
Department of Psychology
University of Pittsburgh

Randall L. Morrison, Alan S. Bellack
Eastern Pennsylvania Psychiatric Institute
The Medical College of Pennsylvania

Joanna M. Polefrone
Department of Psychology
University of Pittsburgh

It is generally agreed that essential hypertension is a "multifactorial" disorder quite diverse and involving a complex pathogenesis (Weiner, 1977). Thus, although many etiologic factors have been proposed (e.g., salt intake, stress), it is likely that each pertains to some, but not all, hypertensive cases. As noted later in this discussion, mechanisms that are significant at an initial phase of hypertension may differ greatly from those responsible for maintaining elevated pressures in more advanced stages of the disorder.

Considering the contributions of the autonomic nervous system in regulating blood pressure and the well-documented associations between behavioral and cardiovascular adjustments (Obrist, Black, Brener, & DiCara, 1974), it is not surprising that an extensive literature has developed regarding the possible impact of psychosocial factors on the development of essential hypertension. Much of this work may be divided into two largely independent lines of investigation. The first of these has sought to isolate specific personality traits or intrapsychic conflicts typifying hypertensive patients. The second major focus of research has examined individual differences in cardiovascular reactivity, as exhibited in

Research described here was supported, in part, by NIH HL29028, NIH BRSG Grant S07 RR07084-14 and by MHCRC Grant MH30915.

response to behavioral stressors. Several investigators have proposed, in particular, that repeated episodes of acute cardiovascular arousal caused by stress may, over time and in persons who are most reactive to such influences, lead to a more sustained or established hypertensive state. Despite the large number of studies included in this literature, findings to date have revealed little convincing evidence that behavioral variables contribute substantially to the *development* of hypertension. In addition, certain hypotheses, such as that implicating a heightened cardiovascular responsivity in the origin of the disorder, remain controversial. However, these areas represent an enduring target of investigation, and each has generated numerous findings of a "suggestive" nature. It is likely that the rather weak and inconsistent findings characterizing many earlier studies are attributable more to poorly contrived experimental procedures and/or inadequate conceptualization of psychogenic factors than to the absence of significant relationships.

One purpose of this chapter is to summarize briefly, and in a somewhat selective and critical fashion, the research that seeks to establish associations between essential hypertension and two dimensions of individual differences: behavioral attributes (especially as related to anger) and psychophysiologic response characteristics. An additional purpose is to suggest possible avenues for further investigation. We have attempted to integrate the behavioral and psychophysiologic approaches discussed above into a more general model of idiosyncratic cardiovascular response to stress. We further intend to re-examine psychodynamic notions of suppressed hostility (still the most intriguing of psychosomatic hypotheses) within a more objective and operationalized context: namely, as specific and measurable deficits in interpersonal, assertive skill.

PERSONALITY FACTORS IN HYPERTENSION

Unlike coronary heart disease, for which a well established profile of behavioral risk has already been identified (viz., Type A, or coronary-prone behavior pattern) (Matthews, 1982), the search for personality characteristics important in hypertension has continued to frustrate researchers. Some investigators have reported increased anxiety or neuroticism among hypertensive patients, while others examining these same variables have failed to observe significant relationships (Steptoe, 1981). Interestingly, in accord with Alexander's (1939) initial hypothesis, self-reported problems with anger, unexpressed hostility, and "inhibited power motivation" have consistently been found to be associated with either elevated blood pressure or hypertensive status in young adult, middle-aged, and patient populations (Esler, Julius, Zweifler, Randall, Harburg, Gardiner, & DeQuattro, 1977; Hamilton, 1942; Harburg, Blakelock, & Roeper, 1979; Harburg, Erfurt, Hauenstein, Chape, Schull, & Schork, 1973; Harburg, Julius, McGinn, McLeod, & Hoobler, 1964; Kahn, Medalie, Neufeld, Riss & Goldbourt, 1972; Light & Obrist, 1983; McClelland, 1979; Miller & Grim, 1979).

Early studies involving more direct behavioral observations have also reported hypertensive patients to lack appropriate assertiveness, compared to normotensive controls (Harris, Sokolow, Carpenter, Freedman, & Hunt, 1953; Gressel, Shobe, Saslow, DuBois, & Schroeder, 1949; Matarazzo, 1954; Wolff & Wolf, 1951). There is evidence, too, that hypertensives may misperceive (or deny) the aversive qualities inherent in threatening and "potentially hostile" interpersonal encounters (Handkins & Munz, 1978; Sapira, Scheib, Moriarity, & Shapiro, 1971): a defensive style that may promote submissive, deferential and inhibited behavior in hypertensives by permitting them to give a more benign appraisal to situations which otherwise call for assertive responding. It is noteworthy that the relationship between hypertension and inhibited anger or aggression emerges across studies of widely varying design, including two recent prospective investigations (Kahn et al., 1972; McClelland, 1979). Still, some studies fail to support the preceding findings (Cochrane, 1973; Neiberg, 1957; Ostfeld & Lebovitz, 1959). In fact, a few investigators have found that hypertensives report experiencing greater hostility or behave more aggressively than their normotensive counterparts (Baer, Collins, Bourianoff, & Ketchel; Kaplan, Gottschalk, Magliocco, Rohovit, & Ross, 1961; Mann, 1977; Schachter, 1957). Harburg et al. (1979) recently proposed that an elevated blood pressure may be related to " 'inappropriate assertiveness' . . . as well as 'inappropriate submissiveness' " (p. 199).

It is striking, nevertheless, that most of the available literature specifically identifies problems of anger and assertive expression as characteristic of some hypertensive patients (Weiner, 1977). Reported findings are often quite modest, even when statistically significant; moreover, failure to replicate these results prevents any definitive statement concerning the overall significance of these personality variables. Such limitations may denote the lack of a uniform or robust association, or, as suggested already, may reflect poor methodology common among investigations that contribute to this literature.

Of course, some difficulties are inherent in the study of any chronic or serious medical condition. For example, there are the problems of retrospective observation, which include effects attributable to the condition itself, unknown consequences of the patient's knowledge of his or her diagnostic status and, particularly in the case of hypertension, side effects that may be associated with commonly prescribed medications (e.g., the anxiety reducing actions of beta-adrenergic blocking agents). Many of the preceding studies may also be faulted for non-representative patient sampling and inadequate selection of control subjects, an over-reliance on subjective and global behavioral judgments that are subject to observer bias, and the use of psychometric devices that possess limited or unknown reliability and have, at best, questionable external validity. Most of these criticisms have been discussed at length in other recent reviews (Diamond, 1982; Harrell, 1979) and, therefore, will not be pursued further here. Instead, we wish to briefly draw attention to two aspects of the study of hypertension which, so far, have been neglected by psychosomatic investigations: the natural history of essential hypertension, and the apparent role of the autonomic nervous system (and possibly also, behavioral factors) early in the course of the disorder.

It is often observed that in established hypertension—typically defined as a sustained blood pressure elevation above 160/100 mm Hg—cardiac performance changes, baroreceptor sensitivity decreases, and the structure of the resistance vessels changes (Weiner, 1977). Because of the number and complexity of these secondary adjustments, it is frequently argued that the search for factors that influence initial blood pressure elevations might best focus on " . . . patients very early in the disease process, before (mal)adaptive changes to the high blood pressure itself occur" (Weiner, 1977; p. 2). As a result, studies of mechanism have increasingly examined borderline essential hypertension, which is characterized by blood pressures in the range of 150/90 to 160/100 mm Hg.

Borderline hypertension is prevalent among younger individuals and is often considered a first step toward the development of established hypertension. Although many borderline hypertensives do not experience a progressive rise in blood pressure, relative to normotensive individuals the borderline patients are much more likely to subsequently exhibit a sustained hypertension, suffer an excess mortality rate, and develop coronary heart disease (cf. Julius, 1977; see also Julius, Chap. 6). From a methodologic standpoint, moreover, examination of borderline hypertensive samples is less susceptible to some of the usual problems inherent in retrospective designs. Of obvious benefit to the investigator is the fact that blood pressure elevations in borderline hypertension are still relatively small, readily controlled, and of little immediate prognostic significance, increasing the likelihood that many borderline patients may be unmedicated or safely withdrawn from medications over any brief period of investigation.

Other characteristics of borderline hypertension are also of interest. About 30 percent of these patients show an increased cardiac output, accompanied by a "normal" or only moderately elevated total peripheral resistance (Julius & Esler, 1975).[1] This hemodynamic "portrait" contrasts with that of established hypertension, where it is commonly found that the cardiac output is within normal limits, while the total peripheral resistance is significantly elevated (Dustan, Frohlich & Tarazi, 1972). There is evidence that an increased cardiac output in borderline hypertension is achieved through actions of the autonomic nervous system, because heart rate and stroke volume do return to normal values following autonomic blockade (Julius & Esler, 1975; see also Julius, Chap. 6). Although findings appear somewhat mixed, circulating catecholamines are likewise elevated in at least a large proportion of borderline cases (Kuchel, 1977; Steptoe, 1981). Despite the considerable support for an increased sympathetic drive in borderline hypertension, however, it must be emphasized that the autonomic nervous system cannot be implicated as responsible in all individuals carrying this diagnosis (Kuchel, 1977); hence, the borderline category of hypertension is, itself, heterogeneous.

The foregoing observations have particular significance for psychosomatic investigations because behavioral factors would presumably influence the development of hypertension mainly through autonomic mechanisms. Therefore, in addition to characterizing patients by diagnostic category (e.g., established or borderline hypertension), it may also prove fruitful to attempt identification of hypertensive individuals for whom autonomic events are of importance: the subgroup of hypertensives in whom psychologic factors would be most strongly suspected.

Noting that the sympathetic nervous system may modulate renin secretion by the kidney, it has been proposed that high plasma-renin activity (PRA) may serve as one indicator of borderline hypertensive states that involve more general sympathetic arousal (Esler et al., 1977; Esler, Julius, Randall, Ellis, & Kashima, 1975; Esler & Nestel, 1973). In a study of mild essential hypertensive patients

---

[1] An increase in the cardiac output would ordinarily be offset by a decreased peripheral resistance in order to maintain a relatively constant blood pressure. Thus, Julius and Esler (1975) argue that a "normal" total peripheral resistance in borderline hypertension actually represents "an inappropriate adjustment of the peripheral resistance to the increased tissue perfusion accompanying the increased cardiac output" (p. 689).

differing in remin status, Esler et al. (1971) report that compared to "normal" PRA hypertensive subjects, high renin hypertensives displayed: (a) higher concentrations of resting plasma norepinephrine; and (b) greater decreases in cardiac output and total peripheral resistance, with reductions of blood pressure to normal values, following pharmacologic blockade of the autonomic nervous system. High PRA hypertensive patients also differed significantly from normal renin hypertensives and from normotensive control subjects on measures of "suppressed hostility," as derived from a variety of psychometric indices. The reliable differences obtained between the high and normal PRA hypertensive groups further suggests that characteristics distinguishing the high renin condition were distinct from any behavioral consequences of the hypertension itself. Thus, the authors conclude that mild essential hypertension, when accompanied by an elevated PRA, is maintained by autonomic mechanisms and may be psychogenic in origin (Esler et al., 1977).

It is likely that if psychosocial variables contribute strongly to the development of essential hypertension, such effects occur primarily among patients in whom autonomic mechanisms are of significance in maintaining the hypertensive state. Distinguishing hypertensive samples by biochemical markers for sympathetic activation (such as PRA), by cardiovascular reactions to autonomic blockade, or in relation to psychophysiologic response characteristics (as suggested below), however, has not been done in previous research on the role of personality factors in essential hypertension and may be one of the reasons for inconsistent results. A failure to account for, or to exploit, this aspect of hypertension may dilute or obscure any significant behavioral relationships that exist.

HYPERTENSION, FAMILIAL RISK FOR HYPERTENSION, AND BEHAVIORALLY-INDUCED CARDIOVASCULAR REACTIVITY

As noted previously, a second area of investigation relating behavioral factors to hypertension pertains to a tenet of psychophysiology: namely that individuals vary markedly in their cardiovascular responsivity to behavioral stimuli. When subjected to laboratory stressors, such as shock avoidance or mental arithmetic, for instance, some persons show substantial elevations in heart rate and blood pressure—occasionally attaining values 50-80 percent above resting states. Other, less reactive, individuals exhibit little cardiovascular arousal on exposure to the same experimental procedures. These response differences occur across varying stimulus conditions (Bunnell, 1982; Lawler, 1980; Manuck & Garland, 1980; Obrist, 1981) and appear to generalize from laboratory assessments to "casual" measurements obtained during more naturally occurring activities (Eliot, Buell, & Dembroski, 1982; Manuck, Corse, & Winkelman, 1979). Differences in the relative magnitudes of subjects' cardiovascular reactions to standard behavioral challenges also denote a stable, or enduring, characteristic of individuals, highly reproducible over time, both in children (Giordani, Manuck, & Farmer, 1981) and adults (Manuck & Garland, 1980; Obrist, 1981). That such idiosyncratic cardiovascular reactivity may reflect, in part, an underlying distribution of individual differences in sympathetic-adrenomedullary response is suggested by the significant correlation in plasma catecholamine responses to heart rate and blood pressure reactions during mental arithmetic (Engel, Muller, Munch, & Ackenheil, 1980; Leblanc, Cote, Jobin, & Labrie, 1979).

It is often noted that hypertensive individuals exhibit a greater reactivity to common laboratory stressors than do normotensive controls. In an early study of autonomic response patterning, for example, Engel and Bickford (1961) demonstrated that, across a wide range of experimental stimuli, hypertensives differed consistently from normotensive subjects by their tendency to "overrespond" on a single response measure, systolic blood pressure. Compared to normotensive subjects, hypertensives have also been observed to show larger pressor responses in the following situations: during experimentally induced emotions of fear and anger (Schachter, 1957); in interviews targeted at areas of personal conflict (McKegney & Williams, 1967); in anticipation of aversive stimulation (e.g., hypodermic injection; Shapiro, Moutsos, & Krifcher, 1963); when required to perform a variety of demanding cognitive tasks (Baumann, Ziprian, Godicke, Hartrodt, Nauman, & Lauter, 1973; Lorimer, MacFarlane, Provan, Duffy, & Lawrie, 1971; Nestel, 1969; Shapiro et al., 1963); and occasionally, on exposure to the cold pressor test (Shapiro et al., 1963).

The epidemiologic evidence that the offspring of hypertensives are more likely to develop essential hypertension later in life than persons without positive family histories (Paffenbarger, Thorne, & Wing, 1968; Paul, 1977) has encouraged a number of investigators to contrast the psychophysiologic reactions of currently normotensive individuals who have hypertensive parents with those who have normotensive parents. In general, the findings of these studies demonstrate a significant and consistent relationship between familial risk for hypertension and a heightened cardiovascular responsivity to experimental challenges. Falkner and her colleagues (1979) report, for example, that heart rate and diastolic blood pressure elevations observed during mental arithmetic were greater in normotensive adolescents with hypertensive parents than in age-matched, normotensive control subjects having no parental histories of hypertension. Jorgensen and Houston (1981) report similar results, with differences in the responsivity of children of hypertensive and normotensive parents emerging uniformly across a number of different laboratory stressors. Likewise, Shapiro (1961) notes that, under a variety of stimulus conditions involving both physical and "mental" stressors (e.g., cold pressor test, Stroop word-color interference task), adult, normotensive offspring of hypertensive parents exhibited greater systolic pressor responses when contrasted with subjects having only normotensive parents.

In a series of experiments conducted in our own laboratory, we have also observed that sons of hypertensive parents show greater heart rate and/or pressor responses to various cognitive challenges, as well as to isometric exercise, than do sons of normotensive parents (Manuck, Giordani, McQuaid, & Garrity, 1981; Manuck & Proietti, 1982). And finally, Hastrup, Light, and Obrist (1982) report that young adult males of hypertensive parentage showed larger heart rate and systolic blood pressure elevations than did subjects without histories of parental hypertension when performing a reaction time-contingent shock avoidance task. Unlike Shapiro (1961), Hastrup et al. (1982) found only a marginal relationship between cold pressor reactivity and parental status, and similarly mixed results characterized the early investigations that administered the cold stimulus alone

(Briggs & Overtine, 1937; Dieckman & Michel, 1935; Feldt & Wendstrandt, 1942; Hines & Brown, 1936; Remington, Lambreth, Moser, & Hoobler, 1961).

These findings obviously contribute to our knowledge of the psychophysiologic response characteristics of hypertensives, and of persons with a familial predisposition to hypertension. Yet, are transient episodes of acute cardiovascular arousal, such as those observed in the laboratory, relevant to an understanding of the hypertensive condition? This question is currently the focus of considerable debate, though at least several possible answers may be suggested. First, among hypertensive individuals, behaviorally-elicited pressor responses of 30 or 40 mm Hg (which are not uncommon) may be of significance clinically, because these reactions are superimposed upon an already elevated arterial pressure. If experienced frequently, consequences might include a hastening of vascular and end-organ damage, and, in persons with existing coronary disease, an increased risk of acute clinical events (e.g., angina pectoris, myocardial infarction) (Sime, Buel, & Eliot, Note 1; Sokolow & McIlroy, 1977). In addition, there is some evidence that a heightened cardiovascular reactivity to behavioral stimuli contributes to the development of atherosclerotic lesions (Keys, Taylor, Blackburn, Brozek, Anderson, & Simonson, 1971; Manuck, Kaplan, & Clarkson, 1983).

More controversial is the frequent proposal that a chronic elevation in blood pressure may, itself, arise from the repeated elicitation of large cardiovascular responses to environmental events. A serious challenge to psychosomatic speculations is the need to reconcile an increased cardiac output, such as that often occurring under "stress" and in cases of borderline hypertension, with a causal process climaxing in sustained elevations of the peripheral resistance (i.e., in established hypertension). In perhaps the most recent statement of this hypothesis, Obrist (1981) suggests that large increases in the cardiac output exhibited by highly reactive individuals in certain behavioral contexts may, over protracted intervals, raise resistance in the vasculature through ensuing structural changes in the arterioles (e.g., smooth muscle hypertrophy) or through intrinsic autoregulatory processes serving to stem an over-perfusion of body tissues. Obrist argues that the latter mechanism may be especially relevant because, in many behavioral situations, a highly elevated cardiac output may supply O_2 levels in excess of concurrent metabolic demands (Gliner, Bedi, & Horvath, 1979; Langer, Obrist, & McCubbin, 1979).[2]

No matter how the secondary cardiovascular effects of established hypertension are achieved, Obrist's proposal presumes that there is (a) a shift in hemodynamic status between early and later phases of hypertension (i.e., from

---

[2] The status of autoregulation as a "transitional" mechanism between the borderline and established phases of hypertension is a subject of much debate. In borderline hypertensives, O_2 consumption is often elevated, as well as the cardiac output, suggesting that output is not in disproportion to metabolic demand (e.g., Julius & Conway, 1968). Obrist, Langer, Light & Koepke (1983) note in reply that (a) such findings are generally derived from studies of resting state hemodynamics (i.e., where behaviorally relevant, sympathetic effects on the heart are minimal); and (b) even among individuals who show an increased cardiac output and higher O_2 consumption, the arterio-venus O_2 content difference—an index of relative O_2 extraction—may still be appreciably reduced (e.g., Gorlin, Brachfeld, Turner, Messer, Salazar, 1959; Stead, Warren, Merrill & Brannon, 1945).

an elevated cardiac output to increased total peripheral resistance), and (b) a behaviorally-induced cardiovascular hyperreactivity that precedes the elevated pressure and serves as a predictor of eventual hypertension. Longitudinal evidence indicates that in many hypertensives a significant decline in the cardiac output over time occurs along with a progressive increase in the peripheral resistance (Eich, Cuddy, Smulyan, & Lyons, 1966; Lund-Johanson, 1967, 1977, 1979; Safar, Kamienecka, Levenson, Dimitriu, & Pauleau, 1978). Whether a cardiovascular hyperresponsivity to behavioral events represents a "triggering" mechanism in this process as suggested by Obrist (1981), however, remains speculative and will ultimately require longitudinal observations following prehypertensive individuals through the borderline and established phases of hypertension. It is possible that the greater reactivity of hypertensive patients, as well as their elevated blood pressures, are manifestations of a common CNS disruption of autonomic control over the heart and vasculature. In that case, a hyperresponsivity to psychosocial stimuli among younger, normotensive individuals may still be predictive of later hypertension, but plays no direct or causative role in the development of the hypertensive condition.

Before leaving this topic, a final set of observations suggests that psychophysiologic and familial factors may relate to blood pressure in an interactive fashion. On several occasions, we have observed in our own investigations that sons of hypertensive parents often show slightly elevated systolic blood pressure baselines, in addition to their generally increased cardiovascular responsivity. However, these systolic elevations occur only in persons who have a positive family history *and* exhibit the greatest heart rate elevations to experimental stressors (Manuck et al., 1981; Manuck & Proietti, 1982). Although this relationship has not emerged in all of our studies (Manuck, Note 2), where it has, an increased systolic pressure has been recorded among these subjects both before and after performance of laboratory tasks, following periods of instructed relaxation, and in casual measurements obtained at "on campus" blood pressure screenings.

Of similar interest, Light and colleagues (Note 3) report that a comparably defined subject group—high heart rate reactive offspring of hypertensive parents—exhibited significant reductions in fluid and sodium excretion when exposed to choice-reaction time and mental arithmetic tasks. Although not showing the elevated pre-task, baseline blood pressures seen in our study (Manuck et al., 1981), recordings made by Light et al. more than half an hour after subjects' completion of the "stress" period did show that resting pressures of these individuals were higher than in persons with a less pronounced heart rate reactivity and/or normotensive parentage. This finding was accompanied, by a continued decrease in sodium and water excretion, relative to other subject groups. Hence, persons having a high cardiac responsivity to stress and a familial predisposition to hypertension may show frequent elevations in blood pressure, even during otherwise calm periods; additionally, these effects may be associated with an unusual retention of sodium and fluid, possibly caused by sympathetic influences on the renal barostatic control of blood pressure. Finally, consistent with these considerations, Falkner, Onesti, and Hamstra (1981) report that, among a large sample of adolescent, borderline hypertensives, individuals who subsequently progressed to a sustained, established hypertension also tended to exhibit heightened cardiovascular responses to "mental stress," together with a positive family history of hypertension.

A MODEL OF IDIOSYNCRATIC CARDIOVASCULAR REACTIVITY

To this point, psychophysiologic and personality characteristics of possible relevance to hypertension have been considered independently. As implied earlier, we discussed these two research areas separately because each has represented a traditionally distinct avenue of investigation. From a conceptual standpoint, however, joining these two literatures is desirable to document the physiologic correlates of any behavioral characteristics implicated in hypertension and to elucidate origins of the cardiovascular hyperresponsivity commonly observed in hypertensive patients and among persons at familial risk for hypertension. Accordingly, our purpose in the present section is to describe a heuristic model for examining determinants of individual differences in behaviorally-induced cardiovascular reactivity, and to suggest how this model may account for data reported in our own investigations and in those of others.

First, any heightened autonomic responsivity that precedes the development of hypertension may conceivably have originated in either hereditary or psychosocial factors, or may reflect an interaction of both of these factors. We have recently collected data on cardiovascular and affective reactions of individuals who are exposed to a distinctly frustrating cognitive task (Manuck, Note 2). The participants in this study were young adult male volunteers, with and without a parental history of hypertension. For each subject, repeated heart rate and blood pressure measurements were obtained under resting (baseline) conditions and during the performance of difficult mental arithmetic problems in the presence of the experimenter (i.e., in an ego-threatening situation). In addition, subjects' immediate feelings of anxiety and anger, as experienced before and during the experimental stressor, were measured by administration of "state" forms of the Spielberger State-Trait Anxiety Inventory (STAI) (Spielberger, Gorsuch, & Lushene, 1970) and State-Trait Anger Inventory (STAgI) (Spielberger, Jacobs, Crane, & Russell, 1982).

In accord with previous investigations, our results demonstrated that sons of hypertensive parents showed greater heart rate and diastolic blood pressure elevations during mental arithmetic, compared to offspring of normotensives. When subjects were subsequently divided into distinct groups of "high" and "low" affect (i.e., anxiety, anger) responders, however, we observed that the heart rate reactions of persons having hypertensive and normotensive parents differed significantly only among those subjects who had reported experiencing the greatest anxiety—and to a slightly lesser extent, anger—when performing the mental arithmetic task. In persons who reported little increase in negative affect over the period of the experimental stressor, the relative heart rate responsivity was thus unrelated to parental hypertension. Although this interaction of parental status and level of affect was not as apparent on measures of blood pressure responsivity, our heart rate findings are suggestive of a two-factor model of behaviorally-elicited cardiovascular reactivity involving both familial and psychosocial variables. Stated more specifically, persons having a positive parental history appear to possess a heightened cardiovascular response "potential," but they express this underlying hyperactivity in a behavioral context, in part, in proportion to accompanying affective (or other psychologic) responses of the individual.

Extrapolating somewhat from these results and reviewing findings of other investigators, we have begun to conceptualize the determinants of idiosyncratic cardiovascular response as illustrated in Figure 1. The vertical axis at the rear of this model denotes the magnitude of an *observed response*. In a psychophysiologic experiment, this is actually recorded on the polygraph, such as a change in heart rate in beats-per-minute. To account for the magnitude of the observed response, we suggest that two variables may be of particular importance. The first variable is a dimension of individual differences reflecting an underlying, or intrinsic, *response potential*. It is proposed that parental hypertensive and normotensive status represent "markers" for differences in such a response potential; that is, persons with a parental history of hypertension possess a greater response potential than do offspring of normotensives. Although the exact nature of this potential remains unclear, it conceivably has a significant genetic basis. Indeed, there is now increasing evidence for the heritability of idiosyncratic heart rate and pressor responses, as recorded under varying stimulus conditions (Rose, Miller, & Grim, Note 4; Shapiro, Nicotoro, Sapira, & Scheib, 1968; Theorell, DeFaire, Schalling, Adamson, & Askevoid, 1979); and in an animal model, rats bearing a genetic susceptibility to hypertension (spontaneously hypertensive rats) similarly show increased sympathetic reactivity to experimental stressors (Hallback & Folkow, 1974; McCarty, Chiueh, & Kopin, 1978).

Yet the manifestation of an individual's response potential as an actual or observed response of some specific magnitude is dependent, in any particular situation, on certain behavioral characteristics of the individual. Several years ago, Singer (1974) proposed that individual differences in autonomic and neuroendocrine response might be understood behaviorally in terms of coping styles, or habitual levels of transactional "engagement." Persons who encounter

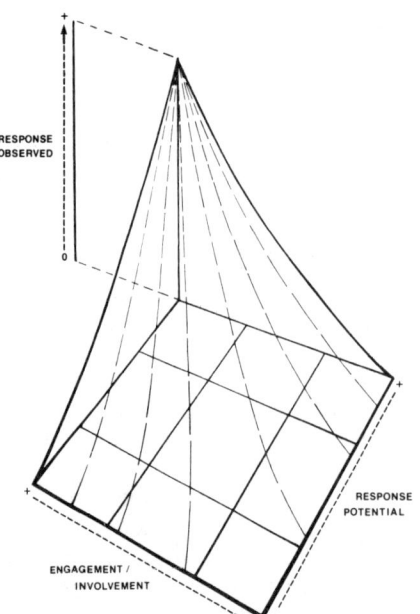

Figure 1 A model of determinants of individual differences in behaviorally-elicited cardiovascular reactivity.

situations with more immediate and active patterns of involvement, Singer concluded, would also prove more reactive physiologically than individuals who are typically less engaged, or who are more passive in regard to their environments. Following Singer, the third axis of our model is labelled a continuum of relative *engagement/involvement* experienced by the individual when subjected to the various experimental stressors employed in our laboratory studies (and through generalization, when facing challenges of the natural environment).

A number of factors may determine the degree of engagement/involvement that an individual will experience in relation to a given stimulus or set of stimuli. These are not depicted in Figure 1, but familiar factors tend to fall into two broad classes: situational and dispositional variables. Obrist (1976, 1981) has argued that situational demands for active coping, especially where the individual is allowed "an opportunity to cope, but not quite successfully" elicit major sympathetic effects on the heart, resulting in an increased cardiac output, with accompanying changes in heart rate, heart contractility, and systolic blood pressure. He has contrasted this with similarly "stressful" conditions for which the subject has no effective or active coping response, and in which sympathetic effects (specifically, beta-adrenergic influences) are much diminished. Task demands for active coping, by their very nature, encourage significant engagement/involvement on the part of the subject. Other situational factors having similar effects might include task-related incentives, as suggested by Elliott (1969), attentional requirements for "sensory rejection" (Williams, 1975), and, perhaps, stimulus novelty (Light & Obrist, 1980).

Turning to behavioral determinants of engagement/involvement, we have previously suggested that the domain of effort-dependent coping activity cited by Obrist (1976) would logically subsume many of the components of the Type A, or coronary-prone behavior pattern (e.g., accelerated work pace, heightened vigilance, increased task involvement) (Manuck & Garland, 1979). Indeed, the coronary-prone behavior pattern might be conceived as behavioral analogue of situational demands for active coping: Type A denoting an individual who characteristically approaches tasks in a more active, effortful and engaged manner than does his or her more placid, Type B counterpart.

We may represent "high" and "low" ends of the engagement/involvement axis, then by thinking in terms of active and passive coping, high and low task incentives, novelty versus familiarity of the stimulus, Type A and Type B behavior pattern, or other contrasting dimensions. We may also infer the degree of engagement/involvement experienced by the individual through retrospective inquiry, as in the state affect measures employed in the study just described (Manuck, Note 2). These affect measures are illustrated in Figure 2, in which we have plotted the heart rate changes observed among our high and low angered subjects, with and without a parental history of hypertension. Note that the "response observed" axis has been replaced by a scale of task-related heart rate change (in beats-per-minute). Parental hypertensive and normotensive status appear as indices of varying response potential, and the high and low anger groups are shown as descriptors of relative engagement/involvement. The height of the embedded columns, projected against the rear axis, represents the *amount* of heart rate change observed during the mental arithmetic task in each of the respective groups. As already noted, these data demonstrate a catalytic interaction of parental history and anger: although offspring of hypertensive parents

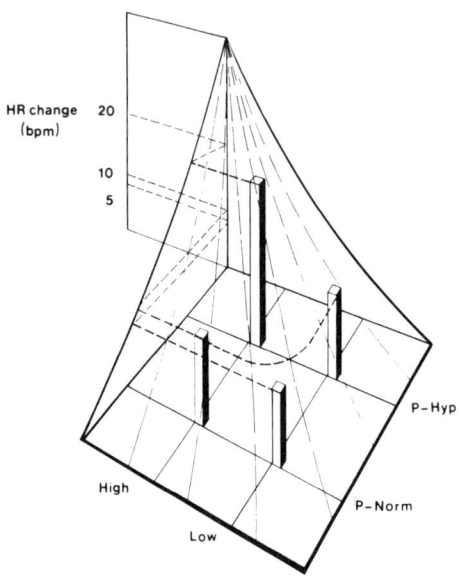

Figure 2 Mean heart rate changes during mental arithmetic of high and low angered subjects, with and without parental histories of hypertension (P-Hyp, P-Norm).

exhibited greater heart rate elevations than subjects of normotensive parentage, this difference was pronounced only among subjects who reported becoming most angered on exposure to the experimental stressor. Similarly, high anger was associated with increased heart rate elevations, yet this relationship was strongest among persons familially predisposed to hypertension.

Focusing now on the coronary-prone behavior pattern, it is frequently reported that elevated heart rate and pressor responses during laboratory stressors are associated with the Type A pattern, as well as with specific components of Pattern A, such as vigorous voice stylistics and anger. While some investigators have failed to find significant associations (Price & Clarke, 1978; Steptoe & Ross, 1981; Jennings & Choi, 1981), most available evidence indicates a greater cardiovascular responsivity among Type A individuals, when compared to Bs, particularly in experiments involving threat of failure (Manuck, Craft, & Gold, 1978; Corse, Manuck, Cantwell et al., 1982; Pittner & Houston, 1980); harassment and/or competition (Glass, Krakoff, Contrada, Giordani, & Matthews, 1980; Van Egeren, 1979); or instructional sets intended to enhance subjects' overall task involvement (Dembroski, MacDougall, Herd, & Shields, 1979; Goldband, 1980).

In the present context, we would predict that any increased physiologic responsivity among Type As would be most apparent in subjects possessing a high response potential, such as offspring or hypertensive parents. Fortunately, several groups of investigators have recently examined psychophysiologic correlates of the coronary prone behavior pattern in relation to family histories of cardiovascular disease (Allen, Note 5; Katkin, Goldband, & Medine, Note 6; Newlin & Levenson, 1982; Williams, Lane, Kuhn, Melosh, White, & Schanberg, 1982). Although Newlin and Levenson (1982) noted only additive effects of these two variables, Katkin et al. (Note 6), Williams et al. (1982) and Allen (Note 5) all report finding that a cardiovascular hyperresponsivity to psychomotor or cognitive challenges occurred, in their experiments, primarily among persons having both a positive family history *and* Type A characteristics. Likewise, in the absence of a positive family history, Pattern A had little influence on measures of task-related reactivity.

An additional observation consistent with the present model is the report of Hastrup et al. (1982) that heart rate and systolic pressor responses to a reaction time-contingent shock avoidance task strongly differentiated offspring of hypertensive and normotensive parents, whereas responses to a cold pressor test did so only slightly. Interestingly, Obrist's (1976) distinction between active and passive coping was initially based on a comparison of cardiovascular adjustments recorded under conditions of avoidance (active coping) and cold immersion (passive exposure to a noxious stimulus). Moreover, to the extent that coping, the behavioral demand implicit in an avoidance task, is indicative of high engagement/involvement, we would expect to find response differences emerging between persons with and without parental histories of hypertension under avoidance procedures; we would also expect these differences to exceed any observed during the cold pressor task, which is characterized by passive coping (in Obrist's terminology) and by low engagement/involvement (in ours). This relationship might further help to explain the largely negative results of studies that have attempted to predict subsequent hypertension based on individual differences in cold pressor reactivity (e.g., Harland, Osborne, & Graybiel, 1964), as well as the somewhat inconsistent findings of investigations contrasting cold pressor responses in hypertensive and normotensive subjects (Boyer, Fraser, & Doyle, 1960; Remington et al., 1960; Shapiro et al., 1963).

To summarize, we suggest that responses observed in our laboratory experiments are the outcome of an interaction between two sets of variables. The first of these is an intrinsic response potential, which varies among individuals and may be registered, in part, by the presence or absence of a family history of cardiovascular disease. Among persons *at* familial risk, response potential may also be related to the strength of this association (e.g., whether one or both parents are affected). The second variable is the relative engagement/involvement of the individual in an ongoing task or activity. Engagement/involvement is a characteristic of the individual's immediate experience (Singer, 1974), but may be influenced by many factors, including situational cues, task demands, and dispositional attributes. Finally, much of the data at hand indicate that these two variables—response potential and engagement/involvement—interact in a partially catalytic manner, as illustrated in Figures 1 and 2.

In one respect, the present discussion reflects a probable oversimplification of behaviorally-induced reactivity because we have ignored likely relationships (and differences) among the various parameters of cardiovascular response. This is because most investigators either treat each of the available response measures independently (e.g., heart rate, systolic blood pressure, diastolic blood pressure) (Manuck & Schaefer, 1978; Lawler, 1980), or focus on the peripheral manifestations of a single, underlying mechanism (e.g., effects of beta-adrenergic stimulation on related aspects of myocardial performance) (Obrist, 1981). More recently, though, greater attention has been paid to the patterns of hemodynamic adjustment which give rise to the cardiovascular responses commonly observed. Eliot et al. (1982) describe, for example, what they believe to be three distinct patterns of individual response to behavioral stressors. In one, relative elevations in blood pressure arise primarily from an increase in the cardiac output; in a second, pressor responses are accouted for by an increased total systemic resistance; and in the third, there occurs a "combined" elevation of the cardiac output and resistance factors. These investigators suggest that these three response patterns may have differential prognostic significance, though little systematic research has yet been reported. If stable dimensions of individual difference are ultimately demonstrated within this classification scheme, however, it will be of interest to determine whether each pattern reflects a unique response potential, and secondly, whether each pattern is similarly influenced by the relative engagement/involvement of the individual. It is conceivable that the expression of each hemodynamic pattern may be sensitive to somewhat different though equally significant, behavioral dimensions.

HYPERTENSION AND SOCIAL COMPETENCE

Having considered cardiovascular response characteristics in hypertension and their possible relationship to behavioral attributes of the individual, we now wish to return to the role of anger and its "suppression" in development of the hypertensive condition. Numerous studies provide thematic support for Alexander's (1939) hypothesis that inhibited aggressive impulses characterize many hypertensive patients, though because of methodologic deficiencies, failures of replication and, occasionally, contradictory findings, this literature remains inconclusive. In addition, many of the interpretations and conclusions drawn in previous work have been highly inferential and speculative. Although hypertensives are purported to have excessive anger that they suppress or deny, concepts such as "suppression" and "denial" are themselves poorly defined and difficult to measure. They are typically inferred on the basis of indirect or symbolic clues, or sometimes, when a lack of concordance exists between self-report and physiologic indices of arousal (i.e., the subject exhibits arousal, but does not report discomfort). Clearly, there is no direct evidence for such intrapsychic processes.

The hypothesis that hypertensives experience excessive anger remains problematic. First, it is non-specific and an overgeneralization. Because human behavior is highly variable and situationally specific (Mischel, 1968; Bandura, 1977; Endler & Magnusson, 1976), it is unlikely that hypertensives are characteristically always angry. Of necessity, their anger must be tied to specific circumstances, such as events, people, and conflicts. Unfortunately, there are presently few objective data regarding the exact manner in which hypertensives behave or react in pertinent situations. An interesting contrast is the Structured Interview for assessment of Type A, or coronary-prone behavior (Dembroski et al., 1977), which seeks to use appropriate interpersonal challenge to elicit specific, construct-relevant behaviors in susceptible individuals. That the Type A pattern has also been found consistently related to an increased risk for coronary heart disease demonstrates not only the strength of this biobehavioral association but also the sensitivity of the assessment device. Anger may well be the critical affect mediating elevated blood pressure among some hypertensive patients, but this hypothesis must ultimately be confirmed by more direct observation.

A critical and rarely addressed question in this literature concerns when and why hypertensive individuals become angry. One answer to this question, we believe, may be found in the behavioral conception of assertiveness. Assertiveness may be broadly defined as the ability to stand up for one's rights, to express feelings, and to avoid mistreatment by others (Jakubowski & Lange, 1978; Linehan & Egan, 1979). It is a social skill, a learned performance capability involving a complex repertoire of responses that includes: (a) non-verbal elements (e.g., gaze, body posture, gestures); (b) verbal content (e.g., statements of compromise, refusal and disagreement); (c) paralinguistic features (e.g., voice tone and volume); and (d) social perception (e.g., sense of timing). In the past several years, an extensive literature has developed on the measurement of assertiveness (Arkowitz, 1981; Bellack, 1979), which is defined operationally and can be assessed systematically and objectively.

Assertiveness is obviously a vital interpersonal skill and indicator of social competence. Low assertive individuals tend to be mistreated, fail to express their feelings, and are frequently unable to have their needs met. A natural consequence of these problems is frustration and anger. These, too, are precisely the difficulties and reactions described by many as attributes of the hypertensive individual. One promising approach to the study of behavioral factors in this disorder, then, may be to characterize hypertensives by a factor which precipitates their negative affect, such as assertiveness deficits. This hypothesis has also been proposed recently by other investigators (Keane, Martin, Berler, Wooten, Fleece, & Williams, 1982; Linden & Feuerstein, 1981) and is consistent with two aspects of the more psychodynamic perspective: (a) that hypertensives suppress or deny anger; and (b) that they experience excessive anger. These statements suggest that hypertensives cannot effectively assert themselves and express feelings. Of course, the literature has not yet clearly demonstrated that these deficits are common in hypertension. And if they are, they may pertain only to particular subsets of hypertensive patients, such as those for whom autonomic mechanisms play an important role in maintaining the elevated blood pressure (Esler et al., 1977).

Direct observation offers the best opportunity to assess the precise nature of interpersonal behavior and social skill (Arkowitz, 1981; Bellack, 1979; Hersen & Bellack, 1977). While subjects can provide a general statement about their inclinations and attempts to perform certain responses, they are often unaware of, and hence unable to report on, their specific social skill deficits and excesses (e.g., problems in paralinguistic and nonverbal response styles). They cannot indicate that when mistreated, they speak loudly or softly, firmly or meekly, clearly or with subtle dysfluencies. At times, they do not even recognize mistreatment by others and cannot report that they are unassertive. This point is especially relevant for hypotheses relating to hypertension. If some hypertensives do "suppress" or "deny" anger and assertive feelings, it is possible that they would not be able to accurately describe their experiences or behavior. Regarding assertiveness generally, such critical response factors as speech dysfluencies, voice volume, response latency, and compliance content are best assessed by careful observation of the subject in interpersonal encounters.

The most desirable strategy for making observations is obviously to assess the subject in his or her natural environment. However, the unpredictable occurrence of assertion situations, combined with the cost and intrusiveness of *in vivo* observation, make this unfeasible. Laboratory-based, analogue observations provide a next-best option. The most widely used analogue procedure is role-playing (Arkowitz, 1981; Bellack, 1979), in which the subject is seated in an interviewing room with an experimental confederate. A narrator first describes an interpersonal scenario calling for assertion. The confederate then provides a prompt to initiate the interaction, and the subject responds as if he or she were really in the described situation. The interaction can also be extended by having the confederate make a series of further responses to the subject, varying the content according to subject behavior.

With these considerations in mind, we recently conducted an investigation of social competence in hypertension, and in the following paragraphs briefly describe some of our preliminary findings (Morrison, Note 7). The specific purpose of this study was to test the hypothesis that some borderline essential hypertensives exhibit difficulty with assertion, and that these behavioral characteristics may be detected when subjects are challenged to respond appropriately in a standard role-play test of assertiveness. A second purpose of this study was to record cardiovascular responses occurring during the role-play procedure in order to examine relationships between levels of assertive behavior and psychophysiologic responsivity. Our subjects were 22 borderline hypertensives and 13 demographically similar normotensive controls. All subjects were males, and no hypertensive subject was currently prescribed any medication directly affecting autonomic function. The role-play test of assertiveness (RPT) was presented during the second of two experimental sessions; thus, the subject was acclimated to the laboratory setting and to aspects of the recording procedures.

The RPT itself consisted of several brief scenarios, each containing (as described above) an implicit demand for assertive behavior (specifically negative assertion) from the subject. Each role-play scene was also acted out against an experimental confederate whose function was to prompt the subject and increase the difficulty to the interactions by thwarting initial efforts at assertive responding. Each subject's role play performance was videotaped for later scoring; measures of cardiovascular response were also obtained during a preceding baseline period and throughout the task. Behavioral ratings were made by trained research assistants kept "blind" to subjects' hypertensive/normotensive status, and involved a variety of response dimensions important for effective assertiveness. Finally, in addition to the RPT, a "significant other" measure of interpersonal skill, termed the Social Performance Survey Schedule (Lowe & Cautela, 1978), was also administered to gather independent data on subjects' social competence.

In analyzing the data of this study, we first focused on relationships between subjects' psychophysiologic responsivity and assertion by computing correlations between two sets of variables: (a) RPT-related blood pressure changes (calculated as percentage rises over baseline values for systolic and diastolic blood pressure and pulse pressure); and (b) behavioral measures of assertiveness, based on RPT performance ratings. These analyses revealed no reliable associations between blood pressure change and behavior in normotensive subjects. In hypertensives, however, we found a positive correlation between overall assertiveness and the magnitude of pulse pressure responses observed during the role-play procedure ($r = 0.52$, $p < 0.02$). This finding is of particular interest to us in view of earlier work in our laboratory demonstrating consistent associations between pulse pressure reactivity and behavioral characteristics of the Type A behavior pattern (viz., verbal response stylistics, perception of time) (Manuck et al., 1979). At first glance, though, the relationship observed here seems to indicate that a heightened physiologic responsivity is associated with greater, not less, assertiveness among hypertensive subjects. The correlation, by itself, does not indicate what relationships may exist between levels of assertiveness in hypertensive and normotensive subjects, or what patterns of cardiovascular response underlie the variations in pulse pressure reactivity.

Considering patterns of response, we noted that hypertensives could be partitioned into two rather distinct sub-groups (designated Groups 1 and 2). Group 1 included hypertensive subjects who had shown the most appreciable increases in pulse pressure during the RPT; these responses were attributable to large systolic elevations, which in these subjects exceeded concomitant diastolic reactions (hence, the increased pulse pressure). Systolic pressor responses among Group 1 subjects were significantly greater than in normotensive subjects. They were also greater than among the remaining hypertensives comprising Group 2, who had exhibited low pulse pressure responses; systolic reactions in Group 2 subjects were largely attenuated, although their diastolic elevations during the RPT were still quite substantial—somewhat more pronounced even than in Group 1. Diastolic pressor responses among Group 2 hypertensives also tended to be larger than those observed among normotensive controls. With respect to the patterning of responses observed here, it is tempting to speculate (especially in relation to the descriptive categories of Eliot et al. [1982]), that Group 1 hypertensives exhibited significant increases in cardiac output during the RPT, whereas pressor responses among Group 2 hypertensive subjects were caused by changes in the peripheral resistance. Though we have no direct data indicating such a specificity of cardiovascular response in the two hypertensive groups, it is consistent with this interpretation that concurrent heart rate elevations were somewhat larger in Group 1, and for all hypertensive subjects the elevation correlated significantly with the relative magnitude of subjects' pulse pressure and systolic pressor responses.

Based on our division of hypertensive subjects, we next contrasted Group 1 and Group 2 hypertensives with normotensive controls on overall and component measures of assertion. For purposes of these analyses, the normotensives were treated as a single group because individual differences in psychophysiologic responsivity had been found to be unrelated to differences in assertive behavior.

For overall assertiveness, Group 1 hypertensives were found to be significantly more assertive than their Group 2 counterparts ($p < .05$) and equal in assertiveness to normotensive subjects. Group 1 hypertensives differed from normotensives, however, in verbal content and expressive mannerisms—behavioral categories in which they showed significantly greater hostility or aggressiveness ($p < .05$). In contrast, Group 2 hypertensives were not only less assertive than subjects in Group 1 but also tended to be less assertive than normotensive controls ($p < .08$). The actual mean score of Group 2 hypertensives also fell well below that point on the scale for overall assertiveness which denotes "appropriate assertiveness," and in this respect may reflect a clinically significant deficit in assertive skill. Consistent with these behavioral ratings, moreover, on the Social Performance Survey Schedule Group 2 hypertensives were viewed by "significant others" (e.g., wife, girlfriend) as being less skilled or effective interpersonally than normotensive subjects. Group 1 hypertensives were also seen as less socially competent than normotensives, though this difference did not reach significance.

We believe that the findings of this initial study provide added support for the hypothesis that problems with anger and assertive expression are implicated in borderline hypertension, and that our role-play instruments of assertiveness are sensitive to these effects. The fact that behavioral differences observed here were corroborated by a "significant other" measure of social competence further suggests that findings based on our role-play procedures generalized beyond the laboratory setting. Interestingly, the distinguishing attributes of hypertensives were of two kinds: heightened hostility in one hypertensive sub-group, and lower assertiveness in the second. This result is consistent with the proposal of Harburg et al. (1979) that elevated blood pressures may be related to extremes of behavior at both ends of the assertiveness dimension. We also found that behavioral characteristics were associated with differences in psychophysiologic responsivity among hypertensives, but not in normotensives: in accord with our earlier report that changes on state measures of negative affect (anxiety, anger) during stress were related to accompanying cardiovascular responses in offspring of hypertensive parents but not among persons of normotensive parentage (Manuck, Note 2).

It should be noted that a second research group (Keane et al., 1982) has recently investigated social skills in hypertensives using a similar methodology, though those authors employed a much smaller hypertensive sample than ours, and did not examine assertive behaviors in relation to the accompanying cardiovascular responsivity of hypertensive subjects. In addition, the results of their investigation differed somewhat from our own. In our present study, no initial overall differences were observed between hypertensive and normotensive subjects. It was only when hypertensives were characterized by the patterning of their psychophysiologic reactions to the RPT that significant group differences emerged. In contrast, Keane et al. (1982) reported less assertive responses among hypertensives generally, compared to healthy, normotensive controls. Furthermore, on measures of social performance, hypertensive subjects in their study were comparable to a second control group composed of chronically ill, but normotensive, patients. Based on these findings, Keane et al. (1982) concluded that the interpersonal deficiencies exhibited by hypertensive patients may actually be a consequence of their chronic disorder, rather than a characteristic specific to (or preceding) the hypertensive condition. The authors speculated further that an individual may behave in a passive and unassertive manner if the emotional correlates of an assertive response are believed to be detrimental to the course of the disorder.

Sapira et al. (1971) have suggested that hypertensive individuals may actively avoid difficult interpersonal encounters, or at least interpret such situations as being less threatening, to protect themselves from their excessive cardiovascular reactivity. Results of the present investigation do not generally support this notion, however, because they do not provide a replication of the overall hypertensive-normotensive differences reported by Keane et al. (1982). Indeed, our data indicate that specific, and quite different, assertion problems occur among hypertensive patients, and vary with the patterning of subjects' cardiovascular responsivity to a social stressor. Given this level of specificity, it is difficult to imagine that the behavioral characteristics we have observed result solely from the disorder itself. Data from a subset of these subjects—namely, the lower assertiveness of our Group 2 hypertensive patients—may nevertheless be seen as consistent with such a hypothesis. Certainly, the questions addressed within our study and in that of Keane et al. (1982) stand in need of further investigation. Yet despite their differences, both studies implicate assertion-related difficulties in hypertension, whatever the origin of these problems or their role in the etiology and/or maintenance of the condition. In each of these studies the measurement procedures used are also behaviorally specific, providing objective and reliable conditions that are frequently lacking in previous studies of this type. Indeed, the specificity of assessed behaviors provides a basis for the design of novel, and even individualized, behavioral interventions for hypertension. Improving identifiable deficits in social skill through training may be a more direct approach to treatment, in contrast to current techniques, which are concerned primarily with achieving a generalized reduction in sympathetic arousal (e.g., biofeedback) (Seer, 1979). Such training could, in effect, modify the behavior on which the expression of a heightened sympathetic arousal may depend.

Based on our findings, "traditional" assertion training emphasizing the components of an effective assertive response would appear to be most appropriate for those hypertensives we have designated as Group 2. The present behavior of these individuals is "unassertive" in the usual sense of passive and submissive responding. Group 1, on the other hand, might benefit most from training programs emphasizing anger reduction, possibly through the application of more effective problem-solving skills. Procedures to reduce negative emotional arousal (anxiety, anger), such as relaxation training, might prove an effective component of assertion training for both groups of hypertensive patients. Overall, then, we believe that conceptualizing the behavioral correlates of hypertension within a social competence model, together with the applicaton of both psychophysiologic and behavioral assessment procedures, may provide valuable new data regarding the role of psychologic factors in this disorder, hopefully leading to more effective interventions.

REFERENCES

Alexander, F. Emotional factors in essential hypertension: Presentation of a tentative hypothesis. *Psychosomatic Medicine,* 1939, *1,* 173-179.

Arkowitz, H. The assessment of social skills. In M. Hersen, & A. S. Bellack (Eds.), *Behavioral assessment: A practical handbook* (2nd ed.). New York: Pergamon, 1981.

Baer, P. E., Collins, F. H., Bourianoff, G. C., & Ketchel, M. F. Assessing personality factors in essential hypertension with a brief self-report instrument. *Psychosomatic Medicine,* 1969, *7,* 653-659.

Bandura, A. *Social learning theory.* Englewood Cliffs, N.J.: Prentice-Hall, 1977.

Baumann, R., Ziprian, H., Godicke, W., Hartrodt, W., Naumann, E., & Lauter, J. The influence of acute psychic stress situations on biochemical and vegetative parameters of essential hypertensives at the early stage of the disease. *Psychotherapy and Psychosomatics,* 1973, *22,* 131-140.

Bellack, A. S. A critical appraisal of strategies for assessing social skill. *Behavioral Assessment,* 1979, *1,* 157-176.

Boyer, J. T., Fraser, J. R. E., & Doyle, A. E. The hemodynamic effects of cold immersion. *Clinical Sciences,* 1960, *19,* 539-550.

Brady, J. V., & Harris, A. H. Behavioral patterns and stress in the etiology of cardiovascular disease. In S. S. Kalter (Ed.), *The use of nonhuman primates in cardiovascular diseases.* Austin: University of Texas Press, 1980.

Briggs, J. F., & Oerting, H. The prognostic value of the cold test in pregnancy. *Minnesota Medicine,* 1937, *20,* 382-384.

Bunnell, D. E. Autonomic myocardial influences as a factor determining inter-task consistency of heart rate reactivity. *Psychophysiology,* 1982, *19,* 442-448.

Cochrane, R. Hostility and neuroticism among unselected essential hypertensives. *Journal of Psychosomatic Research*, 1973, *17*, 215-218.
Corse, C. D., Manuck, S. B., Cantwell, J. D., Giordani, B., & Matthews, K. A. Coronary-prone behavior pattern and cardiovascular response in persons with and without coronary heart disease. *Psychosomatic Medicine*, 1982, *44*, 449-459.
Dembroski, T. M., MacDougall, J. M., Herd, J. A., & Shields, J. L. Effect of level of challenge on pressor and heart rate responses in Type A and B subjects. *Journal of Applied Social Psychology*, 1979, *9*, 209-228.
Dembroski, T. M., Weiss, S. M., Shields, J. L., Haynes, S. G., & Feinleib, M. *Coronary-prone behavior*. New York: Springer-Verlag, 1978.
Diamond, E. L. The role of anger and hostility in essential hypertension and coronary heart disease. *Psychological Bulletin*, 1982, *92*, 410-433.
Dieckman, W. J., & Michel, H. L. Thermal study of vasomotor lability in pregnancy. *Archives of Internal Medicine*, 1935, *54*, 420-430.
Eich, R. H., Cuddy, R. P., Smulyan, H., & Lyons, R. H. Hemodynamics in labile hypertension: A follow-up study. *Circulation*, 1966, *34*, 299-307.
Eliot, R. S., Buell, J. C., & Dembroski, T. M. Bio-behavioral perspectives on coronary heart disease, hypertension and sudden cardiac death. *Acta Medicus Scandinavica, Supplement 7*, 1982, *606*, 203-219.
Elliott, R. Tonic heart rate: Experiments on the effects of collative variables lead to a hypothesis about its motivational significance. *Journal of Personality and Social Psychology*, 1969, *12*, 211-228.
Endler, N., & Magnusson, D. Toward and interactional psychology of personality. *Psychology Bulletin*, 1976, *33*, 956-974.
Engel, B. T., & Bickford, A. F. Response-specificity: Stimulus-response and individual-response specificity in essential hypertensives. *Archives of General Psychiatry*, 1961, *5*, 478-489.
Engel, R. R., Muller, F., Munch, V., & Ackenheil, M. M. Plasma catecholamine response and autonomic functions during short-term psychological stress. In E. Usden, R. Kuentnansky, & I. J. Kopin (Eds.), *Catecholamine and stress: Recent progress*. New York: Elsevier, 1980.
Esler, M. D., Julius, S., Randall, O. S., El Iis, C. N., & Kashima, T. Relation of renin status to neurogenic vascular resistance in borderline hypertension. *The American Journal of Cardiology*, 1975, *36*, 708-715.
Esler, M., Julius, S., Zweifler, A., Randall, O., Harburg, E., Gardiner, H., & DeQuattro, V. Mild high-renin essential hypertension: Neurogenic human hypertension? *New England Journal of Medicine*, 1977, *296*, 405-411.
Esler, M. D., & Nestel, P. J. Renin and sympathetic nervous system responsiveness to adrenergic stimuli in essential hypertension. *The American Journal of Cardiology*, 1973, *32*, 643-649.
Falkner, E., Onesti, G., Angelakos, E. T., Fernandes, M., & Langman, C. Cardiovascular response to mental stress in normal adolescents with hypertensive parents. *Hypertension*, 1979, *1*, 23-30.
Falkner, B., Onesti, G., & Hamstra, B. Stress response characteristics of adolescents with high genetic risk for essential hypertension: A five-year follow-up. *Clinical and Experimental Hypertension*, 1981, *3*, 583-591.
Feldt, R. H., & Wenndstrand, D. E. W. The cold-pressor test in subjects with normal blood pressure. Report of observations on 350 subjects, with special reference to the family history. *American Heart Journal*, 1942, *23*, 766-771.
Giordani, B., Manuck, S. B., & Farmer, J. F. Stability of behaviorally-induced heart rate changes in children after one week. *Child Development*, 1981, *52*, 533-537.
Glass, D. C., Krakoff, L. R., Contrada, R., Hilton, W. F., Kehoe, K., Mannucci, E. G., Collins, C., Snow, B., & Elting, E. Effect of harassment and competition upon cardiovascular and catecholamine responses in Type A and Type B individuals. *Psychophysiology*, 1980, *17*, 453-463.
Gliner, J. A., Bedi, J. F., & Horvath, S. M. Somatic and non-somatic influences on the heart: Hemodynamic changes. *Psychophysiology*, 1979, *16*, 358-363.
Goldband, S. Stimulus specificity and physiological response to stress and the Type A coronary-prone behavior pattern. *Journal of Personality and Social Psychology*, 1980, *39*, 670-679.

Gorlin, R., Brachfeld, N., Turner, J. D., Messer, J. V., & Salazar, E. The idiopathic high cardiac output state. *Journal of Clinical Investigation,* 1959, *38,* 2144-2153.
Gressel, G. E., Shobe, F. O., Saslow, G., DuBois, M., & Schroeder, H. A. Personality factors in essential hypertension. *Journal of the American Medical Association,* 1949, *140,* 265-272.
Hallback, M., & Folkow, B. Cardiovacular responses to acute mental "stress" in spontaneously hypertensive rats. *Acta Physiologica Scandinavica,* 1974, *90,* 684-698.
Hamilton, J. A. Psychophysiology of blood pressure. *Psychosomatic Medicine,* 1942, *4,* 125-133.
Handkins, R. E., & Munz, D. C. Essential hypertension and self-disclosure. *Journal of Clinical Psychology,* 1978, *34,* 870-875.
Harburg, E., Blakelock, E. H., & Roeper, P. J. Resentful and reflective coping with arbitrary authority and blood pressure: Detroit. *Psychosomatic Medicine,* 1979, *41,* 189-202.
Harburg, E., Erfurt, J C., Hauenstein, L. S., Chape, C., Schull, W. J., & Schork, M. A. Socio-ecological stress, suppressed hostility, skin color, and black-white male blood pressure: Detroit. *Psychosomatic Medicine,* 1973, *35,* 276-296.
Harburg, E., Julius, S., McGinn, N. F., McLeod, J., & Hoobler, S. W. Personality traits and behavioral patterns associated with systolic blood pressure levels in college males. *Journal of Chronic Diseases,* 1964, *17,* 405-414.
Harlan, W. R., Osborne, R. K., & Graybiel, A. Prognostic value of the cold pressor test. *The American Journal of Cardiology,* 1964, *13,* 832-837.
Harrell, J. P. Psychological factors and hypertension: A status report. *Psychological Bulletin,* 1980, *87,* 482-501.
Harris, R. E., Sokolow, M., Carpenter, L. G., Freedman, M., & Hunt, S. P. Response to psychologic stress in persons who are potentially hypertensive. *Circulation,* 1953, *7,* 572-578.
Hastrup, J. L., Light, K. C., & Obrist, P. A. Parental hypertension and cardiovascular response to stress in healthy young adults. *Psychophysiology,* 1982, *19,* 615-622.
Hersen, M., & Bellack, A. S. Assessment of social skills. In A. R. Ciminero, K. S. Calhoun, & H. E. Adams (Eds.), *Handbook for behavioral assessment.* New York: Wiley, 1977.
Hines, E. A., & Brown, G. E. The cold pressor test for measuring the reactivity of the blood pressure: Data concerning 571 normal and hypertensive subjects. *American Heart Journal,* 1936, *11,* 1-9.
Jakubowski, P., & Lange, A. J. *The assertive option: Your rights and responsibilities.* Champaign, Ill.: Research, 1978.
Jennings, J. R., & Choi, S. Type A components and psychophysiological responses to an attention demanding performance task. *Psychosomatic Medicine,* 1981, *43,* 475-488.
Jorgensen, R. S., & Houston, B. K. Family history of hypertension, gender, and cardiovascular reactivity and stereotypy during stress. *Journal of Behavioral Medicine,* 1981, *4,* 175-189.
Julius, S. Borderline hypertension: Epidemiologic and clinical implications. In J. Genest, E. Koiw, & O. Kuchel (Eds.), *Hypertension.* New York: McGraw-Hill, 1977.
Julius, S., & Conway, J. Hemodynamic studies in patients with borderline blood pressure elevation. *Circulation,* 1968, *38,* 282-288.
Julius, S., & Esler, M. Autonomic nervous cardiovascular regulation in borderline hypertension. *The American Journal of Cardiology,* 1975, *36,* 685-696.
Kaplan, S., Gottschalk, L. A., Magliocco, E., Rohovit, D., & Ross, W. Hostility in verbal productions and hypnotic dreams in hypertensive patients. *Psychosomatic Medicine,* 1961, *23,* 311-322.
Kahn, H. A., Medalie, J. H., Neufeld, H. N., Riss, E., & Goldbourt, U. The incidence of hypertension and associated factors: The Israel ischemic heart disease study. *American Heart Journal,* 1972, *84,* 171-182.
Keane, T. M., Martin, J. E., Berler, E. S., Wooten, L. S., Fleece, E. L., & Williams, J. G. Are hypertensives less assertive? A controlled evaluation. *Journal of Consulting and Clinical Psychology,* 1982, *50,* 499-508.
Keys, A., Taylor, H. L., Blackburn, H., Brozek, J., Anderson, J. T., & Simonson, E. Mortality and coronary heart disease among men studied for 23 years. *Archives of Internal Medicine,* 1971, *128,* 201-214.
Kuchel, O. Autonomic nervous system in hypertension: Clinical aspects. In J. Genest, E. Koiw, & O. Kuchel (Eds.), *Hypertension.* New York: McGraw-Hill, 1977.

Langer, A. W., Obrist, P. A., & McCubbin, J. A. Hemodynamic and metabolic adjustments during exercise and shock avoidance in dogs. *American Journal of Physiology: Heart and Circulatory Physiology*, 1979, *5*, H225-H230.

Lawler, K. A. Cardiovascular and electrodermal response patterns in heart rate reactive individuals during psychological stress. *Psychophysiology*, 1980, *17*, 464-470.

LeBlanc, J., Cote, J., Jobin, M., & Labrie, A. Plasma catecholamines and cardiovascular responses to cold and mental activity. *Journal of Applied Physiology*, 1979, *47*, 1207-1211.

Light, K. C., & Obrist, P. A. Cardiovascular response to stress: Effects of opportunity to avoid, shock experience and performance feedback. *Psychophysiology*, 1980, *17*, 243-252.

Light, K. C., & Obrist, P. A. Task difficulty, heart rate reactivity and cardiovascular response to an appetitive reaction time task. *Psychophysiology*, 1983, *20*, 301-302.

Linden, W., & Fauerstein, M. Essential hypertension and social coping behavior. *Journal of Human Stress*, 1981, *7*, 28-34.

Linehan, M. M., & Egan, K. J. Assertion training for women. In A. S. Bellack & M. Hersen (Eds.), *Research and practice in social skills training*. New York: Plenum, 1979.

Lorimer, A. R., MacFarlane, P. W., Provan, G., Duffy, T., & Lawrie, T. D. V. Blood pressure and catecholamine response to 'stress' in normotensive and hypertensive subjects. *Cardiovascular Research*, 1971, *5*, 169-173.

Lowe, M. R., & Cautela, J. R. A self-report measure of social skill. *Behavior Therapy*, 1978, *9*, 535-544.

Lund-Johansen, P. Hemodynamics in early essential hypertension. *Acta Medica Scandinavica, (Supplement)*, 1967, *182*, 1-101.

Lund-Johansen, P. Central hemodynamics in essential hypertension. *Acta Medica Scandinavica, (Supplement)*, 1977, *606*, 35-42.

Lund-Johansen, P. Spontaneous changes in central hemodynamics in essential hypertension— A 10 year follow-up study. In G. Onesti & C. R. Klimt (Eds.), *Hypertension—Determinants, complications and intervention*. New York: Grune & Stratton, 1979.

Mann, A. H. Psychiatric morbidity and hostility in hypertension. *Psychological Medicine*, 1977, *7*, 653-659.

Manuck, S. B., Corse, C. D., & Winkelman, P. A. Behavioral correlates of individual differences in blood pressure reactivity. *Journal of Psychosomatic Research*, 1979, *23*, 281-288.

Manuck, S. B., Craft, S., & Gold, K. J. Coronary-prone behavior pattern and cardiovascular response. *Psychophysiology*, 1978, *15*, 403-411.

Manuck, S. B., & Garland, F. N. Coronary-prone behavior pattern, task incentive and cardiovascular response. *Psychophysiology*, 1979, *16*, 136-142.

Manuck, S. B., & Garland, F. N. Stability of individual differences in cardiovascular reactivity: A thirteen month follow-up. *Physiology and Behavior*, 1980, *21*, 621-624.

Manuck, S. B., Giordani, B., McQuaid, K. J., & Garrity, S. J. Behaviorally-induced cardiovascular reactivity among sons of reported hypertensive and normotensive parents. *Journal of Psychosomatic Research*, 1981, *25*, 261-269.

Manuck, S. B., Kaplan, J. R., & Clarkson, T. B. Behaviorally-induced heart rate reactivity and atherosclerosis in cynomolgus monkeys. *Psychosomatic Medicine*, 1983, *45*, 95-108.

Manuck, S. B., & Proietti, J. Parental hypertension and cardiovascular response to cognitive isometric challenge. *Psychophysiology*, 1982, *19*, 481-489.

Manuck, S. B., & Schaefer, D. C. Stability of individual differences in cardiovascular reactivity. *Physiology and Behavior*, 1978, *21*, 675-678.

Matarazzo, J. D. An experimental study of aggression in the hypertensive patient. *Journal of Personality*, 1954, *22*, 423-447.

Matthews, K. A. Psychological perspectives on the Type A behavior pattern. *Psychological Bulletin*, 1982, *91*, 292-323.

McCarty, R., Chiueh, C. C., & Kopin, I. J. Spontaneously hypertensive rats: Adrenergic hyper-responsivity to anticipation of electric shock. *Behavioral Biology*, 1978, *23*, 180-188.

McClelland, D. C. Inhibited power motivation and high blood pressure in men. *Journal of Abnormal Psychology*, 1979, *88*, 182-190.

McKegney, F. P., & Williams, R. B. Psychological aspects of hypertension. II. The differential influence of interview variables on blood pressure. *American Journal of Psychiatry*, 1967, *123*, 1539-1545.

Miller, C., & Grim, C. Personality and emotional stress measurement on hypertensive patients with essential and secondary hypertension. *International Journal of Nursing Studies,* 1979, *16,* 85-93.
Michel, W. *Personality and assessment.* New York: Wiley, 1968.
Neiberg, N. A. The effects of induced stress on the management of hostility in essential hypertension. *Dissertation Abstracts,* 1957, *17,* 1597-1598.
Nestel, P. J. Blood pressure and catecholamine excretion after mental stress in labile hypertension. *Lancet,* 1969, *1,* 692-694.
Newlin, D. B., & Levenson, R. W. Cardiovascular responses of individuals with Type A behavior pattern and parental coronary heart disease. *Journal of Psychosomatic Research,* 1982, *26,* 393-402.
Obrist, P. A. The cardiovascular-behavioral interaction—as it appears today. *Psychophysiology,* 1976, *13,* 95-107.
Obrist, P. A. *Cardiovascular psychophysiology: A perspective.* New York: Plenum, 1981.
Obrist, P. A., Black, A. H., Brener, J., & DiCara, L. V. (Eds.). *Cardiovascular psychophysiology.* Chicago: Aldine, 1974.
Obrist, P. A., Langer, A. W., Light, K. A., & Koepke, J. P. A cardiac-behavioral approach in the study of hypertension. In T. M. Dembroski, T. Schmidt, & G. Bluemchen (Eds.), *Bio-behavioral bases of coronary heart disease.* New York: Karger, 1983.
Ostfeld, A. M., & Lebovitz, B. Z. Personality factors and pressor mechanisms in renal and essential hypertension. *Archives of Internal Medicine,* 1959, *104,* 497-502.
Pfaffenbarger, P. S., Throne, M. C., & Wing, A. L. Chronic disease in former college students. VIII. Characteristics of youth predisposing to hypertension in later years. *American Journal of Epidemiology,* 1968, *88,* 25-32.
Paul, O. Epidemiology of hypertension. In J. Genest, E. Koiw, & O. Kutchel (Eds.), *Hypertension: Physiopathology and treatment.* New York: McGraw-Hill, 1977.
Pittner, M. S., & Houston, B. K. Response to stress, cognitive coping strategies, and the Type A behavior pattern. *Journal of Personality and Social Psychology,* 1980, *39,* 147-157.
Price, K. P., & Clark, L. K. Behavioral and psychophysiological correlates of the coronary-prone personality: New data and unanswered questions. *Journal of Psychosomatic Research,* 1978, *22,* 409-417.
Remington, R. D., Lamberth, B., Moser, M., & Hoobler, S. W. Circulatory reactions of normotensive and hypertensive subjects and the children of normal and hypertensive parents. *American Heart Journal,* 1960, *56,* 58-70.
Safar, M. E., Kamiencka, H. A., Levenson, J. A., Dimitriu, V. M., & Pauleau, N. F. Hemodynamic factors and Rorschach testing in borderline and sustained hypertensives. *Psychosomatic Medicine,* 1978, *40,* 620-631.
Sapira, J. D., Scheib, E. T., Moriarty, R., & Shapiro, A. P. Differences in perception between hypertensive and normotensive populations. *Psychosomatic Medicine,* 1971, *33,* 239-250.
Schachter, J. Pain, fear, and anger in hypertensives and normotensives. *Psychosomatic Medicine,* 1957, *19,* 17-29.
Seer, P. Psychological control of essential hypertension: Review of the literature and methodological critique. *Psychological Bulletin,* 1979, *86,* 1015-1043.
Shapiro, A. P. An experimental study of comparative responses of blood pressure to different noxious stimuli. *Journal of Chronic Diseases,* 1961, *13,* 293-311.
Shapiro, A. P., Moutsos, S. E., & Krifcher, E. Patterns of pressor responses to noxious stimuli in normal, hypertensive and diabetic subjects. *Journal of Clinical Investigation,* 1963, *42,* 1890-1898.
Shapiro, A. P., Nicotoro, J., Sapira, J., & Scheib, E. T. Analysis of the variability of blood pressure, pulse rate and catecholamine responsivity in identical and fraternal twins. *Psychosomatic Medicine,* 1968, *30,* 506-520.
Singer, M. T. Engagement-involvement: A central phenomenon in psychophysiological research. *Psychosomatic Medicine,* 1974, *36,* 1-17.
Sokolow, M., & McIlroy, M. B. *Clinical cardiology.* Los Altos, Calif.: Lange Medical, 1977.
Spielberger, C. D., Gorsuch, R. L., & Lushene, R. E. *Manual for the state-trait anxiety inventory.* Palo Alto, Calif.: Consulting Psychologists, 1970.
Spielberger, C. D., Jacobs, G. A., Russell, S., & Crane, R. S. Assessment of anger: The state-trait anger scale. In J. N. Butcher & C. D. Spielberger (Eds.), *Advances in personality assessment* (Vol. 2). Hillsdale, N.J.: Erlbaum, 1983.
Stamler, J., Stamler, B., Riedlinger, W., Algera, G., & Roberts, R. Hypertension screening of 1 million Americans. *Journal of the American Medical Association,* 1976, *235,* 2299-2306.

Stead, E. A., Warren, J. V., Merrill, A. J., & Brannon, E. S. The cardiac output in male subjects as measured by the technique of arterial catheterization. Normal values with observations on the effects of anxiety and tilting. *Journal of Clinical Investigation,* 1945, *24,* 326–331.
Steptoe, A. *Psychological factors in cardiovascular disorders.* New York: Academic, 1981.
Steptoe, A., & Ross, A. Psychophysiological reactivity and the prediction of cardiovascular disorders. *Journal of Psychosomatic Research,* 1981, *25,* 23–31.
Theorell, T., DeFaire, U., Schalling, D., Adamson, U., & Askevoid, F. Personality traits and psychophysiological reactions to a stressful interview in twins with varying degrees of coronary heart disease. *Journal of Psychosomatic Research,* 1979, *23,* 89–99.
VanEgeren, L. F. Cardiovascular changes during social competition in a mixed-motive game. *Journal of Personality and Social Psychology,* 1979, *37,* 858–864.
Weiner, H. *The psychobiology of essential hypertension.* New York: Elsevier, 1979.
Williams, R. B. Physiological mechanisms underlying the association between psychological factors and coronary disease. In W. D. Gentry & R. B. Williams (Eds.), *Psychological aspects of myocardial infarction and coronary care.* Saint Louis: Mosby, 1975.
Williams, R. B., Lane, J. D., Kuhn, C. M., Melosh, W., White, A. D., & Schanberg, S. M. Type A behavior and elevated physiological and neuroendocrine responses to cognitive tasks. *Science,* 1982, *218,* 483–485.
Wolff, H. S., & Wolf, S. A summary of experimental evidence relating life stress to the pathogenesis of essential hypertension in man. In E. T. Bell (Ed.), *Hypertension: A symposium.* Minneapolis: University of Minnesota Press, 1951.

REFERENCE NOTES

1. Sime, W. E., Buell, J. C., & Eliot, R. Psychophysiological (emotional) stress testing: A potential means of detecting the early reinfarction victim. Presented at the 52nd Annual Scientific Sessions of the American Heart Association, 1979. *Circulation,* 1979, *59* and *60,* 11–56. (Abstract)
2. Manuck, S. B. Parental hypertension, affect, and cardiovascular response to cognitive challenge. Presented at the 22nd Annual Meeting of the Society for Psychophysiological Research, 1982. *Psychophysiology,* 1982, *19,* 545. (Abstract)
3. Light, K. C., Koepke, J. P., Obrist, P. A., Grignolo, A., & Willis, P. W. Effects of behavioral stress on the kidney: A possible mechanism for hypertension development. Presented at the 22nd Annual Meeting of the Society for Psychophysiological Research, 1982. *Psychophysiology,* 1982, *19,* 544–545. (Abstract)
4. Rose, R. J., Miller, J. Z., & Grim, C. E. Familial factors in blood pressure response to laboratory stress: A twin study. Presented at the 22nd Annual Meeting of the Society for Psychophysiological Research, 1982. *Psychophysiology,* 1982, *19,* 583. (Abstract)
5. Allen, M. T. *Individual differences and cardiovascular reactivity in college-age students.* Unpublished doctoral dissertation, University of Tennessee-Knoxville, 1982.
6. Katkin, E. S., Goldband, S., & Medine, B. Cardiovascular responses to stressful and nonstressful reaction time tasks as a function of family history of cardiovascular disease and Type A personality. Presented at the 19th Annual Meeting of the Society for Psychophysiological Research, 1979. *Psychophysiology,* 1980, *17,* 318–319. (Abstract)
7. Morrison, R. L. *The role of social competence in essential hypertension.* Unpublished doctoral dissertation, University of Pittsburgh, 1982.

9
The Health Consequences of Hostility

Redford B. Williams, Jr.
Duke University Medical Center

John C. Barefoot
Duke University Medical Center

Richard B. Shekelle
University of Texas Health Science Center at Houston

The purpose of this volume is to review recent research on the assessment, correlates and treatment of anger. In this chapter we shall review the rapidly growing body of evidence indicating that level of hostility is associated with a wide variety of health outcomes. We shall also consider briefly the possible biologic mechanisms whereby hostility and anger could lead to pathophysiologic alterations in bodily functions.

Before proceeding with this review, however, it is in order to consider how the construct of "hostility" relates to that of "anger." Based on our previous research and a review of the relevant literature, we offer the following definitions to guide the reader. *Hostility* is considered to be an attitudinal set—perhaps even a personality trait—which stems from an absence of trust in the basic goodness of others and centers around the belief that others are generally mean, selfish and undependable. We feel it likely that this attitude is, to a large extent, learned from caregivers early in life. From the developmental perspective, it may reflect an incomplete development of "basic trust," to use Erikson's (1963) term. *Anger,* on the other hand, is an emotional state made up of feelings ranging in intensity from minor irritation to fury and rage. While different from hostility, it seems clear that anger bears some relation to the latter concept; persons with a strong attitudinal set of hostility will be likely to experience the emotion of anger more frequently and intensively than persons low in hostility.

Finally, *aggression* is overt antagonistic behavior motivated by the acts of others, as well as by one's own hostility and anger. In this volume and elsewhere, Spielberger (Spielberger, Chap. 1; Spielberger, Jacobs, Russell and Crane, 1983) has considered issues involved in defining hostility, anger and aggression, and the reader is referred to these writings for a more comprehensive discussion.

Preparation of this chapter was supported in part by grants HL-18589 and HL-22740 from the NHLBI and by a Research Scientist Development Award, MH-70482, from the NIMH.

With regard to assessment, it is fair to say that no single instrument for the measurement of hostility, anger or aggression presently enjoys universal acceptance. Guided by Rosenman and Friedman's initial descriptions (Rosenman et al., 1964) of those characteristics comprising Type A behavior pattern, in which hostility and anger were emphasized along with chronic speed and impatience, we determined early on to assess these characteristics using the best available instruments in our studies of the psychosocial correlates of coronary atherosclerosis. As we shall review in this chapter, this has been a productive approach, and one that has led to new insights not only regarding the relation of hostility to coronary heart disease but to other debilitating and life-threatening diseases as well.

HEALTH CORRELATES OF HOSTILITY

Our own research into the health consequences of hostility and anger began with initial efforts to determine whether Type A patients undergoing diagnostic coronary angiography have more severe coronary atherosclerosis (CAD) than Type B patients. In the first study, we found that over 90% of patients with very severe CAD were judged to be Type A using the structured interview (SI) (Blumenthal, Williams, Kong, Schanberg and Thompson, 1978). Based on this finding, over eight years ago we began to systematically collect data pertaining to a broad range of psychosocial characteristics (see Williams et al., 1980, for a description of data collection procedures) on all patients referred to Duke University Medical Center for diagnostic coronary angiography.

In our next study (Williams et al., 1980), we replicated the earlier finding of more severe CAD among those patients characterized as Type A using the SI (Rosenman, 1978) in a sample of 424 patients. Since we had also collected MMPI data on these patients, we were in a position to investigate the various hostility scales that had been developed from the MMPI item set over the years (see Spielberger, Jacobs, Russell and Crane, 1983, for a review of MMPI hostility scales). Purely by chance, the first such scale we evaluated in relation to CAD levels was the 50-item Ho scale developed by Cook and Medley (1954) on the basis of manifest content and differentiation between teachers with good versus poor rapport with pupils. As shown in Figure 1, scores on the Ho scale were significantly related to Type A behavior as assessed by the SI; the mean Ho scores were 16, 18, 20, and 21 for Types B, X, A2 and A1, respectively.

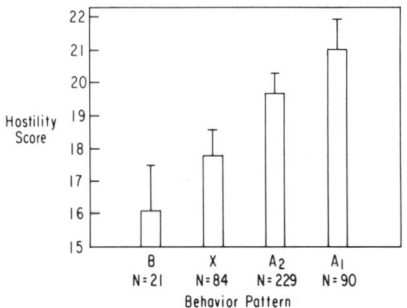

Figure 1 Relationship between scores on the Cook and Medley (1954) Hostility Scale and Type A behavior as assessed by the Structured Interview in patients referred for diagnostic coronary angiography. (Based on data from Williams et al., 1980).

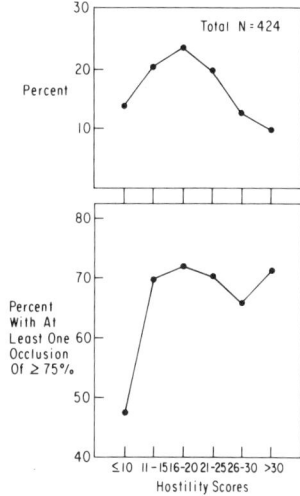

Figure 2 Relationship between Hostility scores and presence of significant (occlusion of 75% or greater) coronary atherosclerosis. (From Williams et al., 1980).

This association between Ho score and Type A behavior provides some support for the construct validity of the Ho scale. Additional support comes from the correlation of 0.59 ($p < 0.0001$) between Ho scores and scores on Spielberger's (Spielberger, Jacobs, Russell and Crane, 1983) Trait Anger Scale. More direct support is provided by a correlation of 0.37 ($p < 0.001$) between Ho scores and behaviorally assessed potential for hostility during the SI among 131 patients in the Duke angiographic sample (Dembroski, MacDougall, Williams, and Haney, Note 2).

In addition to being related to Type A behavior, trait anger and potential for hostility, Ho scores also appear related to the severity of CAD. As illustrated in Figure 2, the relationship between Ho score and prevalence of clinically significant CAD was not linear, but appeared to exhibit a threshold phenomenon; 48% of patients with Ho scores of 10 or less had clinically significant stenosis of at least one coronary artery, whereas, among patients with Ho scores greater than 10, 70% had clinically significant CAD. Thus, in this group of middle-aged patients the prevalence of clinically significant CAD was approximately 1.5 times greater in those with Ho scores higher than 10 as compared to patients with lower scores. Further analysis showed that Type A behavior (SI-assessed), Ho scores and gender were all independently and significantly related to severity of CAD [Figure 3].

It is worth noting, however, that while the significance level of the relation of Ho scores to CAD *increased* from a univariate p-value of 0.02 to a p-value of 0.008 when both gender and Type A were covaried, the significance level of the relation of Type A behavior to CAD decreased from a univariate p-value of 0.01 to a p-value of 0.05 when both gender and Ho score were covaried. A similar decrease in the significance level of the relationship between Type A behavior (SI-assessed) and CAD levels was also observed with statistical adjustment for behaviorally assessed potential for hostility levels. (Dembroski et al., Note 2). These findings suggest that at least some of the variance in prevalence of CAD

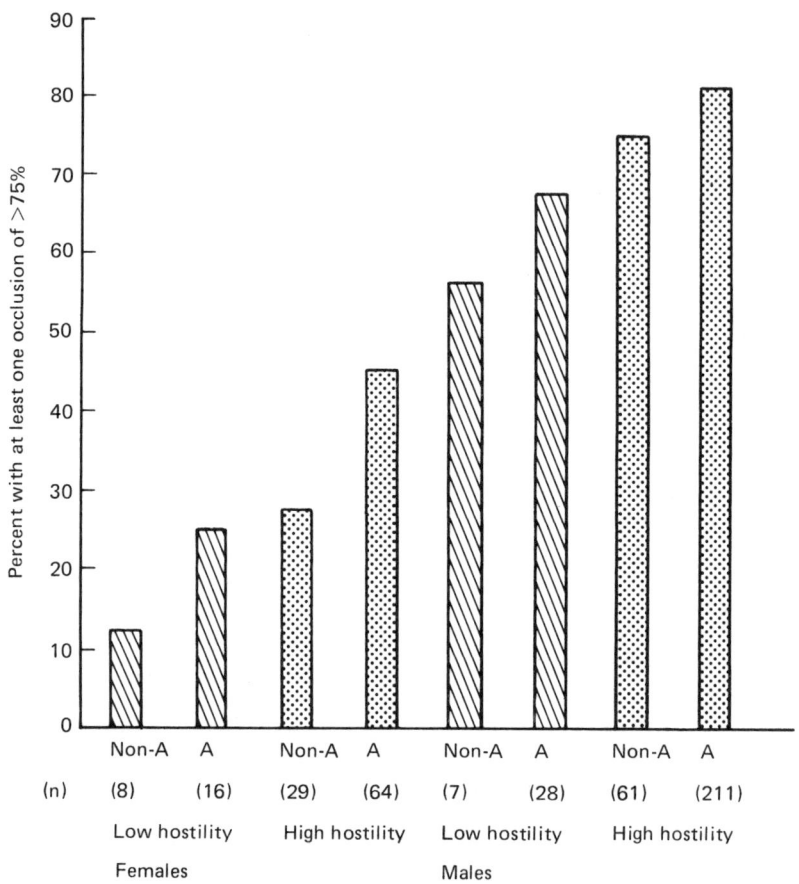

Figure 3 Relationship of Gender, Hostility score and Type A behavior to presence of significant coronary atherosclerosis. (From Williams et al., 1980).

levels associated with Type A behavior is due to the increased Ho levels among Type A patients.

Interpretation of these relationships between hostility and CAD in patients referred for coronary angiography must be qualified by the fact that they are based on concurrent observations in a clinical population with suspected CAD. With respect to the *prospective* relationship between Ho scores and risk of coronary heart disease (CHD), we are fortunate that the Ho scale is based on the MMPI, a psychological test which has been used in previous studies of initially of healthy men whose health status has been followed over periods as long as 25 years after completion of the MMPI.

One such investigation was based on 1877 men in the Western Electric Study. These men, aged 40 to 55 years at time of intake, were employees at the Hawthorne Works of the Western Electric Company in Chicago. They initially completed the MMPI in 1957-58 and again in 1961-62 as part of a larger examination that included blood pressure, cigarette smoking and serum cholesterol. Men continuing in the study were reexamined annually until 1969, primarily to determine the occurrence of new CHD events. The most recent follow up for mortality was carried out in 1978. Following the earlier report of an association between CAD and Ho scores (Williams et al., 1980), Shekelle and colleagues (Shekelle, Gale, Ostfeld and Paul, 1983) used the Western Electric Study to investigate the relationship among Ho scores obtained at the initial examination, subsequent 10-year incidence of CHD, and 20-year mortality;

One important finding was a correlation of 0.84 between Ho scores obtained at the initial examination and again four years later for 1653 men who took the MMPI on both occasions. This suggests that Ho scores may be measuring an unusually stable psychological characteristic, at least in middle-aged men. Another finding (see Figure 4) was that Ho scores were positively associated with increasing age, cigarette smoking and ethanol use. Therefore, these variables, along with systolic blood pressure and serum cholesterol, were included in multivariate analyses to evaluate the independent, prospective relation of Ho scores to risk of CHD and death. Looking first at the 10-year incidence of major coronary events events (myocardial infarction and CHD deaths), higher Ho scores were prospectively associated with increased CHD morbidity (p = 0.004). After adjustment for the variables listed above, the odds of a major CHD event was 1.47 times greater in men with Ho scores greater than 10 compared to men with lower Ho scores. This value is virtually identical to the relative prevalence of clinically significant CAD previously observed by Williams and colleagues (1980). Of equal interest, the shape of the association between level of Ho score and incidence of CHD was nonmonotonic in a manner similar to that noted previously with CAD (see Figure 2). The standardized morbidity ratios for CHD in the Western Electric Study were 0.6, 0.9, 1.5, 1.0, and 0.9, respectively, in the lowest through highest quintiles of the distribution of the Ho score. The cutpoints for these quintiles were 0-8, 9-12, 13-7, 18-23, and 24-44.

The Ho scale was also significantly and positively associated with crude 20-year risk of death from CHD, from malignant neoplasms, and all causes combined (Figure 5). After adjustment for age, cigarette smoking, intake of ethanol, systolic blood pressure, and serum cholesterol level by Cox-type

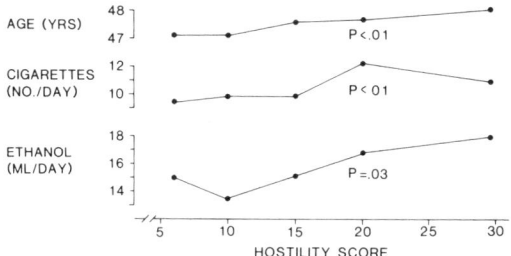

Figure 4 Increasing age, cigarette smoking and ethanol use as a function of Hostility scores in healthy middle-aged men. (Based on data from Shekelle et al., 1983).

20-YEAR MORTALITY,
BY QUINTILE OF MMPI HOSTILITY SCORE,
WESTERN ELECTRIC STUDY, N=1877 MEN

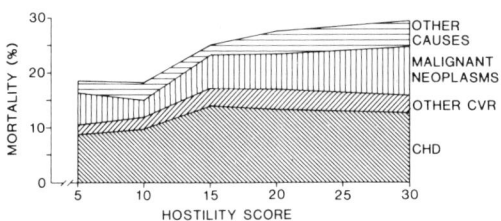

Figure 5 Causes of mortality as a function of Hostility scores in the Western Electric sample. (Based on data from Shekelle et al., 1983).

regression analysis, the Ho scale had a statistically significant (p = 0.001), positive association with 20-year total mortality (Figure 6); a difference of 23 points on the Ho scale, which was the difference between the means of the lowest and higher quintiles, was associated with a 42% increase in the risk of death.

Another opportunity to evaluate the prospective relationship between Ho scores and subsequent morbidity and mortality—in this instance among a younger sample than the Western Electric men—arose when Barefoot, Dahlstrom and Williams (1983) carried out a follow up study of 255 male physicians who had completed the MMPI while in medical school 25 years earlier, when their mean age was 25 years. As in the Shekelle et al. (1983) study, test-retest correlation was remarkably high (.85) among a subsample of 42 students who retook the MMPI one year after the first administration, indicating that the psychological characteristic assessed by the Ho scale is as stable at age 25 as at age 47.

With respect to CHD events over the 25-year follow up period, (Figure 7), men with Ho scores that were at or below the median of 13 experienced a CHD

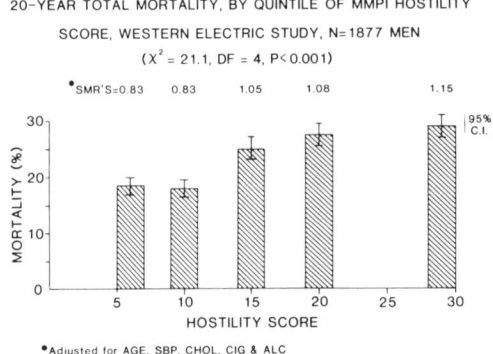

Figure 6 Hostility scores and mortality rates over a 20-year follow up period in healthy middle-aged men. (Based on data from Shekelle et al., 1983).

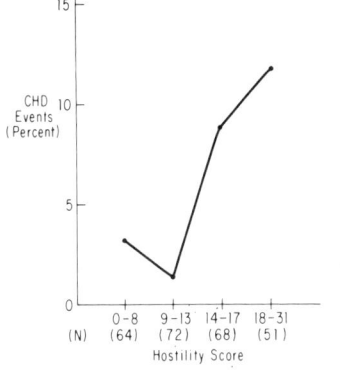

Figure 7 Hostility and coronary heart disease incidence (myocardial infarction or cardiac death) over a 25-year follow up period in 255 physicians who took the MMPI during medical school. (From Barefoot et al., 1983)

incidence (1.5-3%) that was about one-sixth of the incidence (9-12%) observed in men with Ho scores above the median (p < 0.001). A similar curve describes the relationship between Ho scores and total mortality over the 25-year follow-up period. As with the relation of Ho scores to CAD in patients at Duke and to 10-year CHD incidence in the Western Electric study, the shape of the curves relating Ho scores to CHD morbidity and total mortality in this sample of physicians appears to have a "threshold"; with Ho scores up to a certain level–13 in this sample of young men–there was a uniformly low risk of CHD, while above that level the incidence increased rapidly. However, the number of persons in this sample was too small to determine whether or not the level of risk become uniform again at higher levels of Ho.

The most convincing impression of the impact of high Ho scores on subsequent total mortality can be gained by contrasting the survival curve over the 25-year follow up period of those men with initial Ho scores at or below the median with that of those with initial Ho scores above the median (Figure 8). Over the entire 25-year follow up period death came to only 2.2% of those in

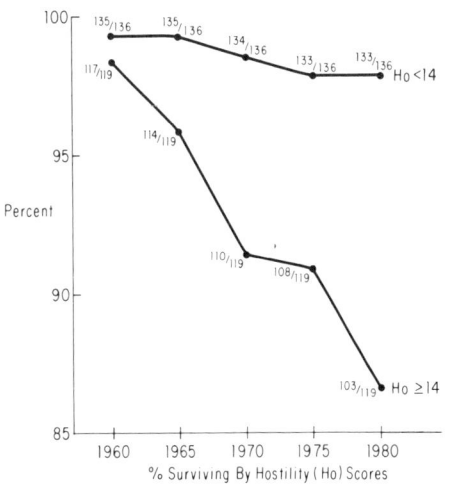

Figure 8 Twenty-five year survival in 136 physicians with Ho scores at or below the median and in 119 physicians with Ho scores above the median on MMPIs completed while they were in medical school. (From Barefoot et al., 1983).

the low Ho group; in marked contrast, 13.4% of those in the high Ho group died. Whereas among middle-aged cardiac patients and Western Electric employees the relative risk of significant CAD or CHD associated with a high Ho score was 1.5, in this sample of healthy young physicians the relative risk of dying in the high versus low Ho group was over 6. Inspection of the survival curve for the high Ho group in Figure 8 suggests one explanation for the lower relative risk associated with a high Ho score among middle-aged persons: by the time middle-age is reached, those who are particularly susceptible to the consequences of high Ho scores will have already died.

What conclusions can we draw from the studies reviewed thus far? First of all, we can have considerable confidence that "something" measured by the Ho scale is in fact associated with a wide range of adverse health consequences. This confidence is based on the observation in three independent studies, one cross-sectional and two prospective, of very reliable associations between high Ho scores and increased prevalence of CAD, increased risk of CHD and increased total mortality over follow up periods of 20-25 years. The similarity of the threshold-type functions relating Ho scores to the various health measures in all three studies further strengthens our conviction that the relationship is real.

Second, with somewhat less confidence, we believe that the "something" being measured by the Ho scale is related to the constructs of hostility and anger and, possibly, aggression, as defined earlier in this chapter. This supposition is based primarily on the evidence cited earlier for the construct validity of the Ho scale, in terms of the strong relationships to Type A, to Spielberger's State Anger scale and to behaviorally assessed potential for hostility in the SI. In addition, it is consistent with some prior findings relating other measures of anger and hostility to adverse health outcomes. Matthews, Glass, Rosenman and Bortner (1977) found that behaviorally rated potential for hostility was the strongest predictor of subsequent CHD events in a subsample of the Western Collaborative Group Study. In the Western Electric Study, results from the Cattell 16PF Questionnaire (Ostfeld et al., 1964) indicated that men who subsequently developed CHD tended to be "more suspicious about the motives of other people." And finally, Harlan, Oberman, Mitchell and Graybiel (1967) found that scores on the Guilford-Zimmerman Temperament Survey that were indicative of an "aggressive personality" were prospectively associated over a 24-year follow up period with increased blood lipid levels among 1,000 naval aviators.

The remarkable stability of Ho scores over periods of one to four years during early adulthood and middle-age suggests that the Ho scale is measuring a rather fundamental psychological characteristic. We have recently completed a principal components factor analysis of the entire MMPI item set in 1500 patients who underwent coronary angiography at Duke (Costa, Zonderman, McCrae and Williams, Note 1). Among the psychometrically valid factors identified was one containing 37 items whose content (e.g., "Most people make friends because friends are likely to be useful to them" and "I have frequently worked under people who seem to have things arranged so that they get credit for good work but are able to pass off mistakes on to those under them") suggested that perhaps a more appropriate label for the psychological construct measured by the Ho scale would be "cynicism."

Also suggesting that cynicism may be the fundamental construct measured by the Ho scale are the results of a replicated split sample principal components factor analysis of the full MMPI that was carried out in a sample of over 11,000 mental health clinic patients by Johsnon, Butcher, Null and Johnson (1983). The third largest factor, in terms of variance explained, after Neuroticism and Psychoticism, contained 20 items and was described by a panel of experienced psychologists as "cynicism." The two cynicism factors emerging from the Costa et al. and the Johnson et al. analyses shared over 50% of items in common. Although there is considerable item overlap between these cynicism scales and the Ho scale, the correlation between them and Ho (above 0.80) is far in excess of that due to item overlap alone.

The fundamental nature of this cynicism characteristic is suggested by its emergence from two independent factor analyses of the full MMPI item set in two quite diverse populations. It is also supported by the central place accorded to early achievement of a sense of basic trust in theories of personality development (Erikson, 1963). Surely, persons in whom this sense of basic trust in others is incompletely developed would be more likely to endorse the type of attitude suggested by the items making up the cynicism scales emerging from these independent studies. Such a lack of basic trust, could also lead to increased hostility. Since these two constructs—hostility and cynicism—are related, further research will be required to determine which label is more accurate.

Nevertheless, the findings point to an attitudinal set (we might even say a rather stable personality trait) consisting of the belief that people in general are selfish, mean and not to be depended upon to treat one well as the fundamental construct which is being assessed by the Ho scale. By implication, it is this psychological characteristic—whether it be termed hostility, cynicism, or lack of basic trust—which is responsible for the adverse health consequences which are so reliably predicted by the Cook and Medley Ho scale.

It now remains to consider the biological mechanisms whereby this psychological characteristic might be translated into pathophysiological processes. While it is possible to describe plausible pathways for these biobehavioral mechanisms, the reader is cautioned that the discussion which follows must be based on a greater level of speculation than has been necessary with respect to the evidence reviewed thus far in this chapter.

HOSTILITY: PATHOPHYSIOLOGICAL MECHANISMS

Based upon a review of a wide range of evidence, Williams (1984) has proposed two major patterns of motor outflow, or physiologic responses, which occur in association with psychosocial environmental challenges. When cognitive appraisal of a given situation results in either a sense of danger or of the need for continuing mental effort to understand or cope with the situation, the pattern of physiological response generated is that which has been described as the "defense reaction," or "fight/flight" response. This pattern is characterized by increased pumping of blood by the heart and by a shunting of this increased cardiac output away from the skin and abdominal viscera to the skeletal musculature. In contrast, where the cognitive appraisal process leads to a decision that the stimuli in the environment are interesting, or that more information about the stimuli is needed, a different pattern ensues. This pattern, which occurs in association with vigilance, or motivated attention to environmental stimuli, is characterized by no change, or even a decrease in cardiac output and by an active vasoconstriction in skeletal muscle.

This hypothesis (that qualitatively distinct patterns of physiological response occur in association with situations requiring defensive or mental work behavior versus those requiring attentive observation of environmental stimuli) was evaluated, along with the associated neuroendocrine response patterns, in a recent study (Williams, Lane, Kuhn, Melosh, White and Schanberg, 1982). Young male subjects were required to perform either a mental arithmetic task (mental work) or a reaction time task (vigilance/sensory intake) while cardiovascular functions were monitored and continuous blood samples were obtained to be assayed for a wide variety of hormones. Responses to the tasks were determined by subtracting baseline levels from levels observed during the tasks. Performance of mental arithmetic was accompanied by an active vasodilation in skeletal muscle, increased heart rate and blood pressure and increased secretion of norepinephrine, epinephrine, cortisol, and prolactin, but *not* of testosterone. In contrast, performance of reaction time tasks was associated with tendency (not significant in this study) to muscle vasoconstriction, and significant increases in norepinephrine and testosterone but *not* in prolactin, epinephrine, and cortisol. Compared to Type B subjects, those subjects characterized as Type A using both the SI and the Jenkins Activity Survey exhibited greater muscle vasodilatation and increases in norepinephrine, epinephrine and cortisol during mental arithmetic, and a greater increase in testosterone during reaction time performance.

Thus, it appears that in situations in which the defense/mental effort response pattern is activated a characteristic response pattern is observed, consisting of increased cardiac output with shunting of blood to skeletal muscle and increased secretion of norepinephrine, epinephrine, cortisol, and prolactin. In contrast, in situations in which vigilant observation of the environmental situation is the outcome of the cognitive appraisal process, the response pattern observed consists of muscle vasoconstriction and increased secretion of norepinephrine and testosterone. Type A persons appear to experience greater arousals of these patterns during specific task performance. How might such excessive cardiovascular and neuroendocrine responses account for the increased CHD risk among Type A and, by implication, hostile/cynical persons?

First of all, being unable to depend upon the good behavior of others and, indeed, being on guard against their bad behavior, the hostile Type A person might be expected to spend a good bit of the waking hours in a state of vigilant observation of others. Since our laboratory study (Williams et al., 1982) suggests that increased secretion of testosterone is one concommitant of such vigilant behavior, it would be expected that cynical persons would excrete more testosterone in their urine during the waking hours (when vigilance would be required) but not while asleep. This prediction was confirmed in a recent study by Zumoff, Rosenfeld, Friedman, Byers, Rosenman and Hellmen (1984) in which Type A men were found to excrete more testosterone in the urine than Type B men during the waking hours but not during the overnight period.

Admittedly, Type A men are characterized by other traits (e.g., time urgency) than hostility/cynicism. But, as reviewed above, it is the hostility/cynicism component which appears most strongly related to their increased CHD risk, and, as we have just hypothesized, it is the hostility/cynicism component which we would expect to be most likely to result (via increased vigilance) in increased testosterone secretion. Supportive of a pathogenic role of testosterone in atherosclerosis is the observation that animal models of atherogenesis are potentiated by administration of exogenous testosterone (Uzunova, Ramey and Ramwell, 1978).

Perhaps even more directly suggestive of testosterone's involvement in human atherosclerosis are the recent observations of increased plasma estradiol levels among male heart attack victims compared to men free of coronary disease (Klaiber et al., 1982; Luria et al., 1982; and Phillips, Castelli, Abbott and McNamara, 1983). Since most of the plasma estradiol in men is derived from testosterone via aromatization (a conversion which is stimulated by norepinephrine), and since Type A men appear to secrete more testosterone and norepinephrine in response to daily challenges, (possibly due to their increased hostility/cynicism), the case is strengthened for a pathogenic role of increased testosterone secretion among hostile/cynical Type A men.

Possibly of equal, if not greater, importance in atherogenesis is the increased secretion of epinephrine and cortisol during the experience of anger, which would be expected to occur with greater frequency and intensity among hostile/cynical persons. Cortisol is known to potentiate both the cardiovascular and metabolic effects of catecholamines, which could accelerate processes involved in endothelial "injury," the most widely accepted model of atherogenesis (Ross and Glomset, 1976). In addition, the administration of corticosteroids has been associated with acceleration of atherosclerosis in patients with rheumatoid arthritis (Kalbak, 1972); and patients with more severe angiographically documented CAD have been found to have higher 9 a.m. cortisol levels than patients with minimal disease (Troxler et al., 1977).

With respect to the possible role of increased levels of hostility/cynicism in other diseases, the evidence from both the Barefoot et al. (1983) and Shekelle et al. (1983) studies is intriguing in that it is suggested that hostility/cynicism predisposes not only to increased risk of coronary disease but to other diseases as well. The increased cancer mortality as a function of higher Ho scores in the Western Electric sample, for example, could be related to the finding by Graves and Thomas (1981) in the Johns Hopkins precursors study that future cancer victims display evidence of a lack of closeness to their parents as well as a relative lack of well-balanced patterns of interaction. These characteristics are attributed to "a linkage to disturbed or otherwise unsatisfactory early human ties." (Graves and Thomas, 1981, p. 224). The same sorts of early experience might also be expected to lead to an incomplete sense of basic trust, and perhaps, increased levels of hostility/cynicism. In view of the growing body of evidence that stress can lead to depression of immune function (Ader, 1982), the same chain of events proposed above for the biological pathways whereby hostility/cynicism might contribute to atherogenesis might also be invoked to explain a contribution to carcinogenesis via effects on immune function that could reduce ability to reject tumors in otherwise susceptible individuals.

Since we would expect hostile/cynical persons both to engage in more vigilance-behavior and to experience more anger in daily life as a result of their hostility/cynicism, the evidence just presented regarding the likely biological correlates of vigilance and anger is strongly suggestive of the existence of biological mechanisms whereby the psychological characteristic of hostility/cynicism *could* be translated into disease processes. While perhaps even highly plausible, the actual participation of these mechanisms in pathogenesis must await further research. Ideally, such research would involve the joint assessment of hostility/cynicism and neuroendocrine responses to both specific laboratory challenges and to the "give and take" of everyday life in several cohorts of young subjects who would then be followed with respect to a variety of disease outcomes. (Although most of the data reviewed has been derived from male samples, undoubtedly at least some of the same mechanisms are relevant to disease processes in women, and studies of female subjects are clearly in order.)

We already know from the studies cited that whatever is being measured by the Ho scale is very reliably predictive of increased rates of developing a wide variety of diseases. It now remains to identify the biological mechanisms responsible for this relationship. Hopefully, the data reviewed and the speculations contained herein will stimulate and guide others toward this end. Ultimately, it is likely that knowledge of the mechanisms responsible for the observed prospective associations will prove most effective in helping to identify the most specific, effective and efficient preventive measures.

REFERENCES

Ader, R. *Psychoneuroimmunology.* New York: Academic, 1982.
Barefoot, J. C., Dahlstrom, G., & Williams, R. B. Hostility, CHD incidence, and total mortality: A 25-year follow-up study of 255 physicians. *Psychosomatic Medicine,* 1983, *45,* 59-63.
Blumenthal, J. A., Williams, R. B., Kong, Y., Schanberg, S. M., & Thompson, L. W. Type A behavior pattern and coronary atherosclerosis. *Circulation,* 1978, *58,* 634-639.
Cook, W. W., & Medley, D. M. Proposed hostility and pharisaic-virtue scales for the MMPI. *Journal of Applied Psychology,* 1954, *38,* 414-418.
Erikson, E. H. *Childhood and society.* New York: Norton, 1963.
Graves, P. L., & Thomas, C. B. Themes of interaction in medical student's Rorschach responses as predictors of mid-life health or disease. *Psychosomatic Medicine,* 1981, *43,* 215-226.
Harlan, W. R., Oberman, A., Mitchell, R. E., & Graybiel, A. Constitutional and environmental factors related to serum-lipid and lipoprotein levels. *Annals of Internal Medicine,* 1967, *66,* 540-555.
Johnson, J. H., Butcher, J. N., Null, C., & Johnson, K. N. A replicated item level factor analysis of the MMPI. *Journal of Personality and Social Psychology,* 1983, *47,* 105-114.
Kalbak, K. Incidence of atherosclerosis in patients with rheumatoid arthritis receiving long-term corticosteroid therapy. *Annals of Rheumatic Disease,* 1972, *31,* 196-200.
Klaiber, E. L., Broverman, D. M., Haffajee, C. I. et al. Serum-estrogen levels in men with acute myocardial infarction. *The American Journal of Medicine,* 1982, *73,* 872-881.
Luria, M. H., Johnson, M. W., Pego, R. et al. Relationship between sex hormones, myocardial infarction, and occlusive coronary disease. *Archives of Internal Medicine,* 1982, *142,* 42-44.
Matthews, K. A., Glass, D. C., Rosenmann, R. H., & Bortner, R. W. Competitive drive, Pattern A, and coronary heart disease: A further analysis of some data from the Western Collaborative Group Study. *Journal of Chronic Disease,* 1977, *30,* 489-498.
Ostfeld, A. M., Lebovits, B. Z., Shekelle, R. B., & Paul, O. A prospective study of the relationship between personality and coronary heart disease. *Journal of Chronic Disease,* 1964, *17,* 265-276.
Phillips, G. B., Kastelli, W. P., Abbott, R. D., and McNamara, P. M. Association of hyperestrogenemia and coronary heart disease in men in the Framingham cohort. *The American Journal of Medicine,* 1983, *74,* 863-869.
Review Panel on Coronary-Prone Behavior and Coronary Heart Disease. Coronary-Prone Behavior and Coronary Heart Disease: A Critical Review. *Circulation,* 1981, *63,* 1199-1215.

Rosenman, R. H. The interview method of assessment of the coronary-prone behavior pattern. In T. M. Dembroski, S. M. Weiss, J. L. Shields, et al. (Eds.), *Coronary-prone behavior.* New York: Springer-Verlag, 1978.

Rosenman, R. H., Friedman, M., Strauss, R., et al. A predictive study of coronary heart disease: The Western Collaborative Group Study. *Journal of the American Medical Association,* 1964, *189,* 15–22.

Ross, R., & Glomset, J. A. The pathogenesis of atherosclerosis. *New England Journal of Medicine,* 1976, *295,* 369–377, 420–425.

Shekelle, R. B., Gayle, M., Ostfeld, A. M., & Paul, O. Hostility, risk of coronary heart disease, and mortality. *Psychosomatic Medicine,* 1983, *45,* 109–114.

Spielberger, C. D., Jacobs, G. A., Russell, S., & Crane, R. S. Assessment of anger: The state-trait anger scale. In J. N. Butcher, & C. D. Spielberger (Eds.), *Advances in personality assessment,* (Vol. 2), Hillsdale, N.J.: Earlbaum, 1983.

Troxler, R. G., Sprague, E. A., Albanese, R. A. et al. The association of elevated plasma cortisol and early atherosclerosis as demonstrated by coronary angiography. *Atherosclerosis,* 1977, *26,* 151–162.

Williams, R. B. Neuroendocrine response patterns and stress: Biobehavioral mechanisms of disease. In R. B. Williams (Ed.), *Perspectives on behavioral medicine: Neuroendocrine control and behavior.* New York: Academic, in press.

Williams, R. B., Haney, T. L., Lee, K. L., Kong, Y., Blumenthal, J. A., & Whalen, R. E. Type A behavior, hostility, and atherosclerosis. *Psychosomatic Medicine,* 1980, *42,* 539–549.

Williams, R. B., Lane, J. D., Kuhn, C. M. et al. Type A behavior and elevated physiological and neuroendocrine responses to cognitive tasks. *Science,* 1982, *218,* 483–485.

Zumoff, B., Rosenfeld, R. S., Friedman, M. et al. Elevated day-time urinary excretion of testosterone glucuronide in men with the Type A behavior pattern. *Psychosomatic Medicine,* 1983, *40,* 223–226.

REFERENCE NOTES

1. Costa, P. T., Zonderman, A. B., McCrae, R. R., & Williams, R. B. Content and comprehensiveness in the MMPI: An item factor analysis in a normal adult sample. *Journal of Personality and Social Psychology,* in press.

2. Dembroski, T. M., MacDougall, J. M., Williams, R. B. et al. Components of Type A, Hostility, and Anger-In: Relationship of Angiographic Findings. *Psychosomatic Medicine,* in press.

10
An Animal Model of Coronary-Prone Behavior

Stephen B. Manuck
University of Pittsburgh

Jay R. Kaplan and Thomas B. Clarkson
Wake Forest University

It is now well-established that behavioral factors are related significantly to the appearance of clinical manifestations of coronary heart disease (CHD). Most extensively investigated in this regard is the Type A, or coronary-prone behavior pattern. Type A individuals are characterized by an intense, hard-driving competitiveness, a persistent sense of time urgency, and easily evoked hostility; a contrasting and, hence, more placid Type B pattern is typically defined by the relative absence of Type A attributes. Retrospective and prospective studies reveal that Type A individuals carry an appreciably greater risk of developing CHD, are more likely to suffer a fatal myocardial infarction, and, among survivors of an initial heart attack, are more susceptible to reinfarction than persons of the Type B pattern (Brand, 1978; Roseman, Brand, Jenkins et al., 1975; Zyzanski, 1978). Additionally, among the various components of Pattern A, a high "potential for hostility" appears to be particularly salient and predictive of CHD, even when assessed apart from the overall Type A construct (Barefoot, Dahlstrom & Williams, 1983). Though available data are somewhat mixed (Dimsdale, Jackett, Hutter, & Black, 1980; Scherwitz, McKelvain, Laman, Patterson, Dutton, Yusim, Lester, Kraft, Rochelle, Leachman, 1983), several investigators also report finding significant relationships between these behavioral characteristics—Type A, hostility—and extent of coronary artery atherosclerosis, both at autopsy (Friedman, Rosenman, Straus, Wurm, & Kositchek, 1968) and on angiographic examination (Frank, Heller, Kornfeld, Sporn, & Weiss, 1978; Williams, Haney, Kong, Blumenthal, & Whalen, 1980; Zyzanski, Jenkins, Ryan, Plessas, & Everist, 1976). Finally, Type A behavior seems to exert a pathogenic influence which is largely independent of effects associated with more "traditional" risk factors, such as serum cholesterol concentration, smoking, blood pressure, and age (Brand, 1978).

What exact role behavior may play in the pathogenesis of atherosclerotic lesions, however, remains unclear. Studies based on examination of angiographic records in selected patient populations are necessarily retrospective, and even

---

Research described here was supported, in part, by grants from the National Heart, Lung and Blood Institute (HL14164, R01 HL26561) and the R. J. Reynolds Industries, Inc.

here, ethical and practical considerations preclude collecting control data from random samples of demographically comparable, asymptomatic individuals. Since significant coronary artery atherosclerosis usually develops over a span of years or decades, any adequate longitudinal investigation with human subjects must also include observations carried out over protracted intervals. For these reasons, we have recently attempted to develop a suitable animal model for examining psychosocial influences on atherogenesis. Among the advantages of studying animals are, of course, the greater experimental control afforded the investigator, and the possibility of creating conditions that accelerate the disease process. In addition, the use of animals permits pathologic observations to be made which are not feasible in *in vivo* studies involving human beings.

We believe that animal models may be useful, not only for studying aspects of lesion development, but also in elucidating the behavioral processes implicated in coronary disease. For example, the Type A construct in human research owes as much to environment and social context as it does to the behavioral characteristics of individuals (Chesney & Rosenman, 1980). Thus, Pattern A is generally defined not as a peronality "trait" but as a constellation of overt behaviors which are exhibited by susceptible individuals when encountering conditions of sufficient challenge or threat (Friedman, 1969; Glass, 1977). Some people may therefore have the appropriate (Type A) predisposition, yet not engage in Type A behaviors—or suffer their consequences—because situational demands or stress are absent. The interaction of behavioral and environmental variables implicit in this definition, however, has not been examined in epidemiologic studies of the Type A-CHD association (Kasl, 1978). Indeed, doing so would require a longitudinal investigation incorporating frequent and detailed assessments of socio-environmental variables (e.g., ongoing life events).

In an animal model, on the other hand, the social environment may be experimentally manipulated and the effects such manipulations analyzed for individual differences in behavioral response (Henry & Stephens, 1977). This is the strategy we have applied in our own work, and in the present chapter we describe results of a recent study examining the influences of stress and social status (environmental and idiosyncratic behavioral characteristics, respectively) on the development of coronary artery atherosclerosis in groups of adult male cynomolgus monkeys (*Macaca fascicularis*) (Kaplan, Manuck, Clarkson, Lusso, & Taub, 1982).

From a behavioral perspective, the value of focusing on non-human primates is readily apparent. Like human beings, other primates live in social groups and solve the recurring problems of life—from reproduction to defense—within a framework of social bonds. Moreover, relationships among individual animals are extremely important in maintaining the stability of primate social groups. Field research of the past several decades has documented the great complexity of primate organization, which encompasses a variety of relational axes such as mother-infant and male-female social bonds, matrifocal sub-units and, of course, dominance hierarchies (Lancaster, 1975). In view of the diverse ecologic niches inhabited by primates, it is not surprising that the specifics of primate behavior also vary widely among species. Between free-ranging rhesus (*Macaca mulatta*), patas (*Erythrocebus patas*), and vervet (*Cercopithecus aethiops*) monkeys, for example, there exist significant differences in typical patterns of agonistic display, as well as in relative rates of affiliative grooming (Kaplan, 1980). These differences aside, however, the common theme of primate life is one of undeniable sociality.

EXPERIMENTAL PROCEDURES

Certain behavioral factors (e.g., crowding, conditions of handling, social perturbations) have previously been found related to development of a variety of arterial lesions in rabbits, mice, birds and swine (Henry & Stephens, 1977; Nerem, Levesque & Cornhill, 1980; Ratcliffe, Yerasimides & Elliot, 1960; Ratcliffe, Luginbuhl, Schnarr & Chacko, 1969). The relevance of these findings to the psychosocial precursors of CHD in human beings is unclear, however, as is the correspondence of arterial changes seen in non-primate models to the characteristics of atherosclerostic lesions in man. The nature of atherosclerosis is highly variable, even among the numerous species of primates. In some species, for example, lesions seldom progress beyond fatty streaks, though in others, fibrous plaques occur quite like those observed in human beings.

The species selected for study here, *M. fascicularis,* is perhaps the most useful of all the macaques in atherosclerosis research. Given an appropriate diet (in the presence of a moderate hypercholesterolemia), cynomolgus monkeys are highly susceptible to development of fatty streaks. These lesions readily progress to fibromuscular plaques, with frequent evidence of necrosis, mineralization, and the pooling of fat droplets or crystalline lipid. Cynomolgus macaques suffer clinical complications in the form of myocardial infarctions more often than do other primate species (Armstrong, Trillo & Prichard, 1980; Clarkson, 1980).

For the purposes of our study, thirty monkeys—all adult feral males—were imported from Malaysia and the Philippine Islands. These animals were housed together in social groups of five members each and fed a moderately atherogenic diet for 22 months. The test diet used was designed to mimic the proportion of calories consumed as saturated fat and cholesterol that is considered usual for urban, North American males (43 percent of calories were present as fat; cholesterol concentration was 0.34 mg cholesterol/Cal., or equivalent to the consumption of about 680 mg cholesterol/day by a human being). At the end of the 22-month experiment, all monkeys were terminated, and the extent and severity of coronary artery atherosclerosis was assessed in each of the study animals.

The primary experimental manipulation employed in this study was suggested by the observation that the introduction of strangers into macaque groups often produces marked social disruption (Bernstein, Gordon & Rose, 1974). The sudden appearance of unfamiliar monkeys poses a threat to existing associations among animals, and, hence, is followed by active attempts to redefine hierarchical, or dominance, relationships, as well as affiliative coalitions. Predictably, such disturbances are accompanied by an intensification of agonistic encounters, and, in particular, by an increased likelihood of direct, or contact, aggression (e.g., hitting, biting, grabbing). To provide a significantly stressful social environment for the present investigation, fifteen animals—those housed in three of the six social groups—were reorganized on a regular basis by redistributing monkeys among the affected groups. This was carried out on a schedule permitting each monkey to be housed with either three or four new animals on every reorganization. Procedurally, the redistribution of monkeys took place once every twelve weeks in the first year of the study, and once every four weeks thereafter. To further increase competition and social uncertainty among these animals, an estrogen-implanted, ovariectomized female was also placed into each of the stressed groups for half of each successive four-week period occurring during the final ten months of the study. Finally, animals assigned to the periodically reorganized groups were designated, for convenience, the *unstable social condition*. The remaining fifteen monkeys were housed in groups of fixed memberships over the entire 22 months of the experiment. These monkeys were thus never exposed to strangers, nor were females introduced as an added source of intra-group competition. Appropriately, these three groups were referred to collectively as the *stable social condition*.

BEHAVIORAL OBSERVATIONS

In order to examine the behavioral effects of our experimental stressor, psychosocial observations were made on each animal on numerous occasions over the course of the study. Fortunately, the behavioral repertoire of macaques is well established, with most social acts classifiable as either aggression, submission, or affiliation, and each behavior characterized by a relatively stereotyped—hence identifiable—motor pattern (e.g., open-mouth threat, lip smack, present, groom) (Sade, 1973; VanHooff, 1969; Wickler, 1969). Technicians recorded the occurrence of each of 21 such behaviors using a focal sampling technique (Altmann, 1974), in conjunction with an electronic data collection device. The focal samples were each 15 minutes long, and 210 samples (or more than 50 hours of observation) were obtained on every monkey during the experiment. All data were transmitted from the recording instruments to a laboratory computer as they were collected and then tabulated by behavior and by animal into matrices of communication (e.g., grooming, aggression, submission, body contact). Rates of performance of specific behaviors were calculated on an "incidents per monkey, per hour" basis, and in the case of certain affiliative acts (viz., passive body contact, sitting alone), as a "percentage of total time" spent in these activities. With respect to agonistic displays, a ratio of aggressive to submissive acts was also computed for each monkey. An overall index identifying the interaction pattern of the animal as either more aggressive or more submissive was based on the more prevalent behavior. A second index reflected the directionality of affiliative interactions and was calculated as a ratio of the frequency with which an animal groomed others to the frequency with which it was itself groomed.

Because status relationships influence the social structure and behavior of macaques, social dominance also represented a primary variable of interest in this experiment. Basically, macaque social groups may be characterized by linear dominance hierarchies, in which the status or rank of an individual animal derives from its ability to defeat other group members in fights (Bernstein, 1970; Sade, 1967; Kawai, 1958). Dominance determinations are, in turn, facilitated among macaques by the fact that such relationships tend to be transitive; that is, if monkey A is dominant to B, and B dominant to C, then A is usually also dominant to C (Sade, 1967). For purposes of the present study, social status assessment was based on outcomes of an animal's aggressive encounters with each of the other monkeys housed within the same social group. Monkeys retaining a high order rank (i.e., judged first or second in their groups) across the majority of social evaluations made over a 20-month period of observation were designated dominant animals in the experiment; the remaining monkeys were identified as subordinates. Interestingly, the relative dominance of individual monkeys remained relatively constant over time, despite the fact that, in the unstable social condition group, memberships were subject to repeated reorganization.

The specific behaviors of dominant and subordinate monkeys in the two experimental conditions differed substantially. First, as expected, dominant animals in the unstable groups tended to show a greater frequency of contact aggression, compared to dominant monkeys assigned to the stable social condition. Among subordinate animals, moreover, those in unstable groups exhibited somewhat higher rates of extreme submission (e.g., fleeing, cowering, grimacing) than did their unstressed (i.e., stable) counterparts. Hence, redistribution of animals in the unstable social condition accentuated agonistic interactions, thereby increasing the frequency of overt fights and, in subordinate monkeys, leading to a more definitive signaling of submission.

Affiliative associations between dominant and subordinate animals also varied significantly between the two experimental conditions. Most notably, in the unstable social groups, dominant monkeys were groomed more frequently than they groomed others, while subordinates groomed other animals more frequently than they were themselves groomed. Grooming relationships in the stable condition also tended to be asymmetric in relation to social status, yet here the direction of the asymmetry was reversed. Although the interpretation of this result is not entirely clear, grooming behavior may represent both an affiliative gesture and, in certain circumstances, an act of appeasement (Seyfarth, 1977; Sparks, 1969). As appeasement, for instance, grooming may serve to alleviate tension among animals housed in stressful social environments that permit little or no avenue for escape. In the unstable groups in this experiment, moreover, grooming may have had instrumental value for subordinate monkeys by allowing them to maintain a non-threatening proximity to dominant animals, and thus retain access to needed resources of food and water.

PATHOLOGIC OBSERVATIONS

The purpose of this experiment was to examine psychosocial influences on the development of atherosclerosis. At the time of necropsy, the thorax of each animal was opened, the heart was then removed, and the coronary arteries perfused with 10 percent neutral buffered formalin at a pressure of 100 mm Hg. After pressure fixation, 15 tissue blocks (each 3 mm in length) were cut perpendicular to the long axis of the coronary arteries. Five of these were serial blocks obtained from the left circumflex, five from the left anterior descending, and five from the right coronary artery. Sections cut from each block were stained with either hematoxylin and eosin or Verhoeff Van Gieson stains. When each of the Verhoeff Van Gieson-stained sections was projected, the area occupied by intima and/or intimal lesion (i.e., the area between the internal elastic lamina and the lumen of the artery) was measured using a *Zeiss* MOP III Image Analyzer. The extent of coronary artery atherosclerosis was then expressed for each animal as the mean intimal area (in mm^2) of 15 sections of coronary artery.

Because two monkeys died during the course of the study, our results are based on 28 animals—six dominant and nine subordinate monkeys in the unstable social condition, and seven dominants and six subordinates in the stable condition. In Table 1, mean intimal areas (±SEM) of monkeys belonging to each of the four groups are presented. For purposes of analysis, a 2-by-2 [Conditions (unstable, stable)-by-Status (dominant, subordinate)] analysis of variance was performed on these data.[1] Although results revealed no overall effects for either the Conditions or Status factors when each was considered alone, this analysis did yield a significant Conditions-by-Status interaction term (p = 0.034). Comparisons between group means further demonstrated that dominant animals housed in the unstable groups had significantly greater atherosclerosis than dominant monkeys from the stable social condition; they also differed significantly from subordinate animals assigned to similar (i.e., unstable) social groups. Parallel analyses based on a second measure of atherosclerosis—lumen stenosis (the ratio of intimal area to total area within the internal elastic lamina) likewise revealed a reliable Conditions-by-Status interation (p = 0.003), with dominant monkeys in the unstable condition again showing the greatest degree of lesion.

For illustration, photomicrographs of sections of left circumflex coronary artery in four monkeys, one animal each from the four groups, are reproduced in Figure 1. The photomicrographs shown were selected to depict the average extent of intimal plaque of the group from which each of these animals was selected. Altogether, the intimal lesions observed here involved numerous foam cells, extracellular lipid, increased collagen and elastin, and occasional mineralization. Medial changes were similar to those found in macaques under comparable dietary conditions, and differences between groups appeared to be quantitative rather than qualitative.

Throughout the experiment, several other physiologic variables of relevance to atherosclerosis were measured at frequent intervals. These included total serum cholesterol (TSC) and high density lipoprotein cholesterol (HDLC) concentrations, systolic and diastolic blood pressures, fasting glucose concentration, and ponderosity. Among these variables, only TSC and HDLC concentrations were

[1] This analysis was performed after an initial data transformation of the form $X' = \sqrt{X} + \sqrt{X + 1}$, as recommended by Sokol and Rohlf (1981) and Freeman and Tukey (1950).

Table 1 Mean coronary artery intimal area measurements (± SEM) among dominant and subordinate monkeys in the stable and unstable social conditions

	Social status	
Social condition	Dominant	Subordinate
Stable	0.32 mm^2 (± 0.13)	0.45 mm^2 (± 0.12)
Unstable	0.74 mm^2 (± 0.12)	0.38 mm^2 (± 0.10)

Kaplan et al., 1982, p. 363. Reprinted by permission of the American Heart Association, Inc.

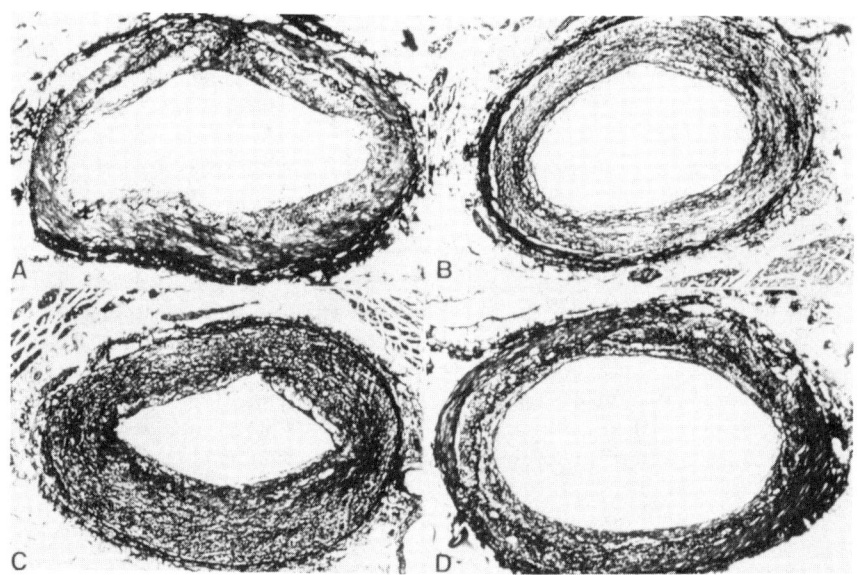

Figure 1 Photomicrographs of sections of left circumflex coronary arteries representing the mean intimal area measured in the socially stable dominant (A), stable subordinate (B), unstable dominant (C), and unstable subordinate (D) groups. All photomicrographs are of paraffin sections stained by the Verhoeff Van Geison method. ×40. Kaplan et al., 1982, p. 364. Reprinted by permission of the American Heart Association, Inc.

significantly related, for all animals, to the degree of atherosclerosis. These lipid effects, however, did not explain the strong behavioral influences on development of coronary lesions. Their statistical independence was demonstrated by re-examination of measurements of intimal area and lumen stenosis using analysis of covariance, with TSC and HDLC entered as covariates; each of these analyses showed, again, a significant Conditions-by-Status interaction term (intimal area: $p = 0.038$; lumen stenosis: $p = 0.004$).

INDIVIDUAL DIFFERENCES IN CARDIAC RESPONSIVITY TO STRESS

Several investigators have recently suggested that recurrent activation of the sympathetic nervous system—like that occurring on elicitation of the so-called "defense reaction"—may promote arterial lesions through accompanying hemodynamic disruptions (e.g., turbulence, sheer stress) (Williams, 1978) or by the influence of circulating catecholamines on lipid metabolism and platelet aggregation (Haft, 1974; Herd, 1981). This line of speculation is also encouraged by two findings frequently reported among studies involving human beings: (a) that individuals vary markedly in their sympathetic responsivity to behavioral stimuli (Manuck & Garland, 1980; McCubbin, Richardson, Langer, Kizer, & Obrist, 1983); and (b) that when exposed to common laboratory stressors, persons behaviorally disposed to CHD exhibit more extensive cardiovascular and catecholamine reactions than do their non-coronary prone, Type B counterparts (Corse,

Manuck, Cantwell, Giordani, & Matthews, 1982; Dembroski, MacDougall, Shields, Petitto, & Lushene, 1978; Friedman, Byers, Diamant, Rosenman, 1975; Glass, Krakoff, Contrada, Hilton, Kehoe, Mannucci, Collins, Snow, & Elting, 1980; Manuck, Craft & Gold, 1978; Williams, Lane, Kuhn, Melosh, White, & Schanberg, 1982).

In an attempted extention of these investigations, the present study further examined relationships between individual differences in behaviorally-elicited cardiac responsivity and severity of atherosclerosis in the coronary arteries (Manuck, Kaplan & Clarkson, 1983). We considered these observations to be of an exploratory nature, however, and wish to emphasize that the psychophysiologic measurements described below are based on somewhat less than our total sample of experimental animals and were obtained at a time near the completion of the overall study.

Procedurally, 26 monkeys were first anesthetized and fitted with small EKG telemetry devices. The heart rates of these animals were then recorded by a portable cardiac monitor under both baseline and stressed conditions. Baseline, or resting, heart rate measurements were taken on a day following the animals' recovery from anesthesia and during a period of relative quiet. Stress-period heart rate measurements were obtained, in contrast, on a subsequent day during the presentation of a laboratory challenge involving threatened capture of the animals. These threats resulted in a mean heart rate acceleration of greater than 90 beats-per-minute across all animals, or an increase in heart rate about 72 percent above resting levels. As with human subjects, the data from individual monkeys differed greatly, permitting identification of clearly differentiated groups of high and low heart rate reactive animals. It was also found that such idiosyncratic reactivity, in monkeys, represents a stable individual characteristic (i.e., is reproducible on retesting) and "generalizes" to other conditions of measurement.

More importantly, those animals identified as *high* heart rate reactors were later found to have developed nearly twice the extent of coronary artery atherosclerosis that *low* heart rate reactive monkeys developed ($p < .05$). This effect was not due to concomitant differences in blood pressure, resting heart rate, body weight or serum lipid concentrations, although HDLC did comprise a slightly smaller fraction of the total cholesterol of high, relative to low, heart rate "reactors." Behaviorally, overt acts of aggression (as observed over the course of the study) were more frequent in high heart rate reactive monkeys, though dominant status per se was not significantly related to the animals' relative heart rate reactivity. The fact that dominant animals in the unstable social condition were not disproportionately represented as high reactive monkeys indicates that differences in heart rate reactivity to our standard laboratory stressor cannot "explain" the interaction of social dominance and environmental stress on lesion development seen in this experiment. Because our heart findings do provide initial support for the hypothesis that a psychophysiologic hyperreactivity under stress may be implicated in atherogenesis, however, it remains plausible that the autonomic events associated with significant psychosocial adjustments may similarly mediate the influences of other behavioral variables on the development of atherosclerosis.

CONCLUDING COMMENTS

Our overall results indicate that for male cynomolgus monkeys fed a moderately atherogenic diet, frequent reorganization of social groups (an experimental stressor) led to an increased severity of coronary artery atherosclerosis, but only for certain experimental animals—namely, those tending to retain dominant social status throughout the study. It is noteworthy that the social behaviors of dominant monkeys assigned to the unstable and stable conditions differed appreciably, as evidenced by the more frequent bouts of contact aggression and the disruption of affiliative bonds (reflected in grooming relationships) in the unstable groups. These results support the hypotheses derived from the study of coronary-prone behaviors in human beings which suggest that the behavioral attributes of individuals (Pattern A) may confer an increased risk for CHD only when in relation to accompanying socio-environmental conditions (e.g., under stress). Also, consistent with epidemiologic evidence pertaining to the Type A-CHD association in humans, the effects of behavioral factors on lesion development in this experiment could not be attributed to the influences of other variables commonly associated with atherosclerosis (e.g., blood pressure and serum lipids).

In this first study, then, we believe we have had some success in developing an appropriate animal model—at least on behavioral and pathologic grounds—for the study of psychosocial parameters in atherogenesis. Of course, the strength of any animal model lies in its ability to test hypotheses which are either difficult to pursue, or ethically precluded, in human research. In subsequent investigations, we hope to better address questions of a "mechanistic" nature concerning biobehavioral relationships in cardiovascular disease. Certainly, issues pertaining to the role of dietary factors or of possible mediating variables, such as autonomic and hormonal responses to stress, may be more closely examined, as well as manipulated experimentally, in studies of similar design. In our most recently completed work, for example, we have observed that behavioral factors potentiate atherogenesis even in the absence of hypercholesterolemia (Kaplan, Manuck, Clarkson et al., 1983). Previously, only arterial hypertension and immunologic injury to arteries were thought to promote atherogenesis in normocholesterolemic monkeys (McGill, Frank & Geer, 1961; Minick, Murphy & Campbell, 1966; Clarkson & Alexander, 1980). This finding is, therefore, of potential importance because it may help to further explain how significant lesions develop in human beings who exhibit normal, and even low, serum lipid concentrations. Finally, beyond questions related directly to disease processes, such experiments provide an opportunity to examine, under well-controlled conditions, the effects of psychosocial perturbations on important aspects of primate social behavior. Ultimately, we may also gain a greater understanding of the relatioship between environmental demands and the behavioral responses of individuals.

REFERENCES

Altmann, J. Observational study of behavior: Sampling methods. *Behaviour,* 1974, *48,* 1-41.
Armstrong, M. L., Trillo, A., & Prichard, R. W. Naturally occurring and experimentally

induced atherosclerosis in nonhuman primates. In S. S. Kalter (Ed.), *The use of nonhuman primates in cardioavscular disease.* Austin: University of Texas Press, 1980.
Barefoot, J. C., Dahlstrom, W. G., & Williams, R. B. Hostility, CHD incidence, and total mortality: A 25-year follow-up of 255 physicians. *Psychosomatic Medicine,* 1983, *45,* 59-63.
Bernstein, I. S. Primate status hierarchies. In L. A. Rosenblum (Ed.), *Primate behavior: Developments in field and laboratory research* (Vol. 1). New York: Academic, 1970.
Bernstein, I. S., Gordon, T. P., & Rose, R. M. Aggression and social controls in rhesus monkeys (*Macaca mulatta*) groups revealed in group formation studies. *Folia Primatologia,* 1974, *21,* 81-107.
Brand, R. J. Coronary-prone behavior as an independent risk factor for coronary heart disease. In T. M. Dembroski, S. M. Weiss, J. L. Shields, S. G. Haynes, & M. Feinleib (Eds.), *Coronary-prone behavior.* New York: Springer-Verlag, 1978.
Chesney, M. A., & Rosenman, R. H. Type A behaviour in the work setting. In C. L. Cooper & R. Payne (Eds.), *Current concerns in occupational stress.* New York: Wiley, 1980.
Clarkson, T. B. Symposium summary. In S. S. Kalter (Ed.), *The use of nonhuman primates in cardiovascular diseases.* Austin: University of Texas Press, 1980.
Clarkson, T. B., & Alexander, N. J. Long-term vasectomy. Effects on the occurrence and extent of atherosclerosis in rhesus monkeys. *Journal of Clinical Investigation,* 1980, *65,* 15-25.
Corse, C. D., Manuck, S. B., Cantwell, J. D., Giordani, B., & Matthews, K. A. Coronary-prone behavior pattern and cardiovascular response in persons with and without coronary heart disease. *Psychosomatic Medicine,* 1982, *44,* 449-459.
Dembroski, T. M., MacDougall, J. M., Shields, J. L., Petitto, J., & Lushene, R. Components of the Type A coronary-prone behavior pattern and cardiovascular responses to psychomotor performance challenge. *Journal of Behavioral Medicine,* 1978, *1,* 159-176.
Dimsdale, J. E., Jackett, T. P., Hutter, A. M., & Block, P. C. The risk of Type A mediated coronary disease in different populations. *Psychosomatic Medicine,* 1980, *42,* 55-62.
Frank, K. A., Heller, S. S., Kornfeld, D. S., Sporn, A. A., & Weiss, M. B. Type A behavior pattern and coronary angiographic findings. *Journal of the American Medical Association,* 1978, *240,* 761-763.
Freeman, M. F., & Tukey, J. W. Transformations related to the angular and the square root. *Annals of Mathematical Statistics,* 1950, *21,* 607-611.
Friedman, M. *Pathogenesis of coronary artery disease.* New York: McGraw-Hill, 1969.
Friedman, M., Byers, S. O., Diamant, J., & Rosenman, R. H. Plasma catecholamine response of coronary-prone subjects (Type A) to a specific challenge. *Metabolism,* 1975, *4,* 205-210.
Friedman, M., Rosenman, R. H., Straus, R., Wurm, M., & Kositchek, R. The relationship of behavior pattern A to the state of the coronary vasculature: A study of fifty-one autopsy subjects. *American Journal of Medicine,* 1968, *44,* 525-537.
Glass, D. C. *Behavior patterns, stress and coronary disease.* Hillsdale, N.J.: Erlbaum, 1977.
Glass, D. C., Krakoff, L. R., Contrada, R., Hilton, W. F., Kehoe, K., Mannucci, E. G., Collins, C., Snow, B., & Elting, E. Effect of harassment and competition upon cardiovascular and catecholaminic responses in Type A and Type B individuals. *Psychophysiology,* 1980, *17,* 453-463.
Haft, J. L. Cardiovascular injury induced by sympathetic catecholamines. *Progress in Cardiovascular Disease,* 1974, *17,* 73-86.
Henry, J. P., & Stephens, P. M. *Stress, health, and the social environment.* New York: Springer-Verlag, 1977.
Herd, J. A. Behavioral factors in the physiological mechanisms of cardiovascular disease. In S. M. Weiss, J. A. Herd, & B. H. Fox, (Eds.), *Perspectives on behavioral medicine.* New York: Academic, 1981.
Kaplan, J. R. Biomedical implications of behavioral variability in older world monkeys. In S. S. Kalter (Ed.), *The use of nonhuman primates in cardiovascular diseases.* Austin: University of Texas Press, 1980.
Kaplan, J. R., Manuck, S. B., Clarkson, T. B., Lusso, F. M., & Taub, D. M. Social status, environment, and atherosclerosis in cynomolgus monkeys. *Arteriosclerosis,* 1982, *2,* 359-368.
Kaplan, J. R., Manuck, S. B., Clarkson, T. B., Lusso, F. M., Taub, D. M., & Miller, W. W. Social stress and atherosclerosis in normocholesterolemic monkeys. *Science,* 1983, *220,* 733-735.

Kasl, S. V. Epidemiological contributions to the study of work stress. In C. L. Cooper & R. Payne (Eds.), *Stress at work.* New York: Wiley, 1978.
Kawai, M. On the rank system in a natural group of Japanese macaques. *Primates,* 1958, *1,* 84-98.
Lancaster, J. B. *Primate behavior and the emergence of human culture.* New York: Holt, 1975.
Manuck, S. B., Craft, S., & Gold, K. J. Coronary prone behavior pattern and cardiovascular response. *Psychophysiology,* 1978, *16,* 403-411.
Manuck, S. B., & Garland, F. N. Stability of individual differences in cardiovascular reactivity: A thirteen month follow-up. *Physiology and Behavior,* 1980, *24,* 621-624.
Manuck, S. B., Kaplan, J. R., & Clarkson, T. B. Behaviorally-induced heart rate reactivity and atherosclerosis in cynomolgus monkeys. *Psychosomatic Medicine,* 1983, *45,* 95-108.
McCubbin, J. A., Richardson, J. E., Langer, A. W., Kizer, J. S., & Obrist, P. A. Sympathetic neuronal function and left ventricular performance during behavioral stress in humans: The relationship between plasma catecholamines and systolic time intervals. *Psychophysiology,* 1983, *20,* 102-110.
McGill, H., Frank, M., & Geer, J. Aortic lesions in hypertensive monkeys. *Archives of Pathology,* 1961, *71,* 96-102.
Minick, C., Murphy, G., & Campbell, W. Experimental induction of athero-arteriosclerosis by the synergy of allergic injury to arteries and lipid-rich diet: I. Effect of repeated injections of horse serum in rabbits fed a diet cholesterol supplement. *Journal of Experimental Medicine,* 1966, *124,* 635-652.
Nerem, R. M., Levesque, M. J., & Cornhill, J. F. Social environment as a factor in diet induced atherosclerosis. *Science,* 1980, *208,* 1475-1476.
Ratcliffe, H. L., Luginbuhl, H., Schnarr, W. R., & Chacko, K. Coronary arteriosclerosis in swine: Evidence of a relation to behavior. *Journal of Comparative and Physiological Psychology,* 1969, *68,* 385-392.
Ratcliffe, H. L., Yerasimides, T. G., & Elliot, G. A. Changes in the character and location of arterial lesions in mammals and birds in the Philadelphia Zoological Garden. *Circulation,* 1960, *21,* 730-738.
Rosenman, R. H., Brand, R. J., Jenkins, C. D., Friedman, M., Straus, R., & Wurm, M. Coronary heart disease in the Western Collaborative Group Study: Final follow-up experience of 8½ years. *Journal of the American Medical Association,* 1975, *233,* 872-877.
Sade, D. S. Determinants of dominance in a group of free ranging rhesus monkeys. In S. Altmann (Ed.), *Social communication among primates.* Chicago: University of Chicago Press, 1967.
Sade, D. S. An ethogram for rhesus monkeys. I. Antithetical contrasts in posture and movement. *American Journal of Physical Anthropology,* 1973, *38,* 537-542.
Scherwitz, L., McKelvain, R., Laman, C., Patterson, J., Dutton, L., Yusim, S., Lester, J., Kraft, I., Rochelle, D., & Leachman, R. Type A behavior, self-involvement, and coronary atherosclerosis. *Psychosomatic Medicine,* 1983, *45,* 47-57.
Seyfarth, R. M. A model of social grooming among adult female monkeys. *Journal of Theoretical Biology,* 1977, *65,* 671-698.
Sokol, R., & Rohlf, F. J. *Biometry.* San Francisco: Freeman, 1981.
Sparks, J. Allogrooming in primates: A review. In D. Morris (Ed.), *Primate ethology.* Garden City, N.Y.: Doubleday, 1969.
Van Hooff, J. The facial displays of the catarrhine monkeys and apes. In D. Morris (Ed.), *Primate ethology.* Garden City, N.Y.: Doubleday, 1969.
Wickler, W. Sociosexual signals and their intraspecific imitation among primates. In D. Morris (Ed.), *Primate ethology.* Garden City, N.Y.: Doubleday, 1969.
Williams, R. B. Psychophysiological processes, the coronary-prone behavior pattern, and coronary heart disease. In T. M. Dembroski, S. M. Weiss, J. L. Shields, S. G. Haynes, & M. Feinleib (Eds.), *Coronary-prone behavior.* New York: Springer-Verlag, 1978.
Williams, R. B., Haney, T., Lee, K., Kong, Y., Blumenthal, J., & Whalen, R. Type A behavior, hostility and coronary heart disease. *Psychosomatic Medicine,* 1980, *42,* 539-549.
Williams, R. B., Lane, J. D., Kuhn, C. M., Melosh, W., White, A. D., & Schanberg, S. M. Type A behavior and elevated physiological and neuroendocrine responses to cognitive tasks. *Science,* 1982, *218,* 483-495.

Zyzanski, S. J. Coronary-prone behavior pattern and coronary heart disease: Epidemiological evidence. In T. M. Dembroski, S. M. Weiss, J. L. Shields, S. G. Haynes, & M. Feinleib (Eds.), *Coronary-prone behavior.* New York: Springer-Verlag, 1978.

Zyzanski, S. J., Jenkins, C. D., Ryan, T. J., Plessas, A., & Everist, M. Psychological correlates of coronary angiographic findings. *Archives of Internal Medicine,* 1976, *136,* 1234–1237.

III

INTERVENTIONS

The evidence relating anger and hostility to cardiovascular disease, as well as behavioral disorders, has focused attention on the efficacy of biobehavioral interventions aimed at reducing anger and modifying hostility. The chapters in this section discuss various approaches to anger management from the perspective of their applicability to behavioral medicine and to cardiovascular risk reduction.

In "Anger and Its Therapeutic Regulation," Raymond Novaco reviews the clinical intervention programs that have been designed to modify anger and aggression. Psychotherapy for anger and aggression spanned the twentieth century, receiving a boost in the late 1930s when psychosomatic medicine recognized the role played by anger in physical disorders, such as hypertension. Novaco points out, however, that systematic outcome research is a recent development that has accompanied those anger treatments that are focused on behavioral and cognitive-behavioral orientations. He reviews behavioral treatments that train patients in relaxation and assertive behavior as alternative, arousal reducing responses to anger provocation. These treatments also involve teaching patients social skills for more effective handling of conflict situations. Following this review, Novaco presents his model, which emphasizes the individual's perception or "cognitive" appraisal in mediating the relationship between environmental situations and individual responses. Novaco then outlines his treatment approach of both modifying cognitive appraisals of situations as anger provoking and applying the arousal reduction strategies discussed previously, such as relaxation and assertive behavior. Data demonstrating the promise of this treatment approach are presented, and directions for future intervention research are discussed.

Chronic hostility, rather than anger and aggression, is the theme of "An Approach to the Diagnosis and Treatment of Chronically Hostile Individuals" by Michael Hecker and Donald Lunde. A typology of chronic hostility is suggested based upon clinical cases the authors have examined and followed. This typology, while reminiscent of the conceptualization of aggressive behavior presented by Megargee in Chapter 2, draws case examples from behavioral medicine. In this manner, Hecker and Lunde provide a tentative model that relates conceptual definitions discussed in the first section of this book to the health consequences of anger and hostility presented in the second section. Treatment strategies are discussed in terms of the typology. The primary components of these strategies are behavioral and cognitive coping skills and are thus similar to the anger management approach proposed by Novaco. Hecker and Lunde specify which of the different anger management strategies, such as assertive training, cognitive reappraisal, and relaxation, are most applicable for reducing chronic hostility in each of the proposed types.

John Reid and Kate Kavanagh illustrate the complexities of anger management in their chapter, "A Social Interactional Approach to Child Abuse: Risk, Prevention, and Treatment." Beyond the fact that child abuse constitutes a major public health problem in the United States, this problem exemplifies the social context in which most anger and aggression emerge, and dramatically illustrates how these interactional and contextual variables can be woven into an effective treatment approach. The conceptual framework presented by Reid and Kavanagh specifies factors that predict the incidence of abuse, such as the frequency of aversive social interactions and the presence of background stressors. Previous strategies to prevent and treat child abuse are reviewed. Not surprisingly, these strategies reflect the range of approaches typically taken in the treatment of anger: individual and group psychotherapy, modeling, and social skills training. Reid and Kavanagh then demonstrate that, by directing social skills training at the factors that predict anger and aggressive situations, the escalation of social interactions into aggression and violence can be avoided. Although the specific training approach described in this chapter is focused on child abuse, Reid and Kavanagh discuss the approach as a general strategy that would be effective in preventing and treating other problems associated with anger arousal.

In "The Possible Effects of Beta-Adrenergic Blocking Drugs on Behavioral and Psychological Concomitants of Anger," Lynn Durel and David Krantz explore a potential pharmacologic approach to anger management. Their thesis is based on evidence that perception and evaluation of peripheral sympathetic arousal plays a role in generating or facilitating the experience of anger. Anger is thus an outcome of the interaction between physiologic arousal and the individual's anger-related cognitive label of that arousal. By selectively reducing peripheral sympathetic arousal, beta-adrenergic blocking drugs may interfere with this anger-generating interaction between physiological arousal and the individual's perception. The Type A behavior pattern is discussed as a predisposition to interpret arousal as anger; preliminary data from research on Type A behavior, as well as behavioral disorders involving rage and aggressive outbursts, are reviewed in relation to research on the psychophysiology of emotion. The implications of this research for pharmacological intervention are discussed.

In the final chapter in Part III, Margaret Chesney turns to the future, presenting issues that need to be addressed by those behavioral science and medical communities interested in interventions for anger and hostility. Progress in intervention is influenced by developments in the areas of assessment and health correlates of anger. Therefore, Chesney introduces her discussion of treatment issues by first elucidating the need for an approach to the assessment of anger that is more comprehensive than one relying solely on self-report questionnaires. Such an assessment would more accurately reflect the conceptual models explicitly or implicitly present in many of the other chapters in this volume. Among the alternative assessment strategies described is the use of behavioral observation and ambulatory monitoring of physiological responses in the natural or simulated environment. Progress in assessment will undoubtedly improve the effectiveness of interventions. However, as the previous chapters in this section illustrate, intervention efforts to modify hostility, anger and aggression are underway. Chesney discusses issues that include barriers to treatment, conflicting treatment objectives, and individual tailoring of treatments, which if not addressed will handicap these and future therapeutic attempts. Recognition of their potential public health impact has elevated anger and hostility in importance and created a mandate for behavioral science and behavioral medicine to respond to a challenging research agenda encompassing assessment, health correlates, and treatment of anger and hostility.

11

Anger and Its Therapeutic Regulation

Raymond W. Novaco
University of California, Irvine

The arousal of anger has no automatic status as a problem. Anger, experienced as a transient emotion, is part of the human fabric. As a response to an abusive act or a serious injustice, it mobilizes our physical and psychological defenses and inclines us to take corrective action. The experience of anger, in fact, can provide us with important information about the psychological significance of an event, situation, or context. And further, anger can be a force that energizes a social movement to redress societal inequities.

Given these adaptive functions of anger, one might be puzzled about the need for therapeutic interventions designed to reduce it. In contrast to anger control treatments, psychodynamically-oriented therapists have viewed anger as something to be unchained, claiming its restraint, suppression, or repression is generative of clinical disorder. Other views on the treatment of pent-up rage advocate the cathartic value of anger expression. Yet, despite these arguments in favor of anger and its expression, it is clear that the manifestation of anger can be troublesome and that its persistence or chronicity is indicative of maladjustment. Although anger does have adaptive functions, it likewise has maladaptive functions. It can disrupt task performance and problem-solving activities, it can activate injurious behaviors, it can preempt self-scrutiny by externalizing conflict, and it can become a role-defined behavior that is overgeneralized (cf. Novaco, 1976).

Anger and aggression are commonly identified as problems that have detrimental effects on personal and community well-being. The arousal of anger is problematic not only as an antecedent/activator of aggression but also as a condition that can impair psychological adjustment and personal welfare. Moreover, recent research on stress-related medical disorders has identified anger as an etiological factor in a variety of health disturbances, including coronary artery disease, hypertension, back pain, headaches, alcoholism, and rheumatoid arthritis (Appel, Holroyd, & Gorkin, in press).

While basic research on anger and clinical disorders is progressing, as evidenced by this present volume, research on the *treatment* of anger and aggression has lagged far behind other clinical problems, such as anxiety and depression. Numerous articles about these latter two disorders appear in scientific journals regularly and consider variations in treatment strategies, analyses of therapeutic processes, investigations of theoretical variables, and controversies surrounding issues of theory and methodology. Anger, by comparison, is virtually forsaken. The puzzling thing is that this dearth of research is not consistent with the clinical interest in the topic, which is considerable.

This chapter will present and review the range of clinical intervention programs that have been designed to modify anger and aggression. A model of anger and aggression will also be presented that is integrally related to one of these therapeutic approaches, which has been developed by me. As a prelude to this material, I will describe some circumstances that have constrained the progress of research on the treatment of anger and aggression.

FACTORS CURTAILING RESEARCH ON ANGER/AGGRESSION MODIFICATION

A number of experimental programs have been designed to modify anger and aggressive behavior, but intervention studies are not commensurate in number with problem prevalence or clinical interest. This state of affairs has resulted from several constraining circumstances: (1) there are unique difficulties associated with the treatment of angry, aggressive persons; (2) basic research on anger and aggression has ignored matters of clinical relevance; and (3) the populations that are commonly linked with anger and aggression are low in social status. Each of these factors can be seen to have had a limiting influence on therapeutic intervention research.

Difficulties in Treating Angry, Aggressive Persons

There are unique difficulties in treating problems of anger and aggression. This pertains not only to the problem condition itself but also to the development of the therapeutic relationship. It is well known that treatment outcomes for certain populations such as prisoners are notoriously bad. When anger and aggression are part of antisocial behavior patterns established since adolescence or childhood, the prognosis is transparently poor. However, while incarcerated offenders or members of juvenile gangs present distinct difficulties for clinical change efforts, complications in the treatment of anger and aggression are not restricted to these difficult populations.

Therapists and counselors are often uneasy in working with persons identified as being explosive. In the case of violent offenders, the clinician's concern about danger is based upon historical realities. Descriptions and expressions of anger, rage, and aggressive impulses can be alarming. Such revelations may unduly worry the therapist who may inadvertently influence the client to limit or curtail disclosures. The client might even test the therapist by describing angry feelings and hostile fantasies so as to gauge the therapist's familiarity with the problem condition, and his very acceptance of the client. The troubled individual may wonder whether it is safe or even useful to reveal matters of deep personal significance. This, in fact, was a common scenario in treating American Vietnam veterans suffering from "delayed stress syndrome," which has explosive rage as a core component (cf. Figley, 1978). If the client senses that his psychological realities alarm or disturb the therapist, this will most assuredly undermine the helping process.

A second difficulty in doing treatment with persons who are prone to provocation is that they can easily become impatient with the treatment process. Clients are often ambivalent about being in treatment, and some become frustrated prematurely because of poorly defined or unrealistic goals. Those with anger problems may be more inclined to disengage from therapy as their impatience mounts when desired treatment effects are not quickly forthcoming. Sometimes annoyance occurring with regard to minor incidental events can induce the client to abandon treatment. In this regard, it would seem advantageous for treatment programs to be clearly defined, structured, and time-limited, so as to minimize ambiguity and the frustration that can result from vague expectations regarding treatment. Importantly, the therapist or counselor must be able to respond to the negative feelings of the client in an effective manner. In a recent study, Hector et al. (1981) found that counselors could be trained to respond consistently to anger using a procedure of verbal practice with modeling, which was significantly more effective than other component and control conditions.

The proneness to frustration and impatience that are intrinsic to the problem constellation dictates that control group conditions in treatment studies must be thoughtfully designed. Waiting-list control and placebo control conditions have the potential of activating the client's problem responses. That is, the absence of a plausible treatment can easily agitate the client, resulting in higher measured anger in the control groups. It may well be that difficulties associated with constructing preferred experimental designs have contributed to the relative absence of treatment experiments in this area.

A third complication in treating angry, aggressive people is that this action-emotion complex has instrumental value in dealing with aversive situations and can impart a sense of control or mastery. One can overcome constraints, dislodge impediments, and dispatch obnoxious others by becoming angry and acting aggressively. Persons who are so disposed are reluctant to relinquish this sense of effectiveness.

Chronic anger reaction patterns represent a learned style of coping with stressful life demands. The propensity for anger reflects a combative orientation in responding to situations of threat, challenge, pressure, and hardship. This mode of response has been viewed as a core component of the Type A behavior pattern (Friedman & Rosenman, 1974), and recent research has buttressed the claim that anger, aggressiveness, and hostility are important coronary disease risk factors (Carver & Glass, 1978; Glass et al. 1980; Williams et al. 1980). This is to say that anger and aggressivity, as dispositional factors, represent more than transient personality states. Glass conceptualized Type A as a style of response to stressful stimulation that threatens the sense of control. Regardless of whether the person with anger problems also exhibits other attributes of coronary proneness, and could thereby be classified as Type A, chronic anger responses reflect a mode of coping with stress linked to cognitive structures and behavior patterns.

By implication, the treatment of anger/aggression problems must involve the acquisition of a new set of coping strategies. To some extent, training in appropriate assertiveness does provide the client with an adaptive way of handling provocation, but many instances of anger cannot be resolved by interpersonal assertiveness. Therefore, the therapeutic program must offer a comprehensive set of coping strategies that involve the cognitive, physiological, behavioral, and environmental domains.

Neglect of Clinical Relevance in Basic Research

Experimental work on aggression has largely addressed the concerns of personality and social psychology, to the virtual exclusion of matters of clinical relevance. This body of laboratory work in the past three decades has advanced theory and methodology, but the experimental analysis of aggression has largely concerned analogue phenomena investigated with little interest in applied issues. This stands in contrast to the subjects of anxiety and depression, which were clinical topics at the outset. The detachment from naturalistic phenomena and clinical problems may in part account for the waning of interest in the topic of aggression as reflected in journal publications.

There are of course notable exceptions to this point. The study by Patterson, Littman, and Bricker (1967) involved an elaborate naturalistic analysis of aggression which served as the foundation for a very significant clinical approach. More recently, the work of Averill (1982) is another example of theoretically-driven research that has enormous clinical relevance. These research programs stand in sharp contrast to the conventional experimental paradigms and have the capacity to enrich therapeutic methods.

It should be recognized that the experimental analysis of anger and aggression is not an easy undertaking. Anger is not as easy to manipulate as anxiety. Anxiety can be induced by presenting the subject with difficult tasks, negative evaluations, the threat of aversive stimuli, or phobic objects. Anger requires conditions of annoyance or insult, which, in the context of a university laboratory, are difficult to do with credibility. Moreover, troublesome human subjects issues surround the use of relatively strong stimulus conditions required to provoke someone and the inducement to perform harmdoing actions. The identification and selection of subject populations has also been an area of limitation. While there are multiple clinical categories for depression and anxiety, anger and aggression are not formally identified by a diagnostic category. Anger and aggression are intrinsic to "explosive disorder," but this is an extreme condition. Although associated with various pathological conditions, anger and aggression have no disorder category. I am not suggesting that there should be some classification, so much as pointing to factors that have possibly curtailed clinically relevant scientific studies.

The absence of a diagnostic group and established diagnostic criteria has at least two consequences. One consequence is that it is not easy to identify target populations in treatment facilities. However, in some problem areas, such as for conduct disorders of children and adolescents, investigators have more easily obtained access to populations of interest. This is reflected in the work of Feindler and Fremouw (1983) in residential units and also in the work of Patterson and his colleagues with outpatients. A second consequence is that the lack of conventional diagnostic criteria makes it difficult to obtain experimental subjects by pretesting potential subject samples and then selecting those with extreme scores. In research on depression, the Beck Depression Inventory has served this purpose as a validated clinical scale, and there are other clinically validated depression measures, including of course that of the MMPI. In the case of anger, there are a number of self-report measures in the literature, and some new ones are described in this volume. However, these existing scales and inventories remain to be clinically validated by demonstrating their relationship to serious disturbances in cognitive, affective, and behavioral functioning.

The Social Status of Aggressive Persons

Attention to the modification and regulation of aggression may be limited due to the the social status of the populations typically identified as exhibiting aggressive behavior. Incarcerated criminals, low SES minorities, combat veterans, and perpetrators of family violence are probably not among the list of preferred client populations. Not only do these populations present refractory problems for clinical change efforts, they also are considerably discrepant from the YAVIS (young, attractive, verbal, intelligent, and successful) clients desired by clinical practitioners. They tend not to be among the monied class, which certainly lowers the appeal of becoming proficient in treating the problems that disturb them. A cynic might observe that interest in anger has been kindled now that anger has been implicated in the coronary problems of corporate executives.

In this regard, I want to note that violence itself is defined in ways that refer primarily to personal acts, although failing to encompass institutional decisions or policies that result in serious harmdoing. This definitional strategy has discriminatory consequences along the lines of social class. Monahan and Novaco (1980) have argued that corporate violence is a significant social phenomenon and one that, for many reasons, has escaped psychological scrutiny. Behavior producing an unreasonable risk of physical harm to consumers, employees, or other persons as a result of deliberate decision-making or culpable negligence ought to be considered violence, no matter how sanitized. A person is just as dead from corporate self-serving decisions involving the faulty engineering of cars like Pintos or Corvairs as by personal self-serving decisions involving the engineering of a Smith and Wesson.

Although funding may have been provided for therapeutic interventions aimed at reducing aggression among criminals, veterans, and child/spouse abusers, I know of no published experimental study with a control group design on these populations. With the exception of Reid and Taplin (1980) on abusive families, there is a void of evaluative research. To be sure, studies with such populations are difficult and may involve institutional impediments. However, it would be well if researchers more extensively investigated these population groups. Making efforts to determine the psychological deficits related to their anger/aggression problems, as well as developing appropriate treatments.

This comment on the social status of populations identified as having anger/aggression problems raises an interesting issue. In this regard, it might be argued that anger and aggression among persons of lower social strata are best addressed as problems of social structure and not as matters of psychopathology. Various sociological perspectives on deviance and criminal behavior, including social disorganization theory (Shaw & McKay, 1942; Thrasher, 1929), frustrated aspiration or opportunity structure theory (Merton, 1957; Cloward & Ohlin,

1960), and conflict theory (Turk, 1969) would view anger/aggression phenomena as products of the social order. One aspect of this social structural analysis is the implication that anger and aggression cannot be remediated unless conditions of society are modified. Another aspect is that anger and aggression are responses to constraining and inequitable societal circumstances and may serve adaptive functions for certain individuals and groups.

In response to these points, conditions of the social order no doubt have a causal role in the occurrence of anger/aggression phenomena, however, this level of analysis neither addresses the malaise or impairment of the individual nor does it provide for therapeutic change for persons who are so motivated. Given the harmful effects that anger can have on personal well-being, we must develop psychologically-based interventions. Such intervention strategies do not preempt efforts to promote larger changes in the social system, such as reductions in inequality and discrimination against societal groups, changing attitudes towards violence-engendering social practices, and improving criminal justice procedures. With regard to the observation that anger and aggression may be adaptive responses, the present analysis recognizes the potential adaptive functions, as delineated in previous writings (Novaco, 1976). However, judgments about the adaptive versus nonadaptive nature of a response must be made with regard to identified outcomes and in the context of a value system. The theoretical model of anger to be presented next will clarify some of these issues.

In the introduction, I have indicated several factors that have, in my view, curtailed research on the modification of anger and aggression. Difficulties associated with treating angry, aggressive persons, the omission of clinical relevance from basic research, and the social status of the populations commonly linked with anger and aggression have exerted a constraining influence. Work on the treatment of anger and aggression must proceed from a conceptual model of these phenomena that allows one to see that a remedy is desirable. The next section, therefore, presents my working conception of anger and aggression.

ANGER AND AGGRESSION

Anger is commonly recognized as an important psychological state, yet it rarely has been given systematic study. Three quarters of a century ago, G. Stanley Hall stated that "psychological literature contains no comprehensive memoir on this very important and interesting subject" (Hall, 1899, p. 515). Curiously, this statement remained true until the appearance of Averill's (1982) recent volume. As history would have it, behavioral principles favored the study of aggressive behavior over anger which eluded the attention of experimentally minded investigators. This has been particularly true in the fields of personality and social psychology, where anger inducement has been an integral part of the prolific research on aggression, yet interest in anger has been incidental to the study of overt aggressive acts.

The past preference for research on aggression is understandable for reasons other than behavioral traditions. The realities of war, surges of social unrest, and the prevalence of violent crime compel our attention to injurious actions. However, for very good reasons, anger should not be the neglected topic that it now is in psychological research. Anger clearly activates aggressive behavior and has demonstrable links to problems of physical health and psychological adjustment. As a manifestation of psychological stress, chronic anger reactions can be induced by enduring contextual conditions, such as long distance commuting or work pressures, particularly when these ambient conditions shape antagonistic cognitive dispositions. Persons who are prone to provocation not only may suffer impairments to their own well-being but may also negatively affect their families and work organizations.

While neither necessary nor sufficient for aggression to occur, anger does lead to aggression. Extensive research has indeed shown that anger arousal increases the probability of aggression (Rule & Nesdale, 1976). A considerable proportion of acts of aggravated assault and homicide involves an angry perpetrator. Instances of criminal assault have been shown to consist not of discrete events but of an escalating sequence of antagonistic moves (Toch, 1969). Domestic violence, whether between spouses or directed toward children, typically is prompted by unmanaged anger. As another example, rape can be motivated by anger toward females. There is little doubt that interpersonal violence ranging from altercations on freeways to assassinations of government leaders is in large measure driven by the forces of anger.

In addition to the aggression-inducing effects of anger at the interpersonal level, violence at the societal level is fomented by the anger that exists among communities. Urban rioting has arisen from the anger of disadvantaged minorities. The racial rioting in the sixties and the occurrence of renewed hostilities, as indicated by the recent turmoil in Miami, is unmistakably rooted in the anger of black people. While enraged communities can often be driven to destructive actions, it is also the case that such anger can promote group unity, as in the nation's response to the embassy takeover in Tehran, and can energize constructive social action, as it did with civil rights legislation. These latter examples again illustrate that anger can have adaptive functions.

The association of anger with aggression engenders the belief that anger is negative or harmful because it is expected to result in harmdoing. This expectation is fortified by our awareness of incidents in which fits of rage have had tragic consequences. The view of anger as a passion by which the person is "gripped," "seized," or "torn" is in fact rooted in ancient philosophical beliefs about the nature of emotion (Averill, 1974). Becoming angry seems to signify that one is out of control, driven by uncivilized forces that ultimately must be checked. Anger is perhaps the prototype of this view of emotions as passions.

There are several difficulties with viewing anger as a passion which takes control of the personality and leads to aggressive acts. One problem is that it implies that anger is not accompanied by reason. As will be delineated later, cognitive operations are centrally involved in the instigation of anger, as well as in its maintenance and dissipation. Anger is by no means a reflexive, automatic response to provoking events. Another difficulty is that we may all too readily attend to the negative aspects of anger and overlook its positive functions. The varied functions of anger in affecting human behavior suggest that anger arousal indeed has adaptive value. A third difficulty is the emphasis that has been given to aggression and its consequences when gauging the harmful effects of anger. Proneness to anger can become a chronic problem for the individual, and the injurious effects of chronic anger go considerably beyond the experience of an unpleasant emotional state that induces aggressive behavior. Many negative effects can result from anger proneness, including impairments to psychological and physical well-being. A fourth problem is that anger is commonly viewed as an emotional state evoked in response to proximate situational events, such as frustrating, annoying, or insulting occasions. This overlooks the possibility that enduring contextual conditions or sequential circumstances may have a cumulative effect of elevating general arousal or tension levels so as to prime the person to experience anger.

In everyday life, only a small proportion of anger instigations result in overt aggression towards others. Such occurrences do have important societal significance. But the point is that by emphasizing the anger aggression relationship we may overlook more subtle and long-term costs associated with anger problems. Psychological research has commonly conducted its analysis of anger by beginning with the exposure to some provoking event and ending with the subject's more or less proximate response to that event. There has been inadequate attention to anger as a style of coping with life problems. The recent work, exemplified in the present volume, that links anger to cardiovascular and other health disturbances is beginning to show that proneness to provocation can have negative consequences other than those that might result from aggressive acts.

The foregoing discussion has argued that research on anger has seriously lagged behind its apparent importance in psychological functioning. It has also been argued that preoccupation with the aggression-inducing properties of anger has obscured the understanding of anger as determined by enduring contextual conditions and the recognition of impairments to well-being that may result from anger as a customary style of coping with life demands. The following section sets forth a model of anger that accommodates the above concerns and which provides for therapeutic interventions at both the individual and socioenvironmental levels.

A Theoretical View of Anger

Provocation to anger has salient manifestations. Anger arousal is marked by physiological activation in the cardiovascular and endocrine systems, tension in the skeletal musculature, antagonistic thought patterns, and, at times, aggressive behavior. The view of anger taken here is that it is an emotional state defined by the presence of physiological arousal and cognitions of antagonism. The cognitive label need not be precisely that of "anger" but may be something semantically proximate, such as "annoyed," "irritated," "enraged," or "provoked." The cognitive labeling may be otherwise viewed as the "subjective affect" dimension of emotional state. Implicit in the cognitive labeling dimension is some impulse to action. That is, the cognitive labeling process inherently involves an inclination on the part of the person to act in an antagonistic or confrontative manner towards the source of provocation. These action impulses in part define the emotional state and are incorporated in the cognitive labeling process. A central proposition is that there is no direct relationship between external events and anger. The arousal of anger is a cognitively mediated process. Expectations and appraisal are designated as the principal classes of cognitions that determine the occurrence of anger.

Another proposition is that anger is neither necessary nor sufficient for aggression, yet it is a significant antecedent of aggression and has a mutually influenced relationship with aggression. This bidirectional causality postulate (Konecni, 1975) means that the level of anger influences the level of aggression and vice-versa. Whether or not aggression occurs following provocation is thought to be a function of various social learning factors other than anger, such as reinforcement contingencies, expected outcomes, and modeling influences. These same social learning factors can also influence the occurrence of aggression independent of anger arousal. Thus, it is possible for someone to aggress without becoming angry, as when the infliction of injury or damage is expected to produce personal gain or when the aggressive act is a well-learned behavior. This view of aggression allows one to consider certain forms of organizational and corporate behavior as acts of violence (cf. Monahan & Novaco, 1980).

The cognitive factors which determine anger are *expectations* and *appraisals.* Generally speaking, when exposed to environmental demands, individuals hold expectations or anticipations of the demand itself and of their performance in response to that demand. In a temporal sequence, this is the first stage of cognitive activity. When the demand occurs, and following its occurrence, it is appraised or interpreted. Similarly, persons appraise their performance in response to the demand. Expectations and appraisals are interrelated. Expectations, as subjective probabilities about events, are based on previous appraisals of related circumstances. Appraisals are a function of the expectations one holds regarding oneself and others. These cognitive factors have a mutually influenced relationship to anger. That is, becoming angry has feedback effects such that future expectations and appraisals are a function of experienced anger arousal. Likewise, the absence or minimization of anger in conjunction with previously provoking circumstances may lead to changes in cognitive structuring.

The concepts of appraisal and expectation appear throughout the psychological literature. The appraisal concept was first used with regard to emotion by Arnold (1960) and was given extensive treatment by Lazarus (1966) in his landmark work on stress. Lazarus proposed a theoretical model that consisted of an integration of the concepts of threat, appraisal, and coping. He differentiated two levels of appraisal: "primary appraisal," which pertains to the judgment or perception of the severity of the threat, and "secondary appraisal," which refers to the judgment about the consequences of available coping strategies. Despite the considerable research on human stress during the time since the presentation of his model, Lazarus has not altered his concept of appraisal, however, he has placed greater emphasis on coping as a crucial factor in understanding human stress (Lazarus & Launier, 1978). In the present model, what Lazarus would view as secondary appraisal is here viewed as expectation about performance.

Expectancy has been, and continues to be, an important construct in the description, explanation, and prediction of behavior. In psychological theory, expectancy is a central construct in Tolman's (1932, 1959) theory of learning, Rotter's theory of personality, and Atkinson's (1964) theory of motivation. Expectancies have been viewed as mediators of environment and behavior relationships in both macro (Lewin, 1951; Tolman & Brunswik, 1935) and micro (MacCorquodale & Meehl, 1953) theories of behavior, and they have often been used to explain behavior in work organizations (Lawler, 1973; Vroom, 1964). Recent theory pertaining to psychological disorder and behavior change that utilizes expectation constructs includes the work of Bandura (1977) on self-efficacy and Seligman (1975) on learned helplessness. The extensive inclusion of expectation in efforts to explain behavior suggests its value as a psychological variable, even though it may seem prosaic to hold to its importance.

Specific to the arousal of anger, there is considerable theory and research in support of the appraisal and expectation concepts. A review of this work can be found in Novaco (1979). The idea that anger results from the appraisal of aversive events can be found in the writings of the Roman period stoic philosophers, as well as in the theories of aggression set forth by Berkowitz (1962), Feshbach (1964, 1970), and Bandura (1973). Ample research has demonstrated that the appraisal of provocation influences the magnitude of aggressive behavior. Aggression has been found to increase with antagonistic appraisals, such as perceived intent to harm, and to decrease with adaptive appraisals, such as benign reinterpretation of the provoking experience.

The attention given to expectation as a determinant of anger and aggression has been relatively less than that given to the appraisal process. However, much of the research on frustration and aggression, beginning with the ideas of Dollard, Doob, Miller, Mowrer, and Sears (1939) can be viewed in terms of expectancies. That is, interferences with goal-directed behavior are easily interpreted as thwartings of outcome expectancies that induce arousal and associated behavioral reactions. Aside from the frustration literature, investigations concerned with expectation effects on aggression have principally concerned (a) the performance of aggression in accord with the values of observers, and (b) the inhibition of aggression due to expected retaliation or due to sex role expectations.

In the present model, expectations are viewed as determinants of anger by virtue of several psychological circumstances which involve the combinations of induced arousal and the presence of contextual cues that lead to the experience or labeling of the arousal as anger. When one's experience is discrepant from expectations, arousal accompanies the disturbance in equilibrium, as the person seeks to adjust to the demands of the situation. The magnitude of the discrepancy between obtained outcomes and expected outcomes will influence the level of arousal. This arousal is experienced as anger when there are contextual cues that signify thwarting or antagonism, as the person may attempt to account for the disturbance in equilibrium in terms of external factors that have antagonistic properties. Here, appraisal processes come into play as the person seeks to account for the arousal induced by the discrepancy between the obtained and the expected. Some preliminary evidence for the operation of the disconfirmed expectations arousal anger mechanism has been found in a study by Novaco and Hayes (1980).

Another way in which expectations influence anger arousal is with regard to the anticipation of aversive events. When one expects an antagonistic experience and when the prepotent appraisals of the events in question are anger-inducing, the expectation of annoyance can lead to selective perception of situational cues so that anger more readily occurs. When one confronts an antagonist, certain words and gestures can have a greater salience than they otherwise might, and anger occurs in conjunction with their appraisal as insulting, thwarting, or annoying.

A third way in which expectations lead to anger is when anger arousal is expected to be instrumental in achieving desired outcomes. In this case, anger may be an adaptive emotional response to a conflict as it energizes problem solving behavior. However, at times, anger occurs because one has unnecessarily low expectations for resolving conflict by nonantagonistic means and attempts to achieve control over the aversive experience through anger and aggression.

Beyond the considerations linked to the study of aggression, anger can be understood as an affective stress reaction. That is, anger arousal is one kind of response that occurs in conjunction with exposure to environmental demands or stressors (Novaco, 1979). Anger is incorporated into the stress theory framework for several reasons. First, one defining property of anger is physiological arousal, and it is unquestionably the case that arousal is activated by exposure to stressors, such as noise, heart, traffic congestion, crowding, difficult tasks, and high pressure job environments. The importance of this is that both acute and prolonged exposure to such conditions may induce arousal that is experienced by the individual in conjunction with other events that pull for the cognitive label "anger." Exposure to certain stressors may produce arousal or excitation that decays slowly, leaving a residual that can subsequently transfer to other experiences (Zillman, 1971). This residual arousal then adds in a nontrivial way to arousal induced by subsequent events appraised in terms of anger. Thus, anger should be understood in terms of contextual conditions, as well as more immediate identifiable provoking agents. The stress framework provides theoretical guidelines for the disaggregation and analysis of contextual factors (environmental demands and moderators) that may act as determinants of anger and aggression.

Analysis of the functional properties of anger (Novaco, 1976a) indicates that it should not automatically be viewed as a negative or undesirable condition of the organism. The determination of anger as a clinical problem is a matter to be evaluated in terms of various response parameters (frequency, intensity, duration, and mode of expression) by which the severity of anger reactions can be gauged with regard to effects on performance, health, and personal relationships.

Concepts of stress and adaptation can be useful for understanding the enduring or long-term effects of anger. Recent research is finding that anger is associated with impairments to health and psychological functioning, particularly in the area of cardiovascular disease (Barefoot, Dahlstrom, & Williams, 1983; Gentry et al., 1982; Williams et al., 1980; Novaco, Sarason, Robinson & Cunningham, 1982). Early writings in the field of psychosomatic medicine (Alexander, 1939; Miller, 1939; Saul, 1939) implicated suppressed anger in the development of essential hypertension. Large-scale epidemiological research (Harburg, Erfurt, Hauenstein, Chape, Schull, & Schork, 1973; Haynes, Levine, Scotch, Feinleib, & Kannel, 1978) has indeed found suppressed anger to be associated with elevated blood pressure. Although the nature of the relationship between anger and hypertension is neither simple nor clear, there is some reason to believe that one's style of coping with provocation may have some etiological significance. It as consistently been found in experimental studies that blood pressure increases when subjects are made angry. Across many published experiments, increases in systolic pressure of 10-21 mm and in diastolic pressure of 3-22 mm have been reported in conjunction with anger arousal manipulations. Recovery time to baseline levels has also been found to be prolonged when anger is not expressed. However, what is not clear is how transient increases in blood pressure become converted to chronically elevated levels. Despite some early hypothesizing about hits question (Buss, 1961), neither the biological nor psychological mechanisms have been identified.

The involvement of anger in the coronary prone behavior pattern (Type A), has been consistently observed clinically but experimental analysis has been sparse. Some experimental evidence of the aggressiveness of Type As has been reported (Carver & Glass, 1978), and other research has linked catecholamine responses to provocation (Glass et al., 1980). Epidemiological work by Haynes, Feinleib, and Kannel (1980), in a prospective study, found that suppressed anger was significantly related to the incidence of coronary artery disease but community-wide studies are extremely rare. While the association between anger and heart disease remains to be untangled, there is good reason to believe that some relationship exists, particularly in view of the longitudinal research of Barefoot, Dahlstrom, & Williams (1982) and Williams et al. (1980). On a more literary, albeit tragic note, Dr. John Hunter, a famous eighteenth century British surgeon, once remarked, "My life is in the hands of any rascal that chooses to annoy me ...." He died suddenly while attending a hospital board meeting (Jenkins, 1978).

In summary, the stress framework can inform us about the extended and unanticipated costs of anger proneness. Stress research can improve our identification of the range of circumstances that engender anger and the varied impacts that anger can have on well-being. With this theoretical background, I now turn to research on therapeutic interventions.

RESEARCH ON THE MODIFICATION OF ANGER AND AGGRESSION

Psychotherapy for anger/aggression problems has a history dating to the work of Witmer (1908), who reported the treatment of an 11 year-old boy prone to "outbursts of uncontrollable and unreasoning anger" and to "mean moods." Witmer, who started the first psychological clinic in 1896 (cf. Levine & Levine, 1970), adopted an educational approach to therapy, and his procedure is characterized by problem-solving methods. However, psychoanalysis dominated the treatment field during the first half of the century, perhaps constraining the development of the approach that Witmer pioneered, which fell into obscurity. Surprisingly, it is not until the work of Redl and Wineman (1951 & 1952) that we find a psychoanalytic account of a treatment approach to aggression-related problems. These authors devised a residential program for aggressive children based upon principles of ego psychology and their ideas of internal control mechanisms. Despite the salience of the concept of aggression in the writings of Freud, as well as that of Adler, Fenichel, Menninger, Fromm, and other prominent psychodynamic theorists, no presentation of procedures for treating the anger/aggression problems of adults appears before the era of behavior therapy. It might also be noted that the field of psychosomatic medicine in the 1930's explicitly recognized the involvement of anger in physical disorders, such as essential hypertension (c.f. Alexander, 1939; Saul, 1939).

Psychotherapeutic interventions that have received research evaluation are exclusively behavioral or cognitive-behavioral in nature. The presentation of this work is classified according to the treatment orientation: (1) behavioral treatments utilizing a counter-conditioning approach; (2) behavioral interventions in social skills or assertion training; (3) behavioral interventions based upon principles of instrumental conditioning; and (4) cognitive-behavioral approaches.

Classical Conditioning Therapies

Following the behavior therapy approach of Wolpe and Lazarus (1966), which is based on a Pavlovian or classical conditioning model, a number of investigators have used systematic desensitization and assertion training techniques in the treatment of anger and aggression. The systematic desensitization approaches typically involve relaxation counter-conditioning, although one study (Smith, 1973) used humor as the incompatible response conditioned to the anger stimuli. The assertiveness training approach, although most commonly used to help individuals who have difficulty experiencing and/or expressing anger (a form of social skills deficit), also has been applied to aggressive persons. The logic in this case is that aggression results from the absence of appropriate alternative response capabilities and that assertion training provides an effective alternative. Wolpe and Lazarus (1966) presented assertion training as a method for treating anger, as well as anxiety.

Significant reductions in anger have been found to result from relaxation counter-conditioning. Experimental studies with student subject populations (Hearn & Evans, 1972 & 1973; O'Donnel & Worell, 1973; Rimm, de Groot, Boord, Reiman & Dillow, 1971) and systematic case studies (Evans, 1971; Herrell, 1971) have shown that desensitization with relaxation can effectively reduce anger. Novaco (1975), however, found that the effects of relaxation counter-conditioning were limited when compared to an attention placebo condition, as significant differences were found only for imaginal mode provocations but not for role play, direct, or real life provocation.

An interesting alternative to relaxation counter-conditioning in the treatment of anger by desensitization was reported by Smith (1973) who, when muscle relaxation proved ineffective, successfully used humor as the incompatible response. However, just as others have questioned the Wolpian model of the therapeutic mechanisms in the desensitization procedure, I interpret Smith's results to be an excellent illustration of cognitive restructuring effects. To use the words of the subject, the humor hierarchy enabled her "to view the anger situations from a new perspective" (p. 580).

Assertiveness training has also received experimental attention as an anger/ aggression therapy, but it is ambiguous whether the family of procedures utilized correspond to the counter-conditioning model of Wolpe and Lazarus (1966), who themselves are unclear about the counter-conditioning process vis-a-vis anger. Although some approaches to assertion training follow a cognitive-behavioral model (Linehan, 1979), those investigators that have used assertiveness training in the treatment of anger and aggression have followed a strict behavioral perspective under the rubric of social skills training. There are a number of studies in this area which are next presented.

Social Skills/Assertion Training

The approach to the treatment of anger and agression views the individual as having deficits in social skills. The person is seen as lacking the ability to deal effectively with interpersonal problems in a socially appropriate manner. By responding to situations of conflict or dispute by avoidance or attack, the person fails to resolve the problem at hand and breeds further antagonism. This approach attempts to teach the client how to respond effectively in situations of interpersonal conflict, thereby minimizing anger and anxiety in preventing aggressive behavior. The training generally consists of modeling, focused instructions, behavioral rehearsal in role play, feedback on target behaviors, and social reinforcement.

The results of the use of this general approach are mixed. The approach as a treatment of anger/aggression problems was first introduced by Kaufmann and Wagner (1972) with their "barb" technique and the case report of its use with an adolescent. Rimm, Hill, Brown, and Stuart (1974) in an experimental project compared an assertion group with placebo controls and found reductions in anger self-report. Yet, several studies (Galassi & Galassi, 1978; Lee, Hallberg & Hassard, 1979; Pentz, 1980) report failures at modifying aggressive behavior through assertion training. The study by Lee et al. was particularly well done methodologically and therapeutically, using the Alberti and Emmons (1974) approach to treatment. Lee et al. (1979) found that the treatment group did not differ from attention placebo or no treatment controls on either peer-rated aggression or self-rated aggression.

In contrast to these studies with non-psychiatric populations, favorable results have been obtained with chronic hospitalized cases. Foy, Eisler, and Pinkston (1975) achieved therapeutic change with a 56-year-old male having a history of explosive anger that was maintained on a six month follow-up. Frederiksen, Jenkins, Foy, & Eisler (1976) also reported the successful use of social skills training in modifying abusive verbal outbursts of two chronic psychiatric patients. These authors performed extensive analyses of behavioral performance (various role play tests and designed, unobtrusive assessments on the ward). Using a multiple baseline design, they found strong improvement and generalization for all target behaviors across measures. Other studies with explosive psychiatric patients using multiple baseline designs have found social skills training to improve role playing performances and reduce fighting and arguing on the ward (Matson & Stephens, 1978; Matson & Zeiss, 1978). Treatment effects were maintained in these latter studies at three month follow-up.

Operant Conditioning Therapies

The work of Gerald Patterson and his colleagues is foremost in this area. Beginning with a monograph that traced the development of aggression in two nursery school groups over two semesters (Patterson, Littman, & Bricker, 1967), Patterson's work views aggression as a high-amplitude response that coerces a reaction from the environment (i.e., forces a particular set of consequences from the social environment). Aggression is viewed as the outcome of specialized socialization processes, whereby the reactions of adults and other children provide reinforcing contingencies that shape aggressive behavior. The basic finding of Patterson et al. (1967) was that children, initially low on rates of aggression, were conditioned by peers to accelerate to high levels of aggression and that this acceleration was a function of the frequency of victimization and successful counterattack. Subsequent research, which focused on the home environment (Patterson, 1976), examined the serial dependencies of family interaction. Aggressive children were found to reside in coercive family systems, whereby they were the frequent recipient of aversive events and also contributed to the acceleration of coercive exchanges by their own performances—by initiating aversive behaviors and by persisting in their behaviors when punished. Reid, Patterson, and Loeber (1982) have extended these analyses to child abuse families, demonstrating that child abuse is part of a pattern of increased aversive interaction between parent and child. These investigators find that both parents and children in abusive families engage in higher levels of aversive behaviors than do those in nondistressed or distressed but non-abusive families. This exposure to negative encounters is one characteristic in their failure to quickly and effectively resolve discipline confrontations (Reid, Taplin & Loeber, 1981).

Following these interactional sequence analyses and principles of instrumental learning, Patterson and his colleagues have developed an intervention program that involves training in parenting skills. The parent training procedure (Patterson, 1975; Patterson, Cobb, & Ray, 1972), which is discussed in detail in Chap. 4, involves several components: a programmed text on child management methods, training in the observation and recording of behavior (e.g., teaching them to pinpoint and track tantrums), and the execution of behavior modification techniques (e.g., use of social and consumable reinforcers for desirable behaviors and of time out for temper tantrums). A number of research reports have demonstrated the effectiveness of these procedures for boys with serious conduct problems (Patterson 1974; Patterson et al., 1972; Patterson, Ray & Shaw, 1968; Patterson & Reid, 1973). The most recent studies (Patterson, 1976; Patterson, Chamberlain, & Reid, 1982) have focused on parental use of effective discipline to reduce the coercive "bursts" or escalating irritable reactions of the aggressive child. The intervention program has demonstrated reductions in the aggressive behavior of the target child and overall reduction in the level of coerciveness for all family members. Fleischman and Szykula (1981) have extended the Patterson intervention program to a community-based facility and have found that the community setting application replicated the results of the Oregon Social Learning Center projects.

Other investigators have instituted change programs based on operant learning principles. Martin and Foxx (1973) implemented a social extinction/social reinforcement procedure in the treatment of a highly aggressive institutionalized retarded female who had been frequently placed in seclusion as an intractable case. The social extinction procedure, whereby the victim-therapist ignored all instances of aggressive behavior of 95 15-minute sessions, was followed by a set of 44 sessions in which the therapist was responsive, and finally the social extinction procedure was reintroduced for 25 sessions. The subject's attacks were reduced to zero during the last 45 sessions of the first extinction phase, escalated to 29 attacks at the end of the responsiveness phase, and again decreased to zero when extinction was reintroduced. This reduction in aggression generalized to the ward environment.

Lastly, a behavioral program for preschool and kindergarten children involving a home-based reinforcement system was implemented and evaluated by Budd, Leibowitz, Riner, Mindell, and Goldfarb (1981). This was an intensive nine week summer program for behavior-problem children. Various indices of disruptive behavior, including aggression and negative statements, were monitored in a multiple baseline design for three groups of children. Parents provided reinforcement contingencies of giving or withholding privileges for two groups, while school-based contingencies were introduced in a third group. The home-based program was highly successful in modifying the target behaviors of nearly all the children except two, who required the use of school setting contingencies.

Cognitive-Behavioral Interventions

Exclusive of the work by Patterson and his colleagues, the majority of intervention programs have been cognitively-based. This reflects the contemporary development in clinical psychology whereby the cognitive-behavioral perspective has become a dominant theoretical system. It might be noted that certain studies discussed earlier (Foy et al., 1975; O'Donnell & Worell, 1973; Smith, 1973), although conducted within a noncognitive behavioral framework, nevertheless incorporated procedures having distinct components of cognitive mediation. To be sure, the critique of Breger and McGaugh (1965) and Bandura's (1969) analysis of behavior change processes long ago led us to question a strict behavioral interpretation of treatment procedures like desensitization. So, the distinction here is not about therapeutic mechanisms of processes but is simply a convenient classification of treatment approaches in terms of their purported framework.

In several studies involving modeling and social learning procedures (Goodwin & Mahoney, 1975; McCullough, Huntsinger, & Nay, 1977; Roback, Frayn, Gunby, & Tuters, 1972) significant improvement has been demonstrated in clients' abilities to cope with provoking events without responding aggressively. While the Goodwin and Mahoney (1975) and McCullough et al. (1977) studies concerned the control of anger directed towards others, Roback et al. (1972) involved a patient that repeatedly self-mutilated when provoked to anger. A multifaced program of medication, cognitive structuring, modeling, role playing, assertion training, psychodrama, and punishment achieved significant reductions in self-mutilation that was maintained over a 4 month follow-up. The dilemma, of course, is that when a complex procedure is used, it is difficult to know which components are the active agents of therapeutic change. Moreover, the case study method obviously does not optimally control for factors confounded with the implementation of treatment and limits inferences to populations.

Cognitive-behavioral interventionists trace their origins to early clinical theorists such as Kelly (1955), Beck (1963 & 1967), and Ellis (1962). Ellis (1977) has extended his rational-emotive approach to the domain of anger, but there is little research on the RET approach as explicitly applied to anger problems. One case study (Hamberger & Lohr, 1980) has been published which found anger reductions in anger related belief systems.

Taking a coping skills approach to the treatment of chronic anger problems, Novaco (1975, 1976b) developed a therapeutic program based on principles of cognitive-behavioral intervention. The treatment approach is linked to a model of anger emphasizing cognitive mediation and reciprocal relationships between environment, cognition, emotion, and behavior. The treatment procedures were experimentally evaluated using control and comparison groups and were demonstrated to be effective as assessed by multiple self-report and physiological measures taken in conjunction with various laboratory provocation procedures and by clinical assessment instruments. The core components of the treatment consisted of (a) cognitive mediation techniques (attentional focus strategies, cognitive restructuring, problem-solving skills, and self-instruction) and (b) arousal reduction methods, primarily relaxation and counter-conditioning. The experimental analysis found that the cognitive interventions were more effective than the relaxation counter-conditioning components, and that the combined treatment was consistently superior to the component conditions, which themselves had significant effects over a self-monitoring control group.

The treatment approach was subsequently reconceptualized in terms of the "stress inoculation" approach suggested by Meichenbaum (1975), as prompted by the author's growing interest in the stress field. The stress inoculation approach for anger regulation was systematically applied to hospitalized patients with severe anger problems (Novaco, 1977a) and to occupational groups at high risk for anger, such as police officers (Novaco, 1977b). In addition, it was then shown in an experimental project involving probation counselors (Novaco, 1980) that those trained in the therapy approach were more proficient in dealing with client anger/aggression problems than were a matched control group. Highly significant differences in proficiencies were maintained at a follow-up testing.

Some studies and case reports by others using the treatment procedures discussed above have begun to appear in the clinical literature. Nomellini and Katz (in press) used the Novaco procedure to treat child abusive parents, obtaining large reductions in parent aversive behavior, parent anger, and child aversive behavior. In an intersting combination of stress inoculation procedures with Patterson-type parent training, Denicola and Sandler (1980) obtained decreases in parent and child aversive behavior, maintained at a three month follow-up. Also, Spirito, Finch, Smith & Cooley (1981) reported the successful application of the stress inoculation approach to the anger problems of a ten-year-old boy. Regarding institutionalized adolescents, significant improvements in anger and aggression following the anger control treatment with groups of institutionalized adolescents have been obtained for residential groups by Schlicter and Horan (1979) and by Schrader et al. (1977). Reporting on a set of studies conducted with adolescents having anger problems, Feindler and Fremouw (1983) have found that the stress inoculation approach is an effective means of controlling adolescent explosive behavior. Feindler et al. (1980) had also found that child care workers in a residential facility could implement an anger control program with beneficial effects for their wards. The work of Feindler and her colleagues holds promise for the further development of the treatment intervention with child and adolescent populations.

In addition to this work on adolescents, cognitive behavioral interventions have successfully been used to modify aggressive behavior for early primary school aged boys. Camp (1977) found that young aggressive boys failed to use verbal mediation (covert) in appropriate situations and thus instituted an intervention program aimed at developing a linguistic control system. Camp, Blum, Hebert, and van Doorninck (1977) present this "think aloud" approach, which involved daily 30-minute individual sessions for six weeks. They experimentally evaluated the program against control groups of aggressive and normal boys (ages six to eight) and found that the treated group differed significantly at post-test from aggressive controls on a variety of cognitive tests. While the aggression groups did not differ in teacher ratings of aggressive behavior, significant differences in prosocial behavior were associated with the treatment program.

Other Intervention: Proposals and Unevaluated Programs

A number of intervention proposals have appeared in the literature that are worthy of mention, as they address anger/aggression for important problem areas or populations. These proposals vary in degree of formal development, and they might best be understood as indications of areas where existing, evaluated approaches could usefully be applied. The selected areas are spouse abuse, post-combat traumatic syndrome, hospital patient care, and cardiovascular disorders.

Marital conflict is certainly one important area for intervention. Patterson and his colleagues have indeed worked in this area, but they have only just begun to address the manifestations of anger that pervade distressed relationships (personal communication). Writings on the management of anger in marital relationships abound, including thoughtful works such as Bach and Wyden (1968) and Ellis (1976), as well as overly simplified approaches (Mace, 1976). An approach that combines the social learning perspective of Patterson with the cognitive-behavioral perspective of Novaco in regard to the treatment of spouse abuse is that proposed by Margolin (1979) who provides a case report of the treatment. The marital conflict area has received extensive clinical-experimental attention, but problems of spouse abuse have not received explicit focus in a treatment study.

Problems of anger and aggression have long been identified as associated with postcombat stress reactions (Novaco & Robinson, 1983). Explosive irritability and unwarranted rage are a central part of the traumatic syndrome that can result from exposure to the harsh circumstances of warfare. The Horowitz and Solomon (1975) concept of "delayed stress syndrome" that arose in conjunction with Vietnam veterans has anger and aggression as a key dimension, but their model offers only meager suggestions about their treatment, despite its supposed therapeutic relevance. It is curious that none of the treatment chapters in the Figley (1978) volume present a systematized intervention program. Moreover, there is no experimental study on psychotherapeutic outcome for Vietnam veterans in the literature. There are some case reports of the use of hypnotherapy, but the dearth of evaluative research is striking, given the salience of the problem during the last decade and the feasibility of conducting the research.

The violent patient gets considerable press in the non-scientific medical literature, and one might think that a staff training program could be developed and evaluated for hospital patient care. The studies presented earlier in the social skills section do involve hospitalized patients, as do those in other intervention models (Novaco, 1977a). However, the concern here is with regard to general patient care and the response of medical personnel to anger and aggression that might arise from assaultive or nonassaultive patients. Rada (1981) offers a number of ideas regarding assessment and management in this broad scope for the general hospital ward and emergency room. For the nursing profession, there have been a number of instructional articles (e.g., Maynard & Chitty, 1979; Thomas, Baker, & Estes, 1970), and one can find trade articles in dealing with patient anger in the areas of gerontology, dermatology, dentistry, burn patients, cardiology, genetics counseling, and veterinary medicine, as well as psychiatry. There would appear to be a manifest interest in patient care techniques that would enable medical personnel to respond effectively to anger and threats of aggression.

OVERVIEW OF INTERVENTION STUDIES AND PREVAILING ISSUES

Although the body of research on interventions is by no means voluminous, there is sufficient evidence from a variety of studies to conclude that problems of anger and aggression can be remediated. Treatment effects have been maintained at follow-up, but this has been demonstrated to a lesser degree. The therapeutic gains have been achieved for young children, adolescents, delinquents, college students, adult outpatients, chronic inpatients, and abusive families. This is indeed a wide range of client populations, yet the density of successful outcome studies in uneven across these groups and is in need of strengthening in nearly all areas.

Much of the evaluative research reviewed here consists of case studies or multiple baseline designs with a small group of subjects. For this reason, we must be more tentative in making empirical generalizations about treatment outcome effects. Until more controlled experimental studies are conducted, our confidence in the available treatments should be tempered. Moreover, experimental designs ought to address questions concerning the match between client and treatment. For example, if a cognitively-oriented investigator were to conduct an intervention study with chronic psychiatric patients, the design should include a social skills training condition, since that approach has been shown to be effective with this population and since cognitive change methods might be unsuitable for chronic patients.

Similarly, treatment conditions can be constructed that allow the investigator to do a component analysis of the treatment. This has been done in several studies in the social skills and the cognitive-behavioral areas. It is not always feasible to add comparison groups to a design that requires a minimal treatment or placebo condition and perhaps a no-treatment group, but it would seem preferable to have a component condition whenever possible.

Across studies, there is considerable variation in the measurements employed. Of course, this is a function of variation in the target problems and theoretical perspective. But it would be fruitful to encourage investigators to utilize a wider range of assessment indices. For example, the measures developed by Patterson and his colleagues have broad applicability to child and adult populations and for both outpatient and residential settings. Also, in studies concerning anger, the investigator should strongly consider the use of physiological measures. Only one study (Novaco, 1975) used physiological assessment, but this would seem to be a key dimension on which therapeutic change should occur in regard to anger problems.

On the topic of assessment, there is a conspicuous lack of a validated self-report scale. There are several self-report instruments in the literature (cf. Biaggio, 1980), but there are two main difficulties: (1) No instrument has been developed from a theory, such that it correspondingly measures dimensions and/or deficits—an anger or hostility scale (it is useful to distinguish scales from inventories) should follow from a theory and assess the theoretically specified problem dimensions; (2) Existing instruments have not been developed systematically, involving painstaking validation procedures. Spielberger has recently developed a state-trait anger scale (Spielberger, Jacobs, Russel, & Crane, 1983), but the validation process is in the early stages. Siegel (1983) has also developed a multidimensional anger scale, but it too is in an early stage of development. Neither of these newly developed instruments follows from a theory of anger.

Beyond these experimental concerns, epidemiological data on anger are needed. Averill's (1982) approach to the assessment of community samples can be very instructive here. However, we need knowledge concerning representative samples of metropolitan and rural communities about how often people get angry and at what level of intensity, what do they do when angry, and how often do they engage in aversive behavior? Importantly, we must learn the relationship between these anger parameters and things such as life events, environmental factors, and impairments to health and adjustment.

Therapeutic interventions for anger problems are being developed by this growing body of research, but the advancement of this field may ultimately hinge on our ability to understand the dynamics of anger/aggression problems. That is, there is a need to identify the kinds of psychological deficits associated with the occurrence of anger disorders. For example, the cognitive processes (thinking styles) and the behavioral tendencies that are linked with anger proneness should be determined. Furthermore, we should not rivet our attention to individual deficit factors and fail to recognize the contextual, environmental determinants of anger, particularly in terms of how prolonged exposure to environmental demands potentiates anger and how anger patterns develop in person-environment transactions. Concerted study of the determinants, manifestations, and consequences of anger in everyday life, as well as in its more problematic forms, is surely needed if we are to improve our therapeutic capabilities.

REFERENCES

Alberti, R. E., & Emmons, M. L. *Your perfect right.* San Luis Obispo, Calif. Impact, 1974.
Appel, M., Holroyd, K. A., & Gorkin, L. Anger and the etiology and progression of physical illness. In C. Van Dyke & L. Temoshok (Eds.), *Emotions in health and illness: Foundations of clinical practice.* New York: Academic, in press.
Averill, J. R. *Anger and aggression: An essay on emotion.* New York: Springer-Verlag, 1982.
Balson, P. M. & Dempster, C. R. Treatment of war neuroses from Vietnam. *Comprehensive Psychiatry,* 1980, *21,* 167-175.
Bandura, A. *Principles of behavior modification.* New York: Holt, 1969.
Bandura, A. *Aggression: A social learning analysis.* Englewood Cliffs, N.J.: Prentice Hall, 1973.
Barefoot, J. C., Dahlstrom, G., & Williams, R. B. Rapid communication: Hostility, CHD incidence, and total mortality: A 25-year follow-up study of 255 physicians. *Psychosomatic Medicine,* 1982, *55,* 59-64.
Biaggio, M. K. Assessment of anger arousal. *Journal of Personality Assessment,* 1980, *44,* 289-298.
Beck, A. T. Thinking and depression. *Archives of General Psychiatry,* 1963, *9,* 324-333.
Beck, A. T. *Depression: Clinical, experimental, and theoretical aspects.* New York: Harper & Row, 1967.
Berkowitz, L. *Aggression: A social psychological analysis.* New York: McGraw-Hill, 1962.
Breger, L. & McGaugh, J. Critique and reformulation of "learning theory" approaches to psychotherapy and neurosis. *Psychological Bulletin,* 1965, *63,* 338-358.
Budd, K. S., Leibowitz, J. M., Riner, L. S., Mindell, C., & Goldfarb, A. Home-based treatment of severe disruptive behaviors. *Behavior Modification,* 1981, *5,* 273-298.

Camp, B. Verbal mediation in young aggressive boys. *Journal of Abnormal Psychology*, 1977, *86*, 145-153.
Camp, B., Blum, G., Hebert, F., & van Doorninck, W. "Think Aloud:" A program for developing self-control in young aggressive boys. *Journal of Abnormal Child Psychology*, 1977, *5*, 157-169.
Denicola, J. & Sandler, J. Training abusive parents in child management and self-control skills. *Behavior Therapy*, 1980, *11*, 263-270.
Ellis, A. *Reason and emotion in psychotherapy*. New York: Stuart, 1962.
Ellis, A. Techniques of handling anger in marriage. *Journal of Marriage and Family Counseling*, 1976, *2*, 305-315.
Ellis, A. *How to live with and without anger*. New York: Reader's Digest, 1977.
Evans, D. R. Specific aggression, arousal, and reciprocal inhibition therapy. *Western Psychologist*, 1971, *1*, 125-130.
Evans, D. R., & Hearn, M. T. Anger and systematic desensitization: A follow-up. *Psychological Reports*, 1973, *32*, 569-570.
Feindler, E. L., & Fremouw, W. J. Stress inoculation training for adolescent anger problems. In D. Merchenbaum and M. Jarenko (Eds.), *Stress reduction and prevention*. New York: Plenum, 1983.
Feindler, E. L., Latini, J., Nape, K., Romano, J., & Doyle, J. *Anger reduction methods for child care workers at a residential delinquency facility*. Paper presented at the 14th Annual Convention of the Association for Advancement of Behavior Therapy, New York, November 1980.
Feshbach, S. Aggression. In P. H. Mussen (Ed.), *Carmichael's manual of child psychology* (Vol. II). New York: Wiley, 1970.
Figley, C. R. (Ed.). *Stress disorders among Vietnam veterans: Theory, research, and treatment*. New York: Brunner/Mazel, 1978.
Fleischman, M. J., & Szykula, S. A. A community setting replication of a social learning treatment for aggressive children. *Behavior Therapy*, 1981, *12*, 115-122.
Foy, D. W., Eisler, R. M., & Pinkston, S. Modeled assertion in a case of explosive rage. *Journal of Behavior Therapy and Experimental Psychiatry*, 1975, *6*, 135-137.
Frederickson, L., Jenkins, J., Foy, D., & Eisler, R. Social-skills training to modify abusive verbal outbursts in adults. *Journal of Applied Behavior Analysis*, 1976, *9*, 117-125.
Freidman, M., & Rosenman, R. *Type A behavior and your heart*. Greenwich, Conn.: Fawcett, 1974.
Galassi, J. P., & Galassi, M. Modifying assertive and aggressive behavior through assertion training: A prelminary investigation. *Journal of College Student Personnel*, 1978.
Gentry, W. D., Chesney, A., Gary, H., Hall, R., & Harburg, E. Habitual anger-coping styles: I. Effect on mean blood pressure and risk for essential hypertension. *Psychosomatic Medicine*, 1982, *44*, 195-202.
Goodwin, S. E., & Mahoney, M. J. Modification of aggression via modeling: An experimental probe. *Journal of Behavior Therapy and Experimental Psychiatry*, 1975, *6*, 200-202.
Hamberger, K., & Lohr, J. M. Rational restructuring for anger control: A quasi-experimental case study. *Cognitive Therapy and Research*, 1980, *4*, 99-102.
Harburg, E., Erfurt, J., Havenstein, L., Chape, C., Schull, W., & Schork, M. Socioecological stress, suppressed hostility, skin color, and black-white male blood pressure: Detroit *Psychosomatic Medicine*, 1973, *35*, 276-296.
Harburg, E., Blakelock, E., & Roeper, P. Resentful and reflective coping with arbitrary authority and blood pressure: Detroit. *Psychosomatic Medicine*, 1979, *41*, 189-202.
Hector, M., Davis, K., Denton, E., Hayes, T., Patton-Crowder, C., & Hinkle, W. Helping counselor trainees to learn to respond consistently to anger and depression. *Journal of Counseling Psychology*, 1981, *28*, 53-58.
Kaufmann, L., & Wagner, B. Barb: A systematic treatment technology for temper control disorders. *Behavior Therapy*, 1972, *3*, 84-90.
Kelly, G. *The psychology of personal constructs* (Vols. 1 and 2). New York: Norton, 1955.
Konecni, V. J. The mediation of aggressive behavior: Arousal level versus anger and cognitive labeling. *Journal of Personality and Social Psychology*, 1975, *32*, 706-712.
Lee, D. Y., Hallberg, E. T., & Hassard, H. Effects of assertion training on aggressive behavior of adolescents. *Journal of Counseling Psychology*, 1979, *26*, 459-461.
Levine, M., & Levine, A. *A social history of the helping services*. New York: Appleton-Century-Croft, 1970.

Linehan, M. M. Structured cognitive-behavioral treatment of assertion problems. In P. Kendall and S. Hollon (Eds.). *Cognitive behavioral interventions.* New York: Academic, 1979.

Margolin, G. Conjoint marital therapy to enhance anger management and reduce spouse abuse. *American Journal of Family Therapy,* 1979, *7,* 13-23.

Martin, P. L., & Foxx, R. M. Victim control of the aggression of an institutionalized retardate. *Journal of Behavior Therapy and Experimental Psychiatry,* 1973, *4,* 161-165.

Matson, J., & Stephens, R. Increasing appropriate behavior of explosive chronic psychiatric patients with a social skills training package. *Behavior Modification,* 1978, *2,* 61-76.

Matson, J. & Zeiss, R. Group training of social skills in chronically explosive, severely disturbed psychiatric patients. *Behavior Engineering,* 1978, *5,* 41-50.

McCullough, J., Huntsinger, G., & Nay, W. Self-control treatment of aggression in a 16 year old male. *Journal of Consulting and Clinical Psychology,* 1977, *45,* 322-331.

Meichenbaum, D. A self-instructional approach to stress management: A proposal for stress inoculation training. In C. Spielberger & I. Sarason (Eds.), *Stress and anxiety* (Vol. 2). New York: Wiley, 1975.

Meichenbaum, D., & Novaco, R. W. Stress inoculation: A preventative approach. In C. Spielberger and I. Sarason (Eds.), *Stress and anxiety* (Vol. 5). New York: Halstead, 1978.

Monahan, J., & Novaco, R. W. Corporate violence: A psychological analysis. In P. Lipsitt & B. Sales (Eds.), *New Directions in psycholegal research.* New York: Van Nostrand, 1980.

Nomelini, S. & Katz, R. Effects of anger control training on abusive parents. *Cognitive Therapy and Research,* in press.

Novaco, R. W. *Anger control: The development and evaluation of an experimental treatment.* Lexington, Mass.: D.C. Heath, 1975.

Novaco, R. W. The function and regulation of the arousal of anger. *American Journal of Psychiatry,* 1976a, *133,* 1124-1128.

Novaco, R. W. Treatment of chronic anger through cognitive and relaxation controls. *Journal of Consulting and Clinical Psychology,* 1976b, *44,* 681.

Novaco, R. W. Stress inoculation: A cognitive therapy for anger and its application to a case of depression. *Journal of Consulting and Clinical Psychology,* 1977a, *45,* 600-608.

Novaco, R. W. A stress inoculation approach to anger management in the training of law enforcement officers. *American Journal of Community Psychology,* 1977b, *5,* 327-346.

Novaco, R. W. Training of probation counselors for anger problems. *Journal of Counseling Psychology,* 1980, *27,* 385-390.

Novaco, R. W., Cook, T., and Sarason, I. G. Military recruit training: An arena for stress coping skills. In D. Meichenbaum & M. Jaremko (Eds.), *Stress reduction and prevention.* New York: Plenum, 1983.

Novaco, R. W., & Robinson, G. Anger and aggression among military personnel. In R. Kaplan, V. J. Konecni, & R. W. Novaco (Eds.), *Aggression in children and youth.* The Hague: Martinus Nijhoff, 1984.

Novaco, R. W. Sarason, I. G., Robinson, G., & Cunningham, F. *Longitudinal analysis of stress and performance among Marine Corps drill instructors.* Washington, D.C.: Office of Naval Research, Report AR-007, 1982.

O'Donnell, C. R., & Worell, L. Motor and cognitive relaxation in the desensitization of anger. *Behavior Research and Therapy,* 1973, *11,* 473-481.

Patterson, G. R. Intervention for boys with conduct problems. Multiple settings, treatments, and criteria. *Journal of Consulting and Clinical Psychology,* 1974, *42,* 471-481.

Patterson, G. *Families: Applications of social learning to family life.* Champaign, Ill.: Research, 1975.

Patterson, G. R. The aggressive child: Victim and architect of a coercive system. In E. Mash, L. Hamerlynck, & L. Handy (Eds.), *Behavior modification and families.* New York: Brunner/Mazel, 1976.

Patterson, G., Chamberlain, P., & Reid, J. B. A comparative evaluation of parent training procedures. *Behavior Therapy,* 1982, *13,* 638-650.

Patterson, G. R., Cobb, J. A., & Ray, R. S. Direct interventions in the classroom: A set of procedures for the aggressive child. In F. W. Clark, D. R. Evans, & L. A. Hamerlynck (Eds.), *Implementing behavior programs for schools and clinics.* Champaign, Ill.: Research, 1972.

Patterson, G. R., Littman, R. A., & Bricker, W. Assertive behavior in children: A step toward a theory of aggression. *Monographs of the Society for Research in Child Development,* 1967, *32*(5).

Patterson, G. R., Ray, R. S., & Shaw, D. A. Direct intervention in the families of deviant children. *Oregon Research Institute Research Bulletin,* 1968, *8*(9).

Patterson, G. R., & Reid, J. B. Intervention for families of aggressive boys: A replication study. *Behavior Research and Therapy*, 1973, *11*, 1-12.
Pentz, M. A. Assertion training and trainer effects on unassertive and aggressive adolescents. *Journal of Counseling Psychology*, 1980, *27*, 76-83.
Rada, R. T. The violent patient: Rapid assessment and management. *Psychosomatics*, 1981, *22*, 101-109.
Redl, F., & Wineman, D. *Children who hate*. New York: Free Press, 1951.
Redl, F., & Wineman, D. *Controls from within: Techniques for the treatment of the aggressive child*. New York: Free Press, 1952.
Reid, J. B., Patterson, G., & Loeber, R. The abused child: Victim, instigator, or innocent bystander. In D. J. Bernstein (Ed.), *Response structure and organization*. Lincoln: University of Nebraska Press, 1982.
Reid, J. B., Taplin, P. S., & Loeber, R. A social interactional approach to the treatment of abusive families. In R. Stuart (Ed.), *Violent behavior: Social learning approaches to prediction, management, and treatment*. New York: Brunner/Mazel, 1981.
Rimm, D. C., deGroot, J. C., Boord, P., Reiman, J., & Dillow, P. V. Systematic desensitization of an anger response. *Behavior Research and Therapy*, 1971, *9*, 273-280.
Rimm, D. C., Hill, G. A., Brown, N. H., & Stuart, J. E. Group-assertive training in treatment of expression of inappropriate anger. *Psychological Reports*, 1974, *34*, 794-798.
Roback, H., Frayn, D., Gunby, L., & Tuters, K. A multifactorial approach to the treatment and ward management of a self-mutilating patient. *Journal of Behavior Therapy and Experimental Psychiatry*, 1972, *3*, 189-193.
Schlichter, K., & Horan, J. *Effects of stress inoculation on the anger and aggression management skills of institutionalized juvenile delinquents*. Paper presented at the meeting of the Educaional Research Association, San Francisco, 1979.
Schrader, C., Long, J., Panzer, C., Gillet, D., & Kornblath, R. *An anger control package for adolescent drug abusers*. Paper presented at the 11th Annual Convention of the Association for Advancement of Behavior Therapy, Atlanta, December 1977.
Smith, R. E. The use of humor in the counter conditioning of an anger response. *Behavior Therapy*, 1973, *4*, 576-580.
Spielberger, C. D., Jacobs, G. A., Russell, S., & Crane, R. S. Assessment of anger: The State-Trait Anger Scale. In J. Butcher and C. D. Spielberger (Eds.), *Advances in personality assessment*. (Vol. 2). Hillsdale, N.J.: LEA, 1983.
Spirito, A., Finch, A. J., Smith, T., & Cooley, W. Stress inoculation for anger and anxiety control: A case study with an emotionally disturbed boy. *Journal of Clinical Child Psychology*, 1981, *10*, 67-70.
Williams, R., Haney, T., Lee, K., Kong, Y., Blumenthal, J., & Whalen, R. Type A behavior, hostility, and coronary atherosclerosis. *Psychosomatic Medicine*, 1980, *42*, 539-549.
Witmer, L. The treatment and cure of a case of mental and moral deficiency. *The Psychological Clinic*, 1908, *2*, 153-179.
Wolpe, J., & Lazarus, A. *Behavior therapy techniques*. Oxford: Pergamin, 1966.
Zillman, D. Excitation transfer in communication-mediated aggressive behavior. *Journal of Experimental Social Psychology*, 1971, *7*, 419-434.

References Added in Proof

Alexander, F. Emotional factors in essential hypertension. *Psychosomatic Medicine*, 1939, *1*, 173-179.
Arnold, M. *Emotion and personality*. New York: Columbia University Press, 1960.
Atkinson, J. W. *An introduction to motivation*. Princeton, N.J.: Von Nostrand, 1984.
Averill, J. R. An analysis of psychosocial symbolism and its influence on theories of emotion. *Journal for the Theory of Social Behavior*, 1974, *4*, 147-190.
Bach, G., & Wyden, P. *The intimate enemy*. New York: Avon, 1968.
Bandura, A. Self-efficacy: Toward a unifying theory of behavior change. *Psychological Review*, 1977, *89*, 191-215.
Buss, A. *The psychology of aggression*. New York: Wiley, 1961.
Carver, C. S., & Glass, D. C. Coronary-prone behavior pattern and interpersonal aggression. *Journal of Personality and Social Psychology*, 1978, *36*, 361-366.
Cloward, R., & Ohlin, L. *Delinquency and opportunity*. New York: Free Press, 1960.
Dollard, J., Doob, L., Miller, N., Mowrer, D., & Sears, R. *Frustration and aggression*. New Haven, Conn.: Yale University Press, 1939.

Feshbach, S. The functions of aggression and the regulation of aggressive drive. *Psychological Review*, 1964, *71*, 257–272.
Glass, D. C. et al. Effect of harassment and competition upon cardiovascular and catecholamine response in Type A and Type B individuals. *Psychophysiology*, 1980, *17*, 453–463.
Hall, G. S. A study of anger. *American Journal of Psychology*, 1899, *10*, 516–591.
Haynes, S., Levine, S., Scotch, N., Feinleib, M., & Kannel, W. The relationship of psychosocial factors to coronary heart disease in the Framingham Study. *American Journal of Epidemiology*, 1978, *107*, 362–383.
Hearn, M., & Evans, D. Anger and reciprocal inhibition therapy. *Psychological Reports*, 1972, *30*, 943–948.
Herrell, J. M. *Use of systematic desensitization to eliminate inappropriate anger.* Proceedings of the 79th Annual Convention of the American Psycological Association, Washington, D.C. American Psychological Association, 1971, 431–432.
Horowitz, M. J., & Solomon, G. F. A prediction of delayed stress response syndromes in Vietnam veterans. *Journal of Social Issues*, 1975, *31*, 67–80.
Jenkins, C. D. Behavioral risk factors in coronary artery disease. *Annual Review of Medicine*, 1978, *29*, 543–562.
Lazarus, R. S. *Psychological stress and the coping process.* New York: McGraw-Hill, 1966.
Lazarus, R. S., & Launier, R. Stress related transactions between person and environment. In L. A. Pervin & M. Lewis (Eds.), *Perspectives in interactional psychology*. New York: Plenum, 1978.
Lawler, E. E. *Motivation in work organizations.* Monterey, Calif.: Brooks, 1973.
Lewin, K. *Field theory in social science.* New York: Harper, 1951.
MacCorquodale, K., & Meehl, P. Preliminary suggestions as to a formalization of expectancy theory. *Psychological Review*, 1953, *60*, 55–63.
Mace, D. R. Marital intimacy and the deadly love-anger cycle. *Journal of Marriage and Family Counseling*, 1976, April, 131–137.
Maynard, C., & Chitty, K. Dealing with anger: Guidelines for nursing intervention. *Journal of Psychiatric Nursing*, 1979, *17*, 36–41.
Merton, R. K. *Social theory and social structure.* Glencoe, Ill.: Free Press, 1957.
Miller, M. L. Blood pressure in relation to inhibited aggression in psychotics. *Psychosomatic Medicine*, 1939, *1*, 162–167.
Novaco, R. W. The cognitive regulation of anger and stress. In D. Kendall & S. Hollon (Eds.), *Cognitive behavioral interventions.* New York: Academic, 1979.
Novaco, R. W., & Hayes, A. *Expectations as determinants of anger arousal and aggressive behavior.* Paper presented at the 59th Annual Convention of the Western Psychological Association, San Diego, April, 1980.
Reid, J. B., & Taplin, P. S. A social interactional approach to the treatment of abusive families. *Journal of Pediatric Psychology*, 1980.
Rule, B., & Nesdale, A. Emotional arousal and aggressive behavior. *Psychological Bulletin*, 1976, *83*, 851–863.
Saul, L. Hostility in cases of essential hypertension. *Psychosomatic Medicine*, 1939, *1*, 153–161.
Seligman, M. *Helplessness: On depression, development, and death.* San Francisco: Freeman, 1975.
Shaw, C. R., & McKay, H. D. *Juvenile delinquency in urban areas.* Chicago: University of Chicago Press, 1942.
Siegel, J. M. *The Multidimensional Anger Inventory.* Unpublished manuscript, University of California, Los Angeles, 1983.
Thomas, M., Baker, J., & Estes, N. Anger: A tool for developing self-awareness. *American Journal of Nursing*, 1970, Dec., 2586–2590.
Thrasher, F. *The gang.* Chicago: University of Chicago Press, 1929.
Toch, H. *Violent men.* Chicago: Aldine, 1969.
Tolman, E. C. *Purposive behavior in animals and men.* New York: Century, 1932.
Tolman, E. C. Principles of purposive behavior. In S. Koch (Ed.), *Psychology: A study of a science* (Vol. II). New York: McGraw-Hill, 1959.
Tolman, E. C., & Brunswik, E. The organism and the causal texture of the environment. *Psychological Review*, 1935, *42*, 43–77.
Turk, A. *Criminality and the legal order.* Chicago: Rand McNally, 1969.
Vroom, V. H. *Work and motivation.* New York: Wiley, 1964.

12
On the Diagnosis and Treatment of Chronically Hostile Individuals

Michael H. L. Hecker
SRI International

Donald T. Lunde
Stanford University Medical Center

According to the social learning theory of aggression, aversive environmental situations, such as interpersonal confrontations, produce a general state of emotional arousal that can facilitate a variety of behaviors (Bandura, 1973). Depending on the individual's cognitive appraisal of environmental conditions and stimuli, the emotional arousal generated may be experienced subjectively as anger. This anger may eventually be expressed as aggressive behavior ranging from a sarcastic remark to a physical attack if the individual has not learned effective skills for coping with stress. Whether or not aggressive behavior occurs, the anger usually diminishes in a matter of minutes, leaving the individual free for new emotional experiences. However, feelings of anger can also be prolonged or regenerated on subsequent occasions by recalling and focusing on provocative situations. In this context, individuals who frequently become angry in the absence of specific external stimuli may be regarded as exhibiting chronic hostility.

Chronic hostility is of considerable interest to behavioral and medical science. Of particular relevance to this volume, chronic hostility has recently been recognized to play a role in the development and progression of physical disorders. Epidemiological studies suggest that chronically hostile individuals are at risk for coronary atherosclerosis, coronary heart disease, and essential hypertension (Diamond, 1982). Whether anger is acknowledged and expressed or denied and suppressed apparently is a critical factor in disease development. For example, among women with metastatic breast cancer, the ability to communicate anger and psychological distress is associated with survival time (Derogatis, Abeloff, & Melisaratos, 1979). Because of such correlations between anger and physical disorders, the assessment of chronic hostility and the design of effective techniques for its treatment have become important topics in behavioral medicine.

Although not recognized as psychopathology, chronic hostility is implicated in a number of psychiatric diagnoses, including Somatization Disorder, Intermittent

Explosive Disorder, Passive-Aggressive Personality Disorder, and Antisocial Personality Disorder (American Psychiatric Association, 1980). Chronically hostile individuals often have deficits in social skills; they may lack sensitivity to interpersonal problems, fail to consider possible consequences of their behavior, and be unable to see a situation from the perspective of another person (Spivack, Platt, & Shure, 1976). In addition, the intense emotional arousal experienced by chronically hostile individuals has been shown to impair their cognitive appraisal of aversive events and facilitate impulsive behavior (Zillmann, 1983). The deficits in social skills, in conjunction with insufficient self-control, can severely limit the social functioning of these individuals.

The etiology of chronic hostility is largely unknown. Many chronically hostile individuals attribute their current attitude to previous stressful events, such as sibling rivalry, frustrated aspirations, occupational disappointments, and contested divorce. Role models, especially parents, can also influence the development of attitudes and behavior patterns. For example, an individual may imitate and adopt the aggressive behavior of a physically abusive father. However, such early experiences and role models cannot be regarded as exclusive causes of chronic hostility because they are also reported by non-hostile individuals. Other factors are undoubtedly involved, including feelings of inadequacy or insecurity, unrealistic views and expectations, and insufficient skills for dealing with stressful situations.

Various therapeutic techniques are available for correcting specific behavioral and cognitive deficits that often underlie chronic hostility. Relaxation training (Jacobsen, 1938) and the technique of systematic desensitization (Rimm, deGroot, Boord, Reiman, & Dillow, 1971) are used to control the physiological correlates of emotional arousal; an individual acquires the ability to deal with perceived challenges without being overwhelmed by physiological symptoms. Techniques emphasizing selfinstruction by means of internalized speech (Meichenbaum & Goodman, 1971; Meichenbaum, 1977) are used to reduce impulsive behavior and modify cognitive appraisals of aversive events. Training in problem solving (D'Zurilla & Goldfried, 1971) often leads to more effective coping in social situations; the individual learns to recognize interpersonal conflicts, generate response alternatives, and make decisions that are consistent with personal goals. The stress inoculation approach to treatment (Novaco, 1979) is a particular combination of many such techniques.

Because chronically hostile individuals do not constitute a clinically homogeneous group, a given individual would be expected to benefit more from certain therapeutic techniques than from others; for this reason, all chronically hostile individuals should not receive the same treatment. Unlike the stress inoculation approach mentioned above, which is applied uniformly to a target population, the authors propose that treatment be tailored to meet the specific needs of each individual. A prerequisite for this approach is the development of a system for identifying and classifying the different forms of chronic hostility. In this chapter, we present a preliminary typology of chronic hostility and discuss intervention strategies that we consider to be particularly well-suited to each of the proposed clinical types. Realizing that our typology is neither unique nor complete, we believe that it can stimulate further efforts toward a more comprehensive diagnostic system.

TYPOLOGY OF CHRONIC HOSTILITY

We conceptualize three main types of chronic hostility, each of which can be divided into two subtypes. This proposed typology is outlined in Table 1. The main types (designated Types I, II, and III) are defined on the basis of two general criteria: the emotional experience of anger, and the ease with which angry feelings are translated into aggressive behavior. The related subtypes (designated A and B) are separated by means of more specific criteria. Each subtype is illustrated by one or two examples of chronically hostile individuals. For the most part, these examples are based on clinical cases that we have examined and followed.

Type I: Undercontrolled Type

According to the proposed typology, individuals who exhibit chronic hostility of the Undercontrolled type experience anger emotionally, that is, they respond to certain situations by *feeling* angry. Furthermore, their angry feelings are readily translated into aggressive behavior. As described by Megargee (1966;

Table 1 Typology of chronic hostility

Type I: Undercontrolled Type		
Anger is experienced emotionally and is readily translated into aggressive behavior.		
Type IA: Impulsive		*Type IB: Deliberate*
Angry feelings lead immediately to aggressive behavior.		Angry feelings lead to a plan for aggressive behavior that is implemented later.
Examples: The Name Caller The Barroom Fighter		Examples: The Prankster The Persistent Avenger
Type II: Overcontrolled Type		
Anger is experienced emotionally but generally is not translated into aggressive behavior.		
Type IIA: Stable		*Type IIB: Unstable*
Stable inhibitions prevent aggressive behavior under all conditions.		Unstable inhibitions may fail under stress, allowing aggressive behavior.
Examples: The Complainer The Martyr		Examples: The Unlikely Killer
Type III: Suppressed Type		
Anger is not experienced emotionally, but its effects are apparent in behavior and health.		
Type IIIA: Normal		*Type IIIB: Psychotic*
Perception of reality is intact; affect is suppressed.		Perception of reality is disturbed; affect is inappropriate.
Examples: The Somatizer The Frantic Worker		Examples: The Paranoid Schizophrenic

1982), these individuals have weak inhibitions against aggressive behavior and exert little or no control over provocations to aggression. Their aggressive behavior may have one or more overt objectives, such as enhancement of self-image, domination of others, acceptance by a peer group, and retaliation. Assuming that these individuals can be identified in a clinical setting, it would be desirable to distinguish between those who act impulsively and those who plan their aggressive behavior.

Type IA: Impulsive Undercontrolled Type

These individuals experience anger emotionally and act impulsively with little or no prior deliberation. Some Type A or coronary-prone individuals who are also hostile are considered to fall into this category. Early descriptions of the Type A behavior pattern emphasize impatience, a sense of time urgency, and aggressiveness (Rosenman, Friedman, Straus, Wurm, Kositchek, Hahn, & Worthessen, 1964). In a more recent study, which confirmed these descriptions, Type A individuals were found to score high on questionnaire scales that measure impulsivity and aggression, and low on scales that measure self control (Chesney, Black, Chadwick, & Rosenman, 1981). Despite these results it should be noted that not all hostile Type A individuals are characterized by impulsive behavior.

When angry, Impulsive Undercontrolled individuals often disregard personal safety and precipitate accidents that result in injuries to themselves or to others. For example, a driver caught in heavy traffic may become so irritated that he ignores a red light and collides with another vehicle. From the perspective of criminal behavior, when these individuals act aggressively, they are often identified and restrained because their impulsive behavior is likely to occur in the presence of others. Two examples of the Impulsive Undercontrolled type are given below.

The name caller. Eric D., a junior in high school, was frustrated by his family situation, his below-average academic achievement, and his limited mechanical aptitude. As he reluctantly performed household chores requested by his mother and step-father, Eric would mutter profanities and call his parents names. Instead of attempting a difficult homework problem, he would slam shut his textbook and curse his teacher. One day, while working on his bicycle, Eric had trouble adjusting the chain; he got so angry that he kicked his bicycle until the rear wheel was severely damaged.

The barroom fighter. Paul H., a 43-year-old bachelor and truck driver, spent long hours on the road driving and listening to the radio. His favorite programs were news commentaries and interviews that dealt with controversial issues. Alone in unfamiliar towns on lay-overs, he would spend his evenings in local bars. He frequently engaged others in conversation, but became agitated and quarrelsome if their opinions differed from his. Although some of these arguments escalated into physical fights, Paul never hurt anyone seriously and was never arrested for disorderly conduct. However, during a recent altercation he experienced severe chest pains, which were subsequently diagnosed as angina pectoris.

Type IB: Deliberate Undercontrolled Type

Deliberate Undercontrolled individuals experience anger that does not lead directly to aggressive behavior. Instead of behaving impulsively, they develop plans for aggressive behavior that can be implemented later. Because the aggressive behavior is separated in time from the provocation, the aggressor is often able to act anonymously. Typical deliberate acts performed by them include conspiring with others to defeat a competitor, plagerism, embezzlement, and homicide. Two examples of this type are presented.

The prankster. Ellen S. worked as a file clerk for a law firm. She felt strongly attracted to a young attorney in the office, but his attitude suggested that he was not interested in a romantic relationship. He was merely polite whenever they spoke about business matters, and he did not initiate any personal conversations with her. Nevertheless, Ellen continued to have fantasies about him until she heard that he was engaged to be married. Rejected and angry, she thought of how she might punish him for loving someone else. Subsequently, she went to the law firm after hours, entered his office, and vandalized his files.

The persistent avenger. George Metesky, an employee of a large utility company, was 28 when he was involved in a boiler accident. He filed a claim for permanent disability pay, alleging that the accident had permanently injured him, but his claim was denied because there was no medical evidence to support it. George wrote a number of angry letters to his former employer and to various government officials demanding that his case be reconsidered. When he received no satisfaction, he planned his revenge. For 16 years, he detonated increasingly powerful and destructive homemade bombs in public places in New York City, effectively terrorizing the populace (Brussel, 1968).

Type II: Overcontrolled Type

Individuals who exhibit chronic hostility of the Overcontrolled type also experience anger emotionally, but their angry feelings are generally not translated into aggressive behavior. Megargee (1966; 1982) describes these individuals as having strong inhibitions against aggressive behavior; they exert enormous control over provocations to aggression. Although their chronic hostility is designated overcontrolled, the inhibitions may be stable or unstable.

Type IIA: Stable Overcontrolled Type

Despite the level of anger experienced by these individuals, their strong and stable inhibitions will prevent them from engaging in aggressive behavior. Even under conditions of extreme stress, they manage to control their responses to nearly all provocations to aggression. When challenged, an individual of this type may adopt a passive stance or withdraw so as to avoid an unpleasant emotional exchange. However, the incident and its resulting frustrations are likely to be remembered for a long time.

Stable Overcontrolled individuals can become so preoccupied with their unexpressed thoughts and feelings that they neglect their health by smoking or eating too much, exercising too little, ignoring early symptoms of physical disorders, or failing to take prescribed medications. These negative health behaviors increase their risk for cardiovascular and cerebrovascular diseases. Two examples of the Stable Overcontrolled type are given below.

The complainer. Joyce R. was a 31-year-old nurse who was dedicated to her profession and emotionally invested in her work. As she performed her duties at a community hospital, she frequently noticed situations that were, in her opinion, potentially harmful to her patients. Joyce was infuriated whenever she discovered an error in a patient's chart or saw poor techniques used by other nurses, but she did not mention her anger to anyone. Instead, she withheld her indignation for days and tried to relieve her anger by indulging herself with food. Sometimes she documented her accumulated complaints in long and tedious memos to her supervisor. Her memos were largely ignored because the situations she described were considered to be insignificant. During her two-year employment at the hospital, she alienated many of her co-workers and gained 45 pounds.

The martyr. Robert B. was a man who lived for his family. When he was 49, he moved his family to another city so that his wife would be closer to her relatives. His new job was not as satisfactory as he had hoped, however, and after an extended search for more suitable employment he finally accepted a lower-status position in a neighboring state. Refusing to leave her relatives, his wife divorced him and was granted custody of their three children. Robert was deeply hurt by these events and blamed his former wife for destroying his family life. He continued to work hard to support his children, who were allowed to visit him regularly, but he never discussed with them how much he resented their mother. When he applied for life insurance to increase their financial security, he learned that he had high blood pressure and that his premiums would be increased because of the additional risk. Robert gradually became an embittered old man who could no longer communicate effectively with others. Shortly after his youngest child finished college, he suffered a stroke and died.

Type IIB: Unstable Overcontrolled Type

Under ordinary conditions, the strong though unstable inhibitions of these individuals are effective in preventing the outbreak of aggressive behavior. But under conditions of extreme stress, the inhibitions suddenly fail for reasons that are not fully understood. Extremely violent, even criminal behavior may occur, including multiple homicides. Individuals who commit such crimes are usually remorseful afterward, and are able to reconstruct their former, unstable inhibitions. An example of this type is given here.

The unlikely killer. At 42, Dan White was known as a crusader against crime. Raised in a large family in San Francisco, he not only served the city as a policeman and then as a fireman but also was elected to the Board of Supervisors. In his campaign for supervisor he stressed law and order, the staple of his law-enforcement career. Ten months after he took office, however, Dan resigned because of extreme stress and exhaustion. His relationships with the other supervisors had deteriorated, his wife had just had a new baby but was forced to work to alleviate their financial problems, and he became quite depressed. As the mayor was about to announce his replacement to the board, Dan asked to be reinstated. His request was denied. Suddenly, he felt overwhelmed and his inhibitions collapsed; he took out his police revolver and killed the mayor and a supervisor who had opposed his reappointment. Then he remorsefully surrendered to the police, waived his rights, and made a tearful confession.

Type III: Suppressed Type

Individuals who exhibit chronic hostility of the Suppressed type do not experience anger emotionally. Their anger is suppressed and functions as a source of anxiety, pain, and maladaptive behavior. Cognitively divorced from their anger, these individuals are often surprised when others call their attitude hostile or their behavior aggressive. They may also suppress other emotions, with the result that their responses to common situations often lack genuine, appropriate affect. The two subtypes within this category are distinguished on the basis of whether perceptions and interpretations of reality are normal or psychotic.

Type IIIA: Normal Suppressed Type

When these individuals encounter difficult or frustrating situations, they generally become anxious and engage in unproductive behavior. Dominant individuals of this type may be so demanding and aggressive in their interpersonal relationships that, while perhaps attaining immediate goals, they compromise their long-term objectives. Submissive individuals, on the other hand, may accommodate themselves to the desires of others at the expense of their own needs. To obtain relief from their psychological distress, individuals of this type immerse themselves in unnecessary work or leisure-time activities that keep them constantly busy.

The emotional detachment of these individuals often leads indirectly to psychosomatic symptoms and physical disorders. According to the early psychoanalytic literature (cf. Alexander, 1939), suppressed anger is thought to be associated with hypertension, migraine headaches, insomnia, bronchial asthma, gastric ulcers, colitis, dermatitis, obesity, and substance abuse. These early hypotheses have recently been the focus of renewed investigation (for reviews see Diamond, 1982, and Appel, Holroyd and Gorkin, in press). With regard to hypertension, survey, clinical, and laboratory research, "though not entirely consistent, supports the view that at least a subset of hypertensives are chronically hostile, conflicted about anger expression and tend to be overly submissive and compliant while nurturing considerable resentment" (Diamond, 1982, p. 428). Two examples of the Normal Suppressed type follow.

The somatizer. Mary B. was rather introverted and shy. When she was 18, she became pregnant and was coerced into marriage by her parents. She viewed mothering, shopping, cooking, cleaning, and washing as unrewarding. After six years of marriage, her husband became inattentive to her and she suspected that he was being unfaithful. Gradually Mary developed various psychosomatic and physical symptoms, including severe headaches, shortness of breath, irregular and painful menstrual periods, blurred vision, and back pain. A thorough physical examination revealed no medical basis for her symptoms, and her husband offered ridicule rather than sympathy for her condition. Although bothered by continued pain and distress, she did not seek further medical treatment.

The frantic worker. Jerome K., 53, managed an engineering group at a large aerospace company but had aspirations to head his own department. He drove himself to put in at least 60 hours per week, including evenings and weekends that could otherwise be spent in leisure activities. By meeting nearly impossible deadlines and struggling to surpass his competition, Jerome led his group to distinction, receiving many company awards and professional citations. In his relationships with his fellow workers, he was cordial but demanding. When others failed to meet his expectations, he would be rather tactless. Whenever he was confronted about his hostile attitude and aggressive behavior, he viewed the allegations as foreign and not pertaining to him. While on a long-delayed vacation with his wife, he suffered a heart attack.

Type IIIB: Psychotic Suppressed Type

Psychotic individuals have distorted perceptions of reality, and their responses to situations and events are often inappropriate. Given their inaccurate view of reality, the diagnosis of chronic hostility among psychotic individuals must be based on behavioral observations. For example, suppressed anger in cases of psychotic depression can be inferred from self-punishing behaviors, such as neglecting personal hygiene, refusing to get out of bed, refusing to eat, and mutilating the body. Some schizophrenics, imagining that they are controlled by hostile outside forces, engage in violent behavior to accomplish "special missions." One example of the Psychotic Suppressed type will suffice.

The paranoid schizophrenic. John Frazier showed no clear indications of mental illness until he was 24. He was fascinated with cars and worked intermittently as an auto mechanic. At the same time, he was concerned about pollution and its effects on the environment. A minor car accident, which caused him no injury, precipitated his first hallucination: He heard the voice of God warn him that he would be killed if he drove again. After this incident, he considered himself ordained to carry out a special mission, saving the world from materialism and pollution. As his ideas became progressively more bizarre, his wife and his mother begged him to seek psychiatric treatment, but he believed that they were part of a conspiracy to prevent him from carrying out his mission. He eventually left his wife and moved into a cow shed. One day, John decided that an elaborately-styled home in the vicinity had to be destroyed in the name of the divinely mandated revolution. He entered the house with a gun, killed its five occupants, and set it on fire (Lunde, 1976).

GOALS AND METHODS OF TREATMENT

The treatment of chronically hostile individuals has several general goals. One goal is to facilitate personal growth and enrichment of life through attenuation of hostility. This often leads to greater self-esteem and creativity, better interpersonal relationships, and more enjoyment of life. A second goal is to prevent physical disorders associated with chronic hostility, or limit their progression. Acquiring non-aggressive coping skills, for instance, appears to reduce a coronary patient's risk of subsequent myocardial infarctions (Thoresen, Friedman, Gill, & Ulmer, 1982). A third goal of treatment is to control violence, especially criminal violence. For example, anger management approaches such as those discussed by Reid and Kavanagh in their chapter in this volume should lower the incidence of child abuse and other crimes that occur primarily among family members.

Different types of chronic hostility have different implications for treatment; therefore, the treatment of a chronically hostile individual must be based on a specific diagnosis. In this section, we describe a general therapeutic approach for each type of chronic hostility, but any treatment plan must also take into account personal and situational factors. Among the personal factors are the individual's intelligence, emotional maturity, social skills, physical health, lifestyle, and long-term goals. The situational factors include the individual's work environment, home environment, social support, and financial resources. In principle, the treatment of chronic hostility is similar to the treatment of other attitudinal and behavioral disorders.

In order to evaluate the effectiveness of treatment, measures of chronic hostility are needed. Questionnaire scales, such as those discussed by Spielberger, Siegel, and Williams and their colleagues in their chapters in this volume, would constitute one alternative. Another approach more akin to behavioral assessment (Ciminero, 1977) would be to develop a measure of the actual frequency and severity of reported or observed aggressive behavior, which would serve as an estimate of the level of hostility. Such an approach would only be appropriate with those types of chronically hostile individuals who engage in aggressive behavior (i.e., Types IA, IB, IIB, and IIIB). Thus, to use the examples given above, the Barroom Fighter would most likely be considered more hostile than the Name Calier, and the Persistent Avenger more hostile than the Prankster. For individuals who do not engage in aggressive behavior (i.e., Types IIA and IIIA), a similar measure could be developed to assess the degree to which the individual's behavior impedes social interaction. An indication of serious problems in interpersonal relationships thought to result from hostility would provide an indirect measure of this underlying attitude. Using such a measure, the Martyr would most likely be considered more hostile than the Complainer, and the Frantic Worker more hostile than the Somatizer. Following treatment, the frequency and severity of reported or observed aggressive behavior, or the degree of social isolation, would be assessed again to evaluate the effectiveness of treatment.

Type IA: Impulsive Undercontrolled Type

Individuals who exhibit chronic hostility of the Impulsive Undercontrolled type are likely to benefit most from intervention techniques that emphasize the acquisition of behavioral coping skills. A fundamental problem of these individuals is their limited repertoire of response alternatives; when they feel angry, they resort to aggressive behavior often because it is the primary coping behavior in their repertoire. In therapy, this problem is dealt with by teaching them a wide variety of non-aggressive response alternatives, including intentional withdrawal from challenging situations, passive observation of the behavior of others, negotiation with potential adversaries, and appropriate humor. While these coping skills are being taught, the individuals are advised to stay away from people and places that are known to arouse their anger.

Another difficulty encountered by these individuals is insufficient impulse control. To provide as much time as possible for the application of newly learned response alternatives, these individuals are trained to recognize the early physiological signs of anger. The perception of these signs becomes a warning that a critical situation has developed and adaptive behavior is called for. Frequently, these individuals experience a rapid escalation of angry feelings before they can apply their coping skills. Anxiety management training can be used to minimize this effect and improve self-control (Hart, 1984). With this approach, individuals are first taught relaxation exercises such as deep breathing and muscle relaxation that are incompatible with physiological arousal (Jacobsen, 1938). Following this training, individuals are taught to imagine stressful, anger-provoking situations and to attend to how they respond to the stress. When individuals are able to experience anger arousal in response to imagined stressful situations, they are taught to induce stress using imagery and practice controlling anger arousal with relaxation exercises. Thus, individuals learn to replace impulsive reactions to stressful events with self-controlled relaxation.

Impulsive Undercontrolled individuals also have a problem communicating. Many cannot express their feelings verbally without offending or alienating others (Bandura, 1973). In therapy, they receive instruction in social skills in order to avoid misunderstandings that result from inaccurate and ineffective communication. These skills are also valuable for resolving interpersonal conflicts through discussion, and for keeping difficult relationships on a superficial and non-aggressive level.

By definition, Impulsive Undercontrolled individuals have poorly developed inhibitions against aggressive behavior. In therapy, efforts are made to strengthen these inhibitions by examining potential consequences of aggressive behavior, including the forfeiture of long-term personal goals. For example, a man may be told that his anger arousal and aggressive behavior could not only have a deleterious effect on his health but could also lead to his losing an important business client, which would jeopardize his position or career. Another technique for strengthening weak inhibitions is social and moral education. This approach may help individuals who have not internalized the social values and attitudes relating to non-aggression.

Type IB: Deliberate Undercontrolled Type

In contrast to the previous group, these individuals benefit more from intervention techniques that provide cognitive coping skills. A major problem of these individuals is that they have many unrealistic views and expectations; they often attach undue personal significance to ordinary events in their life. Therapy focuses on their reassessment of past events that were considered to be threatening or provocative. Their initial interpretation of such an event is evaluated in the context of the situation in which it occurred, using all available facts and information. Other possible interpretations are explored until an alternative, less anger-provoking interpretation is found (Novaco, 1979).

Another problem of these individuals is their tendency to become obsessed with plans for aggressive behavior; they may lose perspective on the present and fail to monitor their current thoughts and activities. Training in self-instruction (Meichenbaum, 1977) is useful to reduce emotional involvement and strengthen inhibitions against aggressive behavior. The individuals develop several personally relevant anger-inhibiting instructions that they are taught to say to themselves whenever a provocation occurs. The following statements are examples of such instructions: "Don't take it personally—it could have happened to somebody else;" "Thinking about this only makes you upset;" "This is not what you should be doing right now," and "You don't really want to hurt this person."

Some of the Deliberate Undercontrolled individuals derive satisfaction from their secret deliberations and anonymous activities. In therapy, they are advised that their aggressive behavior can easily have far more serious results than they intend. For example, the sabotage of production equipment by a disgruntled worker can lead to an accident in which someone is injured.

Type IIA: Stable Overcontrolled Type

Individuals with this type of chronic hostility are taught a variety of behavioral and cognitive coping skills. One of their problems is passive-aggressive behavior that is ineffective in meeting their personal needs. These individuals tend to be insecure, lack self-confidence, and seek recognition. Assertiveness training (Lange & Jakubowski, 1976) is used to define alternative forms of non-aggressive behavior that are more likely to meet their needs. The first step is to identify provocative situations in which the individual tends to be passive. For each of these situations, the therapist working with the individual develops alternative, more assertive responses that will achieve the individual's needs without involving hostility and aggression. The individual first practices the alternative responses in the therapeutic setting, then is assigned to apply the new skill in response to anger-provoking situations in the natural environment.

Stable Overcontrolled individuals tend to have unrealistic expectations of themselves, others, and events. In therapy, they are assisted in reformulating expectations to more realistic levels and encouraged to question their accusations and attributions. For example, these individuals perceive spontaneous, random events such as equipment malfunctions or employee illnesses as the result of negligence or maliciousness. These appraisals are not only often inaccurate, they are destructive. By accepting unavoidable situations instead of getting angry at an imperfect world, these individuals can acquire behavior that is more adaptive and may lose their sense of being controlled or victimized.

Type IIB: Unstable Overcontrolled Type

The problems observed among Type IIA individuals are also exhibited by many Type IIB individuals, and both groups benefit from the same intervention techniques. However, the Type IIB individuals have an additional problem that must be dealt with in therapy: their inhibitions against aggressive behavior are vulnerable under stress. These individuals are instructed to avoid potentially stressful situations as much as possible. Depending on the source and degree of the individual's aggravation, avoiding stress may mean working fewer hours, delegating more responsibility to others, changing jobs, taking a vacation, staying away from certain family members, and even voluntary hospitalization. Consuming alcoholic beverages is strongly discouraged because alcohol generally weakens behavioral inhibitions.

These individuals are taught various skills for managing their feelings, thoughts, and behavior in unavoidable stressful situations. The technique of systematic desensitization (Rimm, deGroot, Boord, Reiman, & Dillow, 1971) works well for stressful situations that are fairly specific. First, the individual describes various critical situations and ranks them according to the level of stress they evoke. Then, the individual receives relaxation training and practices this skill while imagining the least stressful situation. Because relaxation is incompatible with arousal, the individual soon reports an abatement of the initially experienced tension. When the tension is sufficiently reduced, the individual practices relaxation while imagining a more stressful situation. This process is repeated until the individual is able to imagine the most stressful situation without feeling tense.

Systematic desensitization is used in conjunction with cognitive intervention techniques that are designed to modify the individual's views and expectations of stressful encounters. Descriptions of these views and expectations may give the therapist information about the unstable nature of the individual's inhibitions. For example, an individual with a prejudice against certain people or occupations may not apply learned social values and attitudes to all relationships. Inhibitions are likely to be weakened in situations that involve such exceptions. The individual must be taught additional skills for controlling aggressive behavior under such special circumstances.

Type IIIA: Normal Suppressed Type

In general, individuals with this type of chronic hostility do not respond well to treatment because they fail to acknowledge their suppressed anger. These individuals tend to suppress many of their feelings and have difficulties with interpersonal relationships. These problems, in turn, deprive them of social support. Therefore, the focus of treatment is to provide a supportive environment and to assist the individual in identifying and expressing emotions.

Specifically, the therapist can provide social support and guidance for dealing with other relationships. In doing so, he or she serves as a model of an emotionally responsive and expressive person. The therapist also provides systemic reinforcement for the individual's appropriate emotional expressions. These expressions occur both spontaneously in response to the supportive environment and as a result of the modeling. Once individuals are able to recognize their anger, other cognitive-behavioral procedures such as the cognitive-restructuring technique and assertiveness training discussed earlier are applicable. Those procedures can be used to assist the individual in reducing anger arousal and enhance coping skills.

Type IIIB: Psychotic Suppressed Type

Psychotic individuals are poor candidates for psychotherapy. They are not sufficiently aware of their thoughts and behavior to be able to follow logical arguments or understand social injunctions against violence. For them, the treatment of choice is chemotherapy with hospitalization if necessary.

Comparison with Stress-Inoculation Approach

The treatment orientation outlined above differs somewhat from the stress inoculation approach described by Novaco in Chap. 11. The stress inoculation approach, a comprehensive package of many therapeutic techniques, has been shown to be effective with several populations, including law-enforcement officers at high risk for anger provocation, a hospitalized psychiatric patient with severe anger problems, and probation officers who must interact with hostile clients. Although the approach was applied uniformly to all individuals, it is unlikely that they benefited equally from each of the component techniques. The hospitalized psychiatric patient would be expected to derive more benefit from the component of the approach that develops social skills than from the cognitive-restructuring component. On the other hand, the police officers would probably benefit more from the cognitive restructuring than from the social-skills training.

In contrast, the orientation presented here is based on the premise that the particular needs of an individual should determine which therapeutic techniques are applied. These needs are identified in terms of a proposed typology of chronic hostility. Once the individual has been correctly diagnosed, the most effective techniques can be brought to bear on salient anger-related problems. Eventually, the diagnostic categories may specify not only which techniques are to be used, but also their relative importance in achieving a desired result. Both clinical and experimental evaluations of this approach are invited.

REFERENCES

Alexander, F. Emotional factors in essential hypertension. *Psychosomatic Medicine,* 1939, *1,* 173-179.
American Psychiatric Association, Task Force on Nomenclature and Statistics. *Diagnostic and statistical manual of mental disorders* (3rd ed.). Washington, D.C.: American Psychiatric Association, 1980.
Appel, M. A., Holroyd, K. A., & Gorkin, L. Anger and the etiology and progression of physical illness. In L. Temoshok, C. Van Dyke, & L. S. Zegans (Eds.), *Emotions in health and illness: Theoretical and research foundations.* New York: Grune & Stratton, 1983.
Bandura, A. *Aggression: A social learning analysis.* Englewood Cliffs, N.J.: Prentice-Hall, 1973.
Brussel, J. A. *Casebook of a crime psychiatrist.* New York: Grove Press, 1968.
Chesney, M. A., Black, G. W., Chadwick, J. H., & Rosenman, R. H. Psychological correlates of the Type A behavior pattern. *Journal of Behavioral Medicine,* 1981, *4*(No. 2), 217-229.
Ciminero, A. R. Behavioral assessment: An overview. In A. R. Ciminero, K. S. Calhoun, & H. E. Adams (Eds.), *Handbook of behavioral assessment.* New York: Wiley, 1977.
Derogatis, L. R., Abeloff, M. D., & Melisaratos, N. Psychological coping mechanisms and survival time in metastatic breast cancer. *Journal of the American Medical Association,* 1979, *242*(No. 14), 1504-1508.
Diamond, E. L. The role of anger and hostility in essential hypertension and coronary heart disease. *Psychological Bulletin,* 1982, *92*(No. 2), 410-433.
D'Zurilla, T. J., & Goldfried, M. R. Problem-solving and behavior modification. *Journal of Abnormal Psychology,* 1971, *78,* 107-126.
Hart, K. E. Anxiety management training and anger control for Type A individuals. *Journal of Behavioral Therapy and Experimental Psychiatry,* 1984, *15*(No. 2), 1-7.
Jacobsen, E. *Progressive relaxation.* Chicago: University of Chicago Press, 1938.
Lange, A., & Jakubowski, P. *Responsible assertive behavior.* Champaign, Ill.: Research, 1976.
Lunde, D. T. *Murder and madness.* San Francisco: San Francisco Book, 1976.
Megargee, E. I. Undercontrolled and overcontrolled personality types in extreme antisocial aggression. *Psychological Monographs,* 1966, *80*(No. 3), 1-29.
Megargee, E. I. Psychological determinants and correlates of criminal violence. In M. Wolfgang & N. Wiener (Eds.), *Criminal violence.* Beverly Hills, Calif.: Sage, 1982.
Meichenbaum, D. *Cognitive behavior modification.* New York: Plenum, 1977.
Meichenbaum, D., & Goodman, J. Training impulsive children to talk to themselves: A means of developing self-control. *Journal of Abnormal Psychology,* 1971, *77,* 115-126.
Novaco, R. W. The cognitive regulation of anger and stress. In P. C. Kendall & S. D. Hollon (Eds.), *Cognitive-behavioral interventions.* New York: Academic, 1979.
Rimm, D. C., deGroot, J. C., Boord, P., Reiman, J., & Dillow, P. V. Systematic desensitization of an anger response. *Behavior Research and Therapy,* 1971, *9,* 273-280.
Rosenman, R. H., Friedman, M., Straus, R., Wurm, M., Kositchek, R., Hahn, W., & Werthessen, N. T. A predictive study of coronary heart disease: The Western Collaborative Group Study. *Journal of the American Medical Association,* 1964, *189,* 15-22 and Appendix.

Spivack, G., Platt, J. J., & Shure, M. B. *The problem-solving approach to adjustment.* San Francisco: Jossey-Bass, 1976.

Thoresen, C. E., Friedman, M., Gill, J. K., & Ulmer, D. K. The recurrent coronary prevention project: Some preliminary findings. *Acta Medica Scandinavica (Supplementum),* 1982, *660,* 172-192.

Zillmann, D. Arousal and aggression. In R. G. Geen & E. I. Donnerstein (Eds.), *Aggression: Theoretical and empirical reviews* (Vol. 1). New York: Academic, 1983.

13

A Social Interactional Approach to Child Abuse: Risk, Prevention, and Treatment

John B. Reid and Kate Kavanagh
Oregon Social Learning Center

Most of the chapters in this volume deal with the adverse health effects of anger on the individuals who experience excessive and chronic levels of this emotion. While the effect of anger may be on the individual experiencing the emotion, anger often arises in an interpersonal context and has deleterious effects on others besides the individual experiencing the emotion. Thus, interventions to prevent anger and its consequences often involve studying the social antecedents of anger and intervening in a social framework. While research on anger modification is relatively new, the area of child abuse has received systematic study and can serve as a model for effective prevention and intervention. In this chapter, the focus will be on child abuse, a public health problem of staggering proportions that results from anger and hostility. The goals of this chapter are as follows: to present a conceptualization of anger and aggression in the context of child abuse which lends itself to the development of treatment and prevention activities; to review previous treatment strategies and present some preliminary findings relevant to the issues of prevention and treatment of child abuse; and, finally, to discuss implications of this research for treatment of anger and hostility in behavioral medicine.

PREVALENCE OF ABUSE AND PHYSICAL COERCION OF CHILDREN BY THEIR PARENTS

Child abuse gained the attention of the community and public health professionals when its prevalence was recognized during the late 1950s and early 1960s. Estimating the seriousness and extent of child abuse is difficult because statistics on child abuse were not recorded systematically by most states until the 1960s and early 1970s. Depending on the criteria employed and the sampling methodology used, estimates of the incidence of child abuse vary enormously. For example, Gil (1970) estimated that up to four million instances of child abuse occur each year. Kempe (1973) produced an estimate of 60,000 serious incidents for 1972. In 1980, nearly 800,000 cases of child maltreatment were reported in this country (The American Humane Association, 1981). Regardless of the variability among the various estimates, child abuse rates are alarmingly high. As pointed out by Parke and Lewis (1981), there are a number of reasons to expect estimates to vary and to suspect that most underestimate the actual rates of assaults against children. Among other factors, parents who *repeatedly* injure their children may take them to different doctors or hospitals in order to prevent classification as abuse (as opposed to accidents); many types of injuries are difficult to detect or to classify as the result of abuse; it is probable that many doctors under-report abuse instances; and definitions of what constitutes abuse vary widely across public health personnel and from one community or state to another.

An important descriptive fact about the incidence of child abuse that has not received the emphasis it deserves is that the victims of child abuse, particularly serious abuse and injury, are extremely young children. The mean age of child abuse victims is 7.22 years; the mean age for those who die as a result of their injuries is 3.34 years (The American Humane Association, 1981). This is undoubtedly due to the fact that the younger the child, the more easily injury occurs. Although unsettling to consider, this fact has important implications for conceptualizing risk, prevention, and treatment of child abuse. In the case of child abuse, prevention can be considered synonymous with treatment intervention. Families with young children who have patterns of pre-abusive behavior, or even histories of acute abusive behavior, can be treated for a relatively short period of time until the child is old enough to be better able to defend him- or herself using more advanced verbal skills, to learn to avoid conflict with an abusive parent, or to learn to run to a neighbor.

Although the focus in child abuse prevention research and intervention efforts is on high-risk families of young children, aggression is indicated by the prevalence of anger expression in the home and the general acceptance of corporal punishment as a proper form of discipline in Western societies. For example, it is estimated that over 90 percent of parents either consistently employ, or occasionally resort to, spanking or other types of physical coercion to resolve discipline problems (Stark & McEvoy, 1970). In a large and well designed study by Gelles (1979), approximately 2000 parents were interviewed about acts of family aggression that occurred during the previous year. In addition to spanking, over two percent had thrown something at their children more than twice; nearly twenty percent had pushed, grabbed, or shoved their children more than twice; nearly two percent had kicked, bitten, or hit with a fist more than twice; and nearly ten percent had hit their children with objects more than twice. In addition, quite relevant to the issue of the relationship of age of child and severity of risk, nearly 50 percent of the parents interviewed by Stark and McEvoy (1970) agreed that spanking was an appropriate discipline procedure for babies under one year of age.

FACTORS ASSOCIATED WITH ABUSE: A CONCEPTUAL FRAMEWORK

Anger and hostility often surface against a background of psychosocial stress. This is evident in the case of child abuse. Raising a child can be a difficult task that places heavy psychological, social, and financial burdens on parents. Unfortunately, most parents face the task of caring for young children under less than ideal circumstances: when the parents have little financial security, when parents are learning to work together, and sometimes while parents are still in the process of making their own transition from adolescence to adulthood. These sorts of stress have become worse rather than better over the last decade because of increasing inflation and unemployment. In addition, Glick (1979) reported that in 1978, nearly 20 percent of all children under the age of 18 years resided in one-parent families. The number of children living in this situation doubled between 1960 and 1978 (i.e., from nearly 6 to nearly 12 million youngsters). Thus, it is becoming increasingly more common for the hardships of child-rearing to be faced by single parents.

Even well-behaved children in "normal" families present their parents with numerous occasions for discipline. Chamberlain (1980) reported data for 85 families, screened on the basis of their being nondistressed in terms of child-parent relationships. Although reporting harmonious parent-child relationships on a global level, a behaviorally specific interview, coupled with daily reports on the behavior of their children, revealed that in nearly two-thirds of the families, at least one child management problem was chronic. (The most commonly reported problems, in descending order, were arguing, defiance, noncompliance, talking back, whining, and complaining.) These parent-report data are in accord with the direct observation data collected in the homes of nondistressed families, which show that young children behave poorly on the average of three or more times an hour when they interact with their parents (Fawl, 1963; Forehand, King, Peed, & Yoder, 1975; Minton, Kagan, & Levine, 1971; Reid, 1978). Based on these studies, it is reasonable to assume that some time or another during the child-rearing years, most parents experience a great deal of difficulty, stress, and uncertainty in dealing with discipline problems.

In addition to the stresses associated with child rearing, a substantial body of research that strongly implicates background stressors in triggering anger responses and conflict has been documented in the study of child abuse. Wahler and his associates (1978) found that families with severe child-management problems, compared to nondistressed controls, have fewer positive contacts with people in the community, more negative contacts, and that the negative contacts were typically initiated from outside the family. Marital conflict has also been shown to be associated with child abuse (Green, 1976; Reid, Taplin, & Lorber, 1981; Straus, 1980). In addition, situational and financial stress on the family has been found to be implicated in child abuse (Egleland & Brunnquell, 1977; Garbarino, 1976; Justice & Duncan, 1976). Emotional problems, such as depressed mood of parents, have been found to be associated with a decreased ability to deal with discipline situations (Forehand, Wells, & Griest, 1980; Novaco, 1975; Patterson, in press). Finally, it has been found that child-abusive parents, compared to nondistressed controls, tend to become more irritable and angry when dealing with discipline problems and other stressful encounters with their children (Reid, 1983).

IMPLICATIONS FOR THE TREATMENT/PREVENTION OF CHILD ABUSE

Hostility, anger and aggressive behavior often emerge in response to specific challenge. This is discussed frequently in the literature on Type A behavior pattern and is also true in cases of child abuse. Most child abuse occurs in the context of confrontations between the parent and child over discipline issues (Gil, 1969, 1971; Herrenkohl, Herrenkohl, & Egolf, 1983). Moreover, the vast majority of child abusive parents are ineffective and inconsistent in their use of discipline (Elmer & Gregg, 1967; Reid et al., 1981; Reid et al., 1982; Young, 1964), and the children who are abused tend to present parents with more discipline problems than do children who are not abused (Burgess & Conger, 1977; Friedman, 1972; Gil, 1970; Reid et al., 1981). Given these factors, it is clear that successful treatment or prevention procedures to combat child abuse will require a major focus on training abusive parents to deal more effectively with their children around discipline issues.

Given that background and personal stressors are also associated with anger and hostility, it is probable that attempts to train abusive or potentially abusive parents to deal more effectively with child management problems will be unsuccessful unless the background stressors are addressed by counselors and therapists. In research currently underway at our center, Patterson and his associates have found a significant covariation between the number of crises reported by mothers during the previous week and the amount of irritability they demonstrate while engaging in negotiations with their children about discipline issues (Patterson, 1982). Margolin and Christiansen (1981) have reported that parents reporting high marital stress profit little from parent training unless marital stress is dealt with therapeutically. Finally, Dumas and Wahler (1983) recently reported the results of a multiple-regression analysis showing that the insularity and socioeconomic stress experienced by a group of families receiving parent training accounted for 55 percent of the variance in the prediction of treatment outcome, with the families under most stress profiting least from the parent training. Thus, even if background or personal stressors are not directly involved in anger, hostility and their health effects, including child abuse, it is likely that unless significant problems are dealt with, individuals will be unwilling or unable to profit from training and intervention.

TREATMENT OF CHILD ABUSE

Intervention for anger management is relatively new in comparison to interventions for child abuse, where intensive multifaceted and multidisciplinary approaches have been developed and tested (Barnes, Chabon, & Hertzberg, 1974; Savino & Sanders, 1973; Steele & Pollock, 1974). Some approaches have emphasized systematic attempts by therapists to model appropriate parent roles in their treatment of child abusive parents, or to actually assume parent surrogate roles with the parents themselves (Paulson & Chaleff, 1973; Paulson, Savino, Chaleff, Sanders, Frisch, & Dunn, 1974). Other treatment approaches have used group therapy formats (Feinstein, Paul, & Esmiol, 1963; Justice & Justice, 1976); self-help support groups (Armstrong, 1980; Kempe & Helfer, 1972); and more dydactic training programs (Tracy, 1975; Tracy & Clark, 1974). For the most part, reports of intervention programs typically present global or general descriptions of the treatment procedures and, in those studies in which outcome effectiveness data were included, assessment of improvement depended on the uncorroborated self-reports of the therapists and/or parents treated.

SYSTEMATIC PARENT TRAINING FOR ABUSIVE FAMILIES

As stated earlier in this paper and elsewhere (Reid et al., 1981; Reid et al., 1982), specific variables are most immediately and directly involved in aggressive or hostile social interactions. In the case of child abuse, these variables involve discipline confrontations. Specifically, we have argued that abusive behavior is a direct function of the rate of frequency of aversive social interactions engaged in by the individuals involved, that is, parent-child dyads, and of the ability of one of these individuals (the parent) to quickly, nonabusively, and effectively terminate discipline confrontations when they occur. Since the middle of the 1960s, our group at the Oregon Social Learning Center has been developing and evaluating intervention strategies for helping parents to better handle discipline problems and confrontations with their youngsters (Patterson, Chamberlain, & Reid, 1983; Patterson & Gullion, 1968; Patterson & Reid, 1973; Reid & Patterson, 1976). It is only in the last few years that we have focused our attention on the development of intervention procedures assigned specifically for parents who chronically or seriously assault their children (Reid et al., 1981, 1982).

In this section, our general approach to intervention in chronic discipline problems will be described, followed by some additional procedures we have developed for working with child abusive parents. It should be stated at the outset that, although the parenting strategies we prescribe are relatively programmatic and straightforward, we strongly feel that teaching these skills and persuading individuals to use them in a sensible and consistent manner requires (a) clinical skill and flexibility on the part of the therapists, and (b) a significant amount of time and energy in helping individuals deal with the background stresses, personal problems, and situational difficulties in which their anger management problems are embedded. In actual word counts of audio and video tapes of our intervention sessions at OSLC, we have found that about 40 percent of the verbal content making up these sessions does not involve instructional parent training activities, but is focused on helping parents deal with the more general problems of day-to-day living.

The first step in any anger management training program is to establish a working relationship. It is common for individuals to deny or become defensive about their anger. This is particularly important with individuals with anger-exacerbated health problems who are referred by their physicians and of parents who have been court-referred for abuse. The latter group often feels angry and victimized by the state at the time they come for counseling. At least one complete session is devoted to explaining how we will work together to solve their problems. Parents are construed as the experts on their family and therapists are seen as the experts on child-management techniques. With abusive parents, we feel that it is critical to review in detail the episode(s) that led to the referral. Once parents have been able to present their side of the story, and after the therapist has listened without providing judgmental feedback, the violence and anger present in the home become appropriate and "natural" topics of therapy. The last step in the initial phase is to have the parents state what they want to gain from working together. It is necessary to provide parents with a feeling of control over the situation in order to avoid their participating because the court or physician ordered it. If they feel they can gain nothing from the training, then we recommend they seek help elsewhere.

Following this initial stage, we move into teaching specific skills. In interventions for child abuse, these are three core phases: pinpointing and tracking, attention to positive behavior, and punishment of inappropriate behavior. We often find that abusive parents have inconsistent and inappropriate expectations for their children. We attempt to give the parents both normative and individualized information throughout treatment about what they can reasonably expect from their children. We have, for example, worked with parents who thought babies six months of age could understand complicated requests. It is small wonder that such parents would feel their baby is negative and noncompliant. Although these components have been developed for parent training in anger management, it is likely that they have a place in anger intervention generally.

Pinpointing and Tracking

These are two distinct skills that are the basic building blocks of the training programs for improving social interactions. *Pinpointing* is essentially a procedure to separate the emotional and attributional aspects from the concrete, behavioral aspects of problem interactions. The goal of this procedure is to take the emotionality (anger, helplessness, guilt) out of the individual's complaints about others in the situation, such as the child, and to focus instead on the observable and specific behaviors that leave the individual angry and confused. In parent training for child abuse, parents use such labels as "willful," "negative," and "bad attitude" to describe their children. It is the therapist's goal to find out what the parents mean by these labels, translating the labels into behavioral terms. This helps parents and therapist to use a common language. If the child is said to be "willful," the therapist works with the parents to define willful so that specific instances of the behavior can be tracked and reacted to in a systematic fashion. If it can be defined, for example, as not complying to simple requests, then the child's compliance or noncompliance to requests becomes the focus of concern, and it is something that can be observed and counted. In addition to eliciting and pinpointing several problem behaviors that are of concern to the parents, the prosocial opposites of those behaviors are also specified. In the above example, the prosocial opposite might be defined as compliance to a simple request within 15 seconds. The treatment issues are thus expanded to help individuals concentrate not only on the problem behaviors, but on the socially appropriate behaviors as well. In addition to changing the way individuals conceptualize and perceive the situation, pinpointing helps them to think clearly about their behavioral expectations and to more clearly communicate those expectations to others.

Tracking these specific behaviors is the essential second part of this initial phase. In anger management as well as parent training individuals feel they know all that is necessary about the target behaviors and that they will certainly be aware of any improvement. Nevertheless it is the task of the therapist to stress the importance of counting and recording the occurrences of specified behaviors. In parent training, this task is particularly difficult because parents are most often eager to see change, and recording not only does nothing to change the child's behavior, it represents more work. When discussing this procedure with parents, we emphasize its importance as a way to measure our progress together. The therapist needs to know exactly how often the "wilfull" child complies and fails to comply to the parents' requests before and after a procedure is tried in order to evaluate its effectiveness. The collaborative effort between parents and therapist, and the problem-solving nature of our approach, is emphasized. Therapeutically, it is essential to fine-tune and heighten the parents' awareness of each instance of the target behavior so that the parents will later be able to react to the behavior in a consistent fashion. The parents are given a specific task in order to allow them to practice tracking and begin collecting a "data base" against which to measure the effectiveness of subsequent parenting strategies. Each evening for at least a week, the parents actually track three or four pinpointed behaviors for about one hour. The therapist phones each day to get the "data," to encourage the parents, and to trouble shoot if any difficulties are encountered. These phone calls typically take five to ten minutes.

After the parents have collected these tracking data consistently for about one week, we move to the state of active intervention on the parent-child interaction. For most families experiencing parent-child conflict, we begin with attention to positive child behaviors. For seriously abusive families, we begin with discipline strategies, since it is imperative to teach the parents alternatives to physical expressions of anger as quickly as possible.

Attention to the Positive

Active intervention for anger management in social interactions begins with attending to and reinforcing the positive behaviors of others in the social milieu. Most individuals, including abusive parents, have difficulty accepting this, the second phase of the program. Individuals entering this sort of program do so because they want an end to the problems they are experiencing. They typically perceive the solution in terms of others ceasing to engage in the problem behaviors. With this perspective, parents, for example, are often not in the mood to be interested in doing something positive to reward the child for something they think he/she should be doing anyway. The rationale typically provided by the therapist is that others, such as the child, have learned to get the individual's attention by negative behavior; it is important to teach others to attract attention and receive support by acting in a positive fashion.

In parent training, the social context and ages of the parties involved allows us to negotiate a system or contract that specifies for both parties, which reward/praise will be given for which behaviors. Within other social settings, for example, work or business relationships, the individual in training is more likely to develop systems and contracts that do not require the direct involvement of others. However, in the case of parent training, actual direct negotiation is helpful, given parental praise and reward. Chores and other prosocial behaviors that the parents would like to encourage in the child are put on a point chart. Each time the child demonstrates the behavior, the parent is taught to give immediate praise or *encouragement,* and to award a set number of points. At the end of each day, the child is given a small reward (specified in advance during a treatment session) if he or she earns a set number of points. Rewards often taken the form of shared social activities between parent and child such as games, stories, or physical activities. These social rewards should be pleasant for the parent as well as the child. Other types of rewards include money, special desserts, and extra privileges. Although the social and tangible rewards are important to get the positive attention rolling, the real goal is to teach the parent to provide expressive and contingent praise and encouragement when the child behaves in ways appreciated by the parent. Although the points, charts, and rewards are often dropped in favor of a reasonable contingent weekly allowance as the parent-child conflict is reduced, the parents are encouraged to continue the contingent praise indefinitely.

Non-Physical Punishment

The third phase of anger management is to teach individuals alternative responses to challenging situations. In the parent training program, the focus is on teaching parents to use nonphysical punishment for specific instances of misbehavior. With abusive parents, the problem of specifying just what constitutes misbehavior is usually problematic. Often, as stated previously, it is necessary to spend a good deal of time on what children of various ages can be expected to do in terms of such things as impulse control, manners, bladder and bowel control, independent self-help skills, and long-term responses to commands (e.g., some parents feel that a two-year old is defiant if on Thursday the child plays in the ashtray when on Monday the activity was forbidden). Sometimes, then, it is necessary to convince parents to give up unrealistic expectations about the child's ability to exercise good judgment, be responsible, resist temptation, or to use good manners. One cannot write a manual specifying how this is to be accomplished by therapists. A good deal of experience, knowledge of child development, and clinical skills is often required. In addition, a good rapport must be established before one expects to both "educate" a parent about what the child can do, and to convince the parent to enter into precise discipline contracts that might well be *perceived* by the parents as putting limits on their parental prerogatives and authority. Some of them perceive such specificity as downright threatening.

The alternative discipline technique advocated in parent training is called Time Out (TO). Briefly, TO involves putting the child in a room in the house (e.g., the bathroom) that prevents social interaction with other family members for a short time period (e.g., five minutes) *immediately* contingent upon a specified misbehavior. TO is never used as a threat; if an infraction is serious enough to warrant a threat, it is serious enough for TO. The procedure is used quickly to reduce the probability that either the parent or child will escalate before the incident is closed with the brief social isolation. The parents are taught to treat the confrontation as closed after TO. Lecturing or moralizing is discouraged. There are many subcomponents, and a number of potential problems that must be dealt with in teaching parents to use the technique effectivetly. These are dealt with in a videotape recently developed for use with parents (Patterson, 1983).

It is important to note that in our work with families anger management involves more than the instructional sorts of activities just summarized. We are consistently helping parents to reframe or reconceptualize their youngsters' behavior in ways to reduce their anger; we often help them deal with angry feelings by giving them rituals or behavioral prescriptions designed to interrupt the escalation of their anger (e.g., some are instructed to dial time and weather before handling a particularly obnoxious discipline confrontation). We use the parent training exercises to increase inter-parent consistency, to help parents reach mutually agreeable goals and expectations for their child's behavior. The parents are encouraged not only to learn the behaviors necessary to resolve discipline conflicts, but to adopt a general parenting role in which they take on the responsibility for raising, protecting, and socializing their child. It is often necessary to deal with marital and situational irritants and crises as they interfere with the parents' ability to consistently and effectively guide their children's social and psychological development.

In dealing with child-abusive families, the goals are identical to those we have for any parents who have problems in dealing effectively with discipline without resorting to assaultive behaviors. That is, we want the parents to develop reasonable and age-appropriate expectations and goals for their children's behavior. We aim to teach them ways to systematically encourage adaptive and positive social skills, and we attempt to teach them to deal effectively, quickly, and nonviolently with discipline confrontations as they arise. Our emphasis upon an instructional rather than a psychotherapeutic format is by design. Rather than focusing on more general issues such as personality, temperamental, or attitudinal problems of either parent or child, our goal is to specify exactly which child behaviors are difficult for the parent to deal with and to teach them less assaultive ways of dealing with these behaviors as they occur. More general issues relevant to child-abusive situations (e.g., marital problems, socioeconomic problems, environmental stress problems, personal problems of the parent and/or child) are dealt with *only* as they interfere with the parents' acquisition and use of more effective, less coercive parenting techniques.

Outcome Studies: Families with Child Management Problems

Outcome studies based on the treatment approaches described in this chapter were first conducted with families in which interactions between parents and children were problematic and often elicited frustration and anger outbursts. These families were not specifically referred for child abuse, but rather sought treatment to enhance familial relationships. During the 1970s, a number of studies were conducted to evaluate the effects of parent training on such families (Patterson, 1974a; 1974b; Patterson, Cobb, & Ray, 1973; Patterson & Reid, 1973). Each of these studies showed marked and significant reductions in both the rates of aversive behavior directly observed in the home setting, and in the rates per day at which parents reported problem behaviors from pre- to post-treatment. Data from 50 families who both served as subjects in the above-cited studies and who provided from six to 12 months of follow-up data showed that significant treatment effects persisted, as measured by home observation and Parent Daily Report data (Patterson & Fleischman, 1979).

In addition to demonstrating that the parent training had a direct effect on the problem behaviors targeted for treatment, re-analyses of the treatment data showed significant generalization effects on the behavior of siblings who were not directly involved in the treatment process (Arnold, Levine, & Patterson, 1975), to aggressive/aversive behaviors of the referred children which were not targeted specifically in treatment (Patterson, 1974a, b; 1975), and to disruptive and aggressive behavior in the classroom (Patterson, Cobb, & Ray, 1973).

Three outcome studies have been conducted at our center in which families of aggressive/oppositional children were either randomly or otherwise unsystematically assigned to either parent training or to various alternative treatment or waiting-list control groups (Patterson, Chamberlain, & Reid, 1982; Walter & Gilmore, 1973; Wiltz & Patterson, 1974). In each case, parent training demonstrated consistent and positive treatment effects which were consistently superior to those demonstrated by subjects in the control groups.

The dependent variables used in these studies were primarily focused on the molecular behaviors of the child (e.g., total aversive behavior per minute, the number of parent-reported problem behaviors per day). Because of our exceptionally narrow focus on the measurement of child behavior in treatment studies conducted at our center during the 1970s, we rarely carried out analyses of behavioral, emotional, or attitudinal changes in the parents as a function of treatment. However, the few analyses that we did carry out showed significant tendencies for parents to provide more consistent reactions to their child's behavior (Taplin & Reid, 1977), for mothers to report significantly fewer psychological problems as a function of treatment (Patterson, 1982), for parents to express more positive attitudes toward their children as a function of treatment (Patterson, 1982), and for parents to report that their family seemed to be functioning better as a function of treatment (Patterson & Reid, 1973).

These data were highly encouraging and suggested that parent training might be a viable intervention strategy for child-abusive families for the following reasons. First, it is a reasonably short-term intervention which does not require exceptional attributes of the client (e.g., high verbal ability, moderately high anxiety, the ability to self-disclose sensitive material), and the treatment can be successfully employed by sub-doctoral-level therapists (Patterson, Chamberlain, & Reid, 1982). Second, given our assumption that the number or rate of discipline confrontations that a parent must face each day is a significant determinant of the probability of child-abusive encounters, this intervention seemed reasonable as it reliably produced lower rates of child aversive behaviors. Third, there was some evidence that parents referred because of difficulty in handling discipline with their children became less distraught, more kindly disposed toward their children, and more satisfied with their family life after the training.

Outcome Studies: Abusive Families

An examination of case history and intake data, as well as the therapist case notes of 88 cases referred to our center for child management problems, revealed that the parents in at least 27 of the families could have been prosecuted for child abuse under state law (none of these families had been referred because of child abuse). Reid, Taplin, and Lorber (1981) conducted a post hoc analysis comparing the pre- and post-treatment observational data for these 27 "abusive" families; in addition, they compared the pre-treatment observation data for this group with 61 non-abusive families referred for child management problems, and with a group of 27 nondistressed control families. Comparison of the baseline or pre-treatment observation data for the three groups showed that both parents and children in the "abusive" group demonstrated higher rates of molecular aversive behavior during home observations than did their counterparts in the other two groups, thereby lending validity to the post hoc identification of the abusive families on the basis of case file information. Additional pre/post analyses of observation data for the mothers in the abusive group showed a significant reduction in total aversive behavior. The trend was similar for fathers, but was not statistically reliable. Other analyses reported by Reid et al. (1981) and Reid et al. (1982) demonstrated that these unofficially abusive parents differed from nonabusive and nondistressed controls not only in the rate of general aversive behavior but, specifically, they differed in the fact that they demonstrated several times the rates of the most aversive behaviors (i.e., hitting, yelling, humiliating, and threatening).

Although these data were in accord with the idea that microsocial assessment and highly specific parent training might successfully be employed in the treatment of child-abusive families, the subject families were referred because of child management problems, not because of child abuse (thereby creating the possibility that, although these families did abusive things, they could be substantially different in many ways from parents who seriously or chronically assault their children). It was also the case that the assessment and parent training procedures that we had applied up to this point were not designed for work with abusive parents. The focus of our interventions had always been on the child's aggressive or coercive behaviors. It was not assumed that the parents had chronic tendencies to physically assault or discipline their children or that they needed assistance in dealing with their anger.

We are now in the process of completing a three-year study on the effects of parent training with seriously abusive parents. Because of the exploratory nature of the research and the seriousness/acuteness of the problems experienced by these subjects, and because of the limited alternative treatment resources in the community, it was not possible to do a comparative treatment design utilizing no treatment, delayed treatment, or alternative treatment control groups. Instead, a multilevel assessment battery composed of both general and highly specific measures was used to repeatedly assess the experimental treatment group and a nonabusive group who were carefully matched on a large number of demographic variables.[1] The treatment utilized for the abusive families participating in this study was similar to that described previously. However, the specific behaviors of the parents relevant to discipline and other confrontations with the child were more carefully measured. In terms of treatment, parents were not only taught more effective and consistent methods for dealing with discipline and parent-child relationships, the parents were actively discouraged from continuing their

---

[1] Thus, instead of expecting group by occasion interactions in which the two groups begin at the same level on target dependent variables and demonstrate significant differences over time (e.g., both groups high on parental assaultiveness on Occasion 1, with the experimental treatment group showing less parental assaultiveness at Occasion 2), the situation is reversed: that is, we expected the clinical treatment group to look much worse than the comparison group at Time 1 on the parent targeted variables, but to look the same at Time 2 (i.e., after the abusive group has gotten treatment). Although such a design in no way controls for nonspecific treatment effects nor does it adequately substitute for random assignment of abusive families to experimental versus alternative treatments, it serves as an initial step to gain perspective on the measures taken from the abusive group before and after treatment.

patterns of corporal punishment. Additionally, parents' anger was dealt with to the extent that it interfered with their ability to handle conflict with their children in a firm but moderate manner.[2]

Although the data from this project are still being analyzed, some preliminary results have been reported by Reid (1983).[3] As in our previous work with unofficial child abuse cases, observational data collected in the homes showed that before treatment the mothers and fathers in the abusive families demonstrated over twice the rate of physically negative behaviors (e.g., hitting) toward their children as did their counterparts in nonabusive families. During the second set of observations (i.e., following treatment completion for the child-abusive families), the rates of hitting for the abusive and nonabusive parents were nearly identical. The same pattern was demonstrated for threatening commands given by the parents to their children. During baseline, the Parent Daily Report data revealed that parents in the abusive group were reporting spanking their children over three times as often as did parents in the control group (once every three days vs. once every 10 days, respectively); at the second assessment, parents in both groups reported spankings on the average of once every 10 days.

Parents on both groups were given questionnaires on at least five days before and five days after treatment. On each of the 10 days, the parents were asked to describe a discipline confrontation they had had that day with their child. Among other things, they rated their subjective anger during each of the episodes. Before treatment the parents in the abused group rated themselves on the average as significantly more angry during the episodes than did their normal counterparts. After treatment was completed for the abusive groups, there was no difference in subjective anger during discipline confrontations for the two groups.

Even though these data strongly suggest that the abusive parents were becoming less assaultive and threatening over the course of treatment, they were still able to maintain disciplinary control over their children. Table 1 shows the Parent Daily Report data before and after for the two groups. As can be seen, the parents' self-report of the problem behaviors did not increase; in fact, it significantly decreased as they completed treatment. An evaluation of pre- and post-treatment home observation data showed a slight reduction in aversive child behaviors from pre- to post-treatment.

In addition to the clear reduction in abusive behaviors used by the treated group as a function of treatment and the reduction observed in child aversive behaviors, there was an increase in the use of more positive discipline techniques for the abusive group. The Parent Daily Report data showed significant pre-/post-increases in the parents' reliance on such nonabusive punishments as sending the child to his or her room, standing the child in the corner, taking away privileges, assigning work chores, or making the child clean up his or her own mess, as well as an increased reliance on the particular punishments that we teach in parent training (e.g., time-out).

[2] Our clinical staff were actually surprised that in most cases, although parents self-reported a good deal of anger surrounding discipline and other aspects of parent-child relationships at the beginning of or early in treatment, it was not typically necessary to deal with anger as a separate issue. That is, as the parents became more adept at successfully setting and enforcing limits with their children, they became less interested in talking about anger.

[3] This brief report is available from the first author on request.

Table 1 Number of problem behaviors reported by parents each day[a]

	Pre-treatment		Post-treatment	
	Mean	(S.D.)	Mean	(S.D.)
CA group	9.12	(4.80)	5.18	(4.05)
NA group[b]	3.45	(2.06)	2.89	(2.06)

[a] Both main effects and the interaction are significant at p less than .01.
[b] This group never received treatment; the "post-treatment" assessment was an assessment done yoked to the post-treatment assessment for the treated group.

Taken together, these data are quite encouraging in suggesting that a molecular, multilevel assessment of parent-child interaction, coupled with highly specific parent training can be useful in working with serious and/or chronic child abuse cases. On the other hand, there are indications that our treatment resources would be more efficiently deployed if we focused on preventing child abuse rather than on attempts to work most intensively with the most chronic and extreme cases.

First, we experienced a client refusal rate of over twice that encountered in any of our previous work, either with unofficial or self-referred abusive parents or with nonabusive families experiencing parent-child conflict. In this latest sample of officially abusive parents, 45% refused to accept treatment; in work with nonabusive parents, refusal rates have never exceeded 20%. There are obvious reasons for this. People who are referred by child protective agencies or by the courts to receive treatment and who are in the process of litigation because of alleged abuse, or whose children have become wards of the court because of past abuse, are usually reluctant to permit direct home observations or to provide the behavioral descriptive information on their negative encounters with their children that are necessary for such behavioral parent training as described in this paper.

Secondly, the therapists on our project have never before encountered families harder to treat than those in the official abuse sample presented here. Treatment typically takes about eight months for the current officially abusive sample as opposed to about four months for past samples involving non-official cases.

Third, if our goal is to intervene in those abusive families in which serious physical injury or actual death of the child is our focus of prevention, then it is of critical importance to direct our intervention efforts at those families at risk who have very young children. Recall that the American Humane Association (1981) found that the average age of children killed in child-abusive incidents was 2.8 years. This compares to a mean age of 7.3 years for all victims of child abuse and neglect. In another set of analyses by that agency for the same year, over 50% of major physical injuries suffered during child-abusive episodes involve victims of two years of age or less, 70% involving youngsters of five years of age or less. These data clearly show that as the child develops over the course of early childhood, the risk of serious injury and death become less. Babies and toddlers are simply easier to maim and kill than are children who can run away from their parents, or plead with them.

These data suggest a number of things. First, it is possible that by the time a clinician begins to work with a serious child abuse case, the youngster, by simple virtue of increased maturity, strength, and agility, may be significantly less at risk than at the time of the injury which precipitated court action and subsequent referral. Second, such findings are cause for optimism, in that common sense, clinical experience, and a number of research studies show that the younger the child, the easier and more effective it is to conduct parent training. Thus, whatever effects we can show with older and more chronic cases of child abuse are certainly an underestimate of what could be achieved by dealing with families before they achieve a chronic abusive status. The bad news, of course, is our current inability to identify and recruit families of very small children who are a high risk for child abuse. It is imperative that research be conducted which is focused on finding the very earliest predictors, correlates, or risk factors for abusive parent-child interactions.

GENERAL IMPLICATIONS

Most of the work reviewed in this chapter has been joined by a common thread. The intense anger and aggression that result in child abuse are related in significant part to social interactional and situational factors that fluctuate on a moment-to-moment basis. As examples, most physical abuse occurs in the context of discipline confrontations; the longer aversive exchanges persist, the more likely a parent (any parent) will engage in hitting or threatening. Parents behave most aversively toward their children on days of high situational stress.

In the case of child abuse, an attempt has been made to show that parents can be taught that their anger can be reduced if they deal with the stimuli that elicit or exacerbate it on a moment-by-moment basis. For example, they are taught to pinpoint provocative child behaviors and to track them carefully; they are also taught to react quickly and effectively when such situations arise and to record their successes and failures.

Although most of the social and situational factors crucial for dealing with child abuse are conveniently limited to the parent-child interaction in the home settings, the strategy underlying this approach should be useful for other problems associated with anger. Type A individuals with a history of heart disease, for example, are excellent candidates for such an approach. By learning to pinpoint, track, and quickly deal with the elicitors as well as the signs of anger, beneficial results in terms of anger management would be expected by these individuals. For persons living or working in conditions that may increase the risk of heart disease (e.g., Marine drill sargeants; see Novaco, Chap. 11), instruction in systematically tracking and dealing with social or other environmental stressors that are associated with anger arousal may serve a preventive function. Paralleling the advances in micro-social analyses, recent developments in the technology for physiological monitoring of such variables as blood pressure and heart rate, make it feasible to design studies to clarify the moment-to-moment relationships social and environmental situations and cardiovascular activity and potential risk in the natural environment. Research outlining these relationships would enhance our knowledge significantly, and undoubtedly lead, in turn, to clinically effective therapeutic interventions.

REFERENCES

The American Humane Association, Child Protection Division. *Annual Report, 1980: National Analysis of Official Child Neglect and Abuse Reporting.* Denver, Colo.: Author, 1981.

Armstrong, K. A. A treatment and education program for parents and children who are at risk for abuse and neglect. *Child Abuse and Neglect: The International Journal,* 1980, *4,* 119-125.

Arnold, J., Levine, A., & Patterson, G. R. Changes in sibling behavior following family intervention. *Journal of Consulting and Clinical Psychology,* 1975, *43,* 683-688.

Barnes, G. B., Chabon, R. S., & Hertzberg, L. J. Team treatment for abusive families. *Social Casework,* 1974, *55,* 600-611.

Burgess, R. L., & Conger, R. D. Family interaction patterns related to child abuse and neglect: Some preliminary findings. *Child Abuse and Neglect: The International Journal,* 1977, *1,* 269-277.

Chamberlain, P. *Standardization of a parent report measure.* Unpublished doctoral dissertation, University of Oregon, Eugene, 1980.

Dumas, J. E., & Wahler, R. G. Predictors of treatment outcome in parent training: Mother insularity and socioeconomic disadvantage. *Behavioral Assessment,* 1983, *5,* 301-313.

Egleland, R., & Brunnquell, D. *An at-risk approach to the study of child abuse: Some preliminary findings.* Unpublished manuscript, University of Minnesota, Minneapolis, 1977.

Elmer, I. E., & Gregg, G. A. Developmental characteristics of abused children. *Pediatrics,* 1967, *40,* 596-602.

Fawl, C. L. Disturbances experienced by children in their natural habitats. In R. G. Barker (Ed.), *The stream of behavior.* New York: Appleton-Century-Crofts, 1963.

Feinstein, H. M., Paul, N., & Esmiol, P. *Group therapy with infanticidal impulses.* Paper presented at the meeting of the American Psychiatric Association, St. Louis, Mo., 1963.

Forehand, R., King, H. E., Peed, S., & Yoder, P. Mother-child interactions: Comparison of a noncompliant clinic group and a nonclinic group. *Behavior Research and Therapy,* 1975, *13,* 79-84.

Forehand, R., Wells, K., & Griest, D. An examination of the social validity of a parent training program. *Behavior Therapy,* 1980, *11,* 488-502.

Friedman, S. B. The need for intensive follow-up of ab used children. In C. H. Kempe & R. E. Helfer (Eds.), *Helping the battered child and his family.* Philadelphia: Lippincott, 1972.

Garbarino, J. Some ecological correlates of child abuse: The impact of socioeconomic stress on mothers. *Child Development,* 1976, *47,* 178-185.

Gelles, R. J. *Family violence.* Beverly Hills, Calif.: Sage, 1979.

Gil, D. G. Physical abuse of children: Findings and implications of a nationwide survey. *Pediatrics,* 1969, *44,* 857-865.

Gil, D. G. *Violence against children: Physical child abuse in the United States.* Cambridge, Mass.: Harvard University Press, 1970.

Gil, D. G. Violence against children. *Journal of Marriage and the Family,* 1971, *33,* 637-648.

Glick, P. C. *Who are the children in one-parent households?* Paper presented at Wayne State University, Detroit, Mich., 1979.

Green, A. A psychodynamic approach to the study and treatment of child abusing parents. *Journal of Child Psychiatry,* 1976, *15,* 414-429.

Herrenkohl, R. C., Herrenkohl, E. C., & Egolf, B. P. Circumstances surrounding the occurrence of child maltreatment. *Journal of Consulting and Clinical Psychology,* 1983, *51,* 424-431.

Hoffman, D. A. *Parents rate the Family Interaction Coding System: Comparisons of the family interaction of problem and nonproblem boys with parent-derived composites of behavior.* Unpublished doctoral dissertation, University of Oregon, Eugene, 1983.

Jones, R. R., Reid, J. B., & Patterson, G. R. Naturalistic observations in clinical assessment. In P. McReynolds (Ed.), *Advances in psychological assessment* (Vol. 3). San Francisco: Jossey-Bass, 1975.

Justice, B., & Duncan, D. F. Life crisis as a precursor to child abuse. *Public Health Reports,* 1976, *91,* 110-115.

Kempe, C. H. A practical approach to the protection of the abused child and rehabilitation of the abusing parent. *Pediatrics,* 1973, *51,* 804-812.

Kempe, C. H., & Helfer, R. (Eds.). *Helping the battered child and his family.* Chicago: University of Chicago Press, 1972.

Margolin, G., & Christiansen, A. *The treatment of families with marital and child problems.* Paper presented at the annual meeting of the Association for the Advancement of Behavior Therapy, Toronto, Ontario, Canada, 1981.

Minton, C., Kagan, J., & Levine, J. A. Maternal control and obedience in the two-year-old child. *Child Development,* 1971, *42,* 1973-1984.

Novaco, R. W. *Anger control.* Lexington, Mass.: Lexington/Heat, 1975.

Parke, R. D., & Lewis, N. G. The family in context: A multilevel interactional analysis of child abuse. In R. W. Henderson (Ed.), *Parent-child interaction–Theory, research, prospects.* New York: Academic, 1981.

Patterson, G. R. Interventions for boys with conduct problems: Multiple settings, treatments, and criteria. *Journal of Consulting and Clinical Psychology,* 1974, *42,* 471-481. (a)

Patterson, G. R. Retraining of aggressive boys by their parents: Review of recent literature and follow-up evaluation. In F. Lowey (Ed.), Symposium on the severely disturbed preschool child. *Canadian Psychiatric Association Journal,* 1974, *19,* 142-149. (b)

Patterson, G. R. Multiple evaluations of a parent training program. In T. Thomson & W. S. Dockens, III (Eds.), *Applications of behavior modification.* New York: Academic, 1975.

Patterson, G. R. *Coercive family process.* Eugene, Ore.: Castalia, 1982.

Patterson, G. R. The unattached mother: A process analysis. In W. Hartup & Z. Rubin (Eds.), *Social relationships: Their role in children's development,* in press.

Patterson, G. R., Chamberlain, P., & Reid, J. B. A comparative evaluation of parent training procedures. *Behavior Therapy,* 1982, *13,* 638-650.

Patterson, G. R., Cobb, J. A., & Ray, R. S. A social engineering technology for retraining the feamilies of aggressive boys. In H. E. Adams & I. P. Unikel (Eds.), *Issues and trends in behavior therapy.* Springfield, Ill.: Thomas, 1973.

Patterson, G. R., & Fleischman, M. J. Maintenance of treatment effects: Some considerations concerning family systems and follow-up data. *Behavior Therapy,* 1979, *10,* 168-195.

Patterson, G. R., & Gullion, M. E. *Living with children: New methods for parents and teachers.* Champaign, Ill.: Research, 1968.

Patterson, G. R., McNeal, S. A., Hawkins, N., & Phelps, R. Reprogramming the social environment. *Journal of Child Psychology and Psychiatry,* 1967, *8,* 181-195.

Patterson, G. R., Ray, R. S., Shaw, D. A., & Cobb, J. A. Manual for coding of family interactions, 1969 revision. Unpublished manuscript, Oregon Research Institute, Eugene, 1969.

Patterson, G. R., & Reid, J. B. Intervention for families of aggressive boys: A replication study. *Behavior Research and Therapy,* 1973, *11,* 383-394.

Paulson, M. J., & Chaleff, A. Parent surrogate roles: A dynamic concept in understanding and treatment abusive parents. *Journal of Clinical Child Psychology,* 1973, *11,* 38-40.

Paulson, M. J., Savino, A. B., Chaleff, A. B., Sanders, R. W., Frisch, F., & Dunn, R. Parents of the battered child: A multidisciplinary group therapy approach to life-threatening behavior. *Life Threatening Behavior,* 1974, *4,* 18-31.

Reid, J. B. *Reciprocity in family interaction.* Unpublished doctoral dissertation, University of Oregon, Eugene, 1967.

Reid, J. B. (Ed.). *A social learning approach to family intervention: Observation in home settings.* (Vol. 2). Eugene, Ore.: Castalia, 1978.

Reid, J. B. *Final Report: Child abuse: Developmental factors and treatment* (Grant No. MH 37938, NIMH, U.S. PHS). Oregon Social Learning Center, Eugene, 1983.

Reid, J. B., & Arkes, S. *The relationship between aversive and abusive behavior by abusive and nonabusive mothers.* Manuscript in preparation.

Reid, J. B., & Patterson, G. R. Follow-up analyses of a behavioral treatment program for boys with conduct problems: A reply to Kent. *Journal of Consulting and Clinical Psychology,* 1976, *44,* 297-302.

Reid, J. B., Patterson, G. R., & Loeber, R. The abused child: Victim, instigator, or innocent bystander? In D. Bernstein (Ed.), *Response structure and organization.* Lincoln: University of Nebraska Press, 1982.

Reid, J. B., Taplin, P. S., & Lorber, R. A social interactional approach to the treatment of abusive families. In R. Stuart (Ed.), *Violent behavior: Social learning approaches to prediction, management, and treatment.* New York: Brunner/Mazel, 1981.

Savino, A. B., & Sanders, R. W. Working with abusive parents: Group therapy and home visits. *American Journal of Nursing,* 1973, *73,* 482-484.

Stark, R., & McEvoy, J. Middle class violence. *Psychology Today,* 1970, *4,* 52-65.

Steele, B. F., & Pollock, C. B. A psychiatric study of parents who abuse infants and small children. In R. E. Helfer & C. H. Kempe (Eds.), *The battered child* (Rev. ed.). Chicago: University of Chicago Press, 1974.

Straus, M. A. Social stress and marital violence in a national sample of American families. In F. Wright, C. Bain, & R. W. Rieber (Eds.), Forensic psychology and psychiatry. *Annals of the New York Academy of Sciences* (Vol. 347), 1980.

Taplin, P. S., & Reid, J. B. Changes in parent consequation as a function of family intervention. *Journal of Consulting and Clinical Psychology,* 1977, *4,* 973-981.

Tracy, J. J. Child abuse project: A follow-up. *Social Work,* 1975, *20,* 398-399.

Tracy, J. J., & Clark, E. H. Treatment for child abusers. *Social Work,* 1974, *19,* 338-342.

Wahler, R. G., Leske, G., & Rogers, E. S. The insular family: A deviance support system for oppositional children. In L. A. Hamerlynck (Ed.), *Behavioral systems for the developmentally disabled: School and family environments* (Vol. 1). New York: Brunner/Mazel, 1978.

Walter, H. I., & Gilmore, S. K. Placebo versus social learning effects in parent training procedures designed to alter the behavior of aggressive boys. *Behavior Research and Therapy,* 1973, *4,* 361-377.

Wiltz, N. A., Jr., & Patterson, G. R. An evaluation of parent training procedures designed to alter inappropriate aggressive behavior of boys. *Behavior Therapy,* 1974, *5,* 215-221.

Young, L. *A study of child neglect and abuse.* Princeton, N.J.: McGraw-Hill, 1964.

14
The Possible Effects of Beta-Adrenergic Blocking Drugs on Behavioral and Psychological Concomitants of Anger

Lynn A. Durel and David S. Krantz
Uniformed Services University of the Health Sciences

The role of bodily activity in the occurrence and experience of emotion has been the subject of psychological theorizing for over a century (James, 1884). Two major questions bearing on this issue have received the most attention: (1) can various emotions be differentiated from one another in terms of distinct patterns of physiological responses (Ax, 1953; J. Schachter, 1957); and (2) to what extent do either peripheral sympathetic or visceral responses contribute to the intensity of emotional experience (Cannon, 1927; James, 1884; Leventhal, 1980; S. Schachter & Singer, 1962). Although both questions remain subject to controversy, this chapter will focus on the second question—the role of perception and evaluation of peripheral sympathetic responses—as these processes contribute to the occurrence and maintenance of the emotion of anger.[1]

Pharmacologic agents that selectively block or stimulate sympathetic responses allow us to examine in a new way the role of bodily responses in generating emotional experience. The effects of drugs that differ in properties such as site of action and degree of penetration into the central nervous system can be compared. That is, if peripheral reactions of the sympathetic nervous system are important for generating the subjective experience of certain emotions, a blockade of these physiologic responses should reduce psychological and behavioral correlates of emotion. Similarly, stimulation of peripheral sympathetic responses should tend to increase emotional reactions.

Portions of this chapter relating to Type A behavior were adapted from an article by Krantz and Durel (1983). Preparation of this chapter was assisted by NIH grant HL31514 and USUHS grant R07233.

[1] The differences and controversies among various peripheral and central theories of emotion are beyond the scope of this chapter. (See Leventhal, 1980 for such a review and discussion). Throughout the chapter when referring to "peripheral feedback," we only assume that visceral reactions can summate with other aspects of emotional experience, and thereby contribute to the intensity of emotion. We also will not be concerned with whether the processing of information about peripheral responses is automatic or involves conscious awareness (cf. Leventhal, 1980).

In this chapter, we will describe some recent work suggesting that aspects of the Type A behavior pattern—a construct with anger and hostility as major components—may be decreased by beta-adrenergic blocking drugs. We will present these data in the broader context of a review of the role of peripheral sympathetic responses and their interaction with cognitive factors in generating or facilitating the experience of anger, and suggest research directions for investigating possible applications of beta-adrenergic blocking drugs in anger control.

EVIDENCE THAT PERIPHERAL SYMPATHETIC RESPONSES CAN INFLUENCE ANGER AND AGGRESSION

According to theories of emotion such as those of James (1884) and Lange (1885), emotional feeling depends on the perception of visceral, skeletal, and muscular responses. Schachter and Singer (1962) later proposed a two-factor theory that suggested that emotional experience arose not only from the perception of sympathetic responses, but also from the cognitive interpretation of these responses based on cues derived from the social environment or other situational variables. It was alleged that there was considerable plasticity in the type of emotion that could result from a given state of physiological arousal. When individuals injected with epinephrine had no ready explanation for why they were aroused, they labeled this state in terms of the cognitions available to them. Thus, individuals so aroused and exposed to an angry confederate displayed an increase in their angry behavior in the situation (Schachter & Singer, 1962).

The Schachter two-factor theory has provided the basis for a number of research programs investigating the determinants of aggressive behavior. For example, in a series of studies, Zillman demonstrated that residual or undissipated physiological arousal generated by strenuous physical exercise or exposure to sexual stimuli led to increased aggressive behavior in subjects who had previously been provoked, but not in individuals who were not provoked (Zillman, 1971; Zillman, Johnson & Day, 1974). When subjects knew that their arousal was due to physical exertion, aggressiveness was unaffected. But with lower levels of exercise-induced arousal that held no cues to link physiological state with the exertion, the magnitude of residual arousal was related to aggressive behavior following provocation.

In a related line of research, Konecni (1975a; 1975b) has shown that aggressive behavior could be increased by exposure to physiologically arousing noxious stimuli among individuals who had previously been provoked. Individuals not provoked showed no such increase in aggressive behavior when aroused. The point here is that autonomic arousal induced by exogenous environmental stimuli does not by itself facilitate anger or aggressive behavior; the subject must attribute or explain this arousal in terms of provocation or some other anger-related cognitions. Taken together, these data emphasize the interactive role of *both* physiological arousal and cognition in facilitating anger and aggression. It should be noted that, though the aforementioned research has primarily been concerned with aggressive behavior, other research by Geen and associates (Geen, Rakosky & Pigg, 1972) suggests that self-rated anger can also be manipulated by varying the explanation that subjects attach to a particular state of physiological arousal. The previous studies reviewed in this section have dealt with laboratory-induced instances of anger and aggression. Several field studies reinforce the notion that peripheral autonomic reactions (e.g., cardiovascular, respiratory, gastrointestinal, or muscular) are very much a part of the naturalistic experience of anger (Averill, 1982; Gates, 1926; Davitz, 1969). For example, data suggest that a significant percentage of individuals experience anger in terms of symptoms such as quickened and forceful heartbeat, tense musculature, and rapid breathing (Davitz, 1969; Gates, 1926). Although some would argue that there is little specificity and considerable individual variability in the actual and experienced autonomic correlates of anger (Averill, 1982), these naturalistic data do reinforce the idea that autonomic responses play a role in the experience of anger—at least for some people. In conjunction with the notion that anger is the interactive outcome of physiologic arousal and an anger-related cognitive label, we might also suggest that some individuals may be cognitively predisposed to interpret certain autonomic changes in terms of anger, rather than other emotions such as anxiety. Recent research we have conducted on physiological antecedents and correlates of the Type A behavior pattern provides some preliminary support for this notion.

ASSESSMENT OF TYPE A BEHAVIOR: DISSECTING ATTITUDINAL AND STYLISTIC COMPONENTS

Research indicates that the Type A or "coronary-prone" behavior pattern consists of several dimensions which can be empirically separated from one another. The Rosenman structured interview or SI constitutes the primary technique for assessment of Type A behavior (Rosenman, 1978). Studies reveal that, in this interview, speech stylistics and the subject's manner of responding to questions are heavily weighted in arriving at an assessment, and that response content is considered to a lesser extent (Matthews, Krantz, Dembroski, & MacDougall, 1982; Schucker & Jacobs, 1977; Scherwitz, Barton & Leventhal, 1977). In addition to classification into one of four categories ranging from Type B to extreme Type A, the interview can be reliably scored for various speech behaviors along dimensions such as loud/explosive, rapid/accelerated, response latency, potential-for-hostility, and verbal competition (Dembroski, 1978; Matthews et al., 1982). Scoring the individual interview questions for content of responses is also possible. Data presented in Table 1, taken from a study in which we component analyzed measures of Type A behavior, demonstrate the relatively higher correlations of interview assessment with "stylistic," rather than "content" components.

Several self-administered questionnaires have also been developed to measure Type A behavior. Of these, the Jenkins Activity Survey or JAS (Jenkins, Zyzanski & Rosenman, 1971) is by far the most widely used. JAS assessments, based solely on self-reports of competitiveness, impatience, and other Type A characteristics (see Table 1), correlate with "content" components but only minimally with stylistics measured in the interview.

We note these assessment issues here for two interrelated reasons. First, the

Table 1 Correlations of selected interview components with SI and JAS assessments

	Interview component	Interview Type A (n = 163)	JAS Type A (n = 144)
Selected "clinical ratings"	Promptness	.67	.16
	Explosive speech	.68	.19
	Hurrying	.66	.22
	Potential-for-hostility	.63	.36
	Energy level	.51	.27
Selected "response content"	Describes self as harddriving	.38	.51
	Feels sense of time urgency	.09	.37
	Feels time passing too rapidly	.12	.35
	Resents being kept waiting	.29	.19

Note: Copyright 1982 by the American Psychological Association. Reprinted by permission of the publisher.

assumption is often made that similar descriptive and psychological constructs are being measured by the SI and JAS, but the data suggest that they are tapping different components of behavior. Though SI and JAS do classify people similarly above chance levels, they also classify substantial proportions of people differently (cf. Jenkins, 1978). Comparisons of assessments rated on continuous scales indicate only a moderate and often disappointing degree of concordance, that is, correlations ranging between .25 and .40 (Chesney, Black, Chadwick, & Rosenman, 1981; Matthews et al., 1982). This lack of high concordance indicates that SI and JAS are measuring observably different facets of the Type A pattern: the SI tapping speech style and observer-rated potential-for-hostility, and the JAS measuring self-reports of competitiveness, impatience, and others. A second reason we emphasize the relative independence of these assessment instruments here is because research described below also reveals some independence between the two techniques in their correlation with physiological end points (Brand et al., 1978; Dembroski, MacDougall, Shields et al., 1978), and in their susceptibility to pharmacologic agents (Krantz, Durel, Davia, Shaffer, Arabian, Dembroski, & MacDougall, 1982). If the cognitive and self-report components of Type A are empirically separable from the psychomotor/behavioral manifestations, it is possible that, just as anger has both cognitive and physiological bases, so might Type A behavior. Evidence we will present later suggests that this may indeed by the case.

PHYSIOLOGICAL CORRELATES OF TYPE A BEHAVIOR

Situational/Environmental Elicitors

Figure 1 illustrates a possible model for relationships among Type A behavior, physiological response, and coronary heart disease. The preponderance of research has built upon the model moving from left to right. Situations perceived as psychologically stressful or challenging are thought to elicit Type A behavior in susceptible individuals and, in turn, evoke sympathetic neuroendocrine responses which act upon the cardiovascular system to promote or precipitate ischemic heart disease. Implicit in this model is the assumption that there is a set of psychological constructs underlying A-B differences in behavioral and physiological responses. For example, it has been suggested that Type A behaviors may represent attempts to assert and maintain control over stressful aspects of the environment (cf. Glass, 1977), or that achievement striving and impatience derive from childhood socialization experiences characterized by ambiguous standards of evaluation (Matthews, 1982).

Regarding situational elicitors, it has been repeatedly emphasized in the literature (Friedman & Rosenman, 1959; Glass, 1977) that Type A behaviors emerge in the presence of certain challenges or stresses. Thus, in a series of studies, Glass and his coworkers have demonstrated that given appropriate environmental elicitors, Type As display exaggerated achievement strivings, are impatient and irritable, and are more hostile and aggressive than Type Bs when delayed or provoked interpersonally (Glass, 1977; Matthews, 1982). Evidence also suggests that, compared to their Type B counterparts, Type A subjects display greater sympathetic nervous system responsivity, but again these differences are most pronounced when specific situations are encountered (Chesney & Rosenman, 1983; Glass & Contrada, 1984; Krantz, Glass, Schaeffer, & Davis, 1982a; Matthews, 1982). Of particular relevance to anger, conditions of hostile competition are among the most potent of the situational elicitors of A-B differences in cardioavscular and plasma catecholamine responses (Glass et al., 1980).

In addition to the effects of situationally-elicited psychological factors on sympathetic nervous system responsivity, there is emerging evidence that peripheral sympathetic responsivity might influence manifestations of Type A behavior in accordance with reasoning presented in the opening discussion of emotional behavior. We will describe evidence for such a reciprocal relationship between Type A and cardiovascular responsivity at a later point in this chapter.

A-B differences in physiological responsivity appear to be most pronounced when psychological—rather than purely physical—demands are encountered. For example, one study (Dembroski, MacDougall, Herd, & Shields, 1979) manipulated the instructions given to subjects exposed to tests of cold water immersion and reaction time in order to vary the degree of psychological challenge inherent in the task. Results indicated only minimal A-B differences in the condition where instructions were not challenging, and considerably larger differences when subjects were sternly told the tasks were difficult and were provoked to do well.

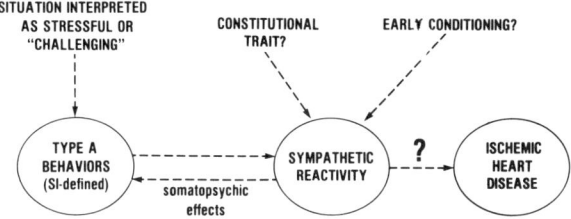

Figure 1   Model illustrating bi-directional relationships between Type A behavior and sympathetic nervous system reactivity. (From Krantz & Durel, 1983). Reprinted with permission.

Additionally, analyses of various Type A components (subjects' voice characteristics and content of responses to questions) were coded from the structured interview and related to magnitude of cardiovascular responses. These analyses revealed that (1) observer ratings of speech hostility and competitiveness were related to cardiovascular responses[2] even in the low challenge conditions, and (2) JAS-defined (i.e., self-reported) Type A behavior was less strongly correlated with physiologic responses than SI-defined assessments, which are based on speech and other observed behavioral mannerisms. These results were interpreted by the study's investigators to suggest that subjects exhibiting high hostility and competitiveness have lower thresholds for perceiving environmental challenge. An alternative interpretation of these data (see below) is that, rather than reflecting lower perceptual thresholds for challenge, hostility detected in the interview reflects an underlying physiological responsiveness that can be elicited by stressors which have minimal psychological components (see Krantz & Durel, 1983; Krantz et al., 1982c).

Coronary Bypass Studies: Re-evaluating the Role of Full Conscious Mediation

As we have noted, most studies have found that Type A behaviors and physiological correlates emerge only in specific situations viewed by an awake individual as challenging or stressful. A recent study (Kahn, Kornfeld, Frank, Heller, & Hoar, 1980) by contrast found that even while under general anesthesia for coronary artery bypass surgery (before maintenance on the heart-lung pump), Type As compared to Bs evidenced greater increases over admission blood pressure. Admission measurements were taken by a physician upon entry into the hospital when patients were fully awake.

These results suggest that there may be, in part, a nonconsciously mediated or "constitutional" basis for A-B differences in cardiovascular reactivity because these responses are observed among patients under general anesthesia. However, the calculation of peak operative increases over admission blood pressure used in this study places some qualification on this conclusion. It is not possible to determine from these data whether increases were accounted for by elevations occurring entirely during surgery (when patients were anesthetized), as opposed to increases over admission blood pressure occurring prior to surgery when patients were fully awake.

Given the tantalizing nature of these findings, we (Krantz et al., 1982b) undertook to replicate and extend this study, obtaining an additional measure of blood pressure at onset of surgery (first operative blood pressure). Three measures were calculated: (1) peak operative increase over admission as in the Kahn et al. (1980) study; (2) peak operative increase over first operative; and (3) preoperative increase from admission to first operative. Figure 2 presents the findings. It is clear that intensity of Type A behavior was positively related to

---

[2] Although several studies have corroborated a positive relationship between interview-derived hostility ratings and physiologic response other research has not (Glass, Lake, Contrada et al., submitted). However, the Glass et al. study did find a positive relationship between self-reported state anger and cardiovascular reactivity, and suggests that overtly expressed anger and potential-for-hostility rated in the SI may have different cardiovascular concomitants.

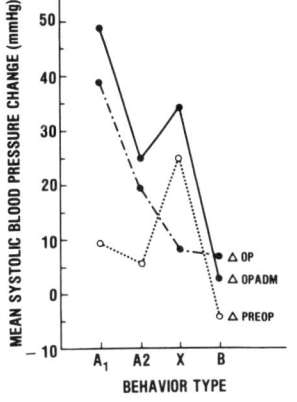

Figure 2 Relationships between 4-point ratings of intensity of interview-defined Type A behavior and systolic blood pressure (SBP) changes among patients undergoing coronary bypass surgery, ΔPREOP: first operative minus hospital admission SBP; ΔOP: peak operative SBP minus first operative SBP; ΔOPADM: peak operative minus admission SBP. (Data adapted from Krantz et al., 1982b; figure from Krantz & Durel, 1983). Reprinted with permission.

intraoperative increases in systolic blood pressure occurring during surgery when patients were anesthetized (ΔOP). In contrast, Type A behavior was *not* related to changes occurring prior to surgery (Δ PREOP).

The Kahn et al. (1980) finding of a positive relationship of Type A intensity to operative increases over admission (ΔOPADMN) was also replicated, and the new findings indicated that the structured interview but not the JAS Type A assessment, was related to intraoperative physiologic changes.

Pharmacologic Studies: Decreasing Sympathetic Reactivity and Type A Behavior

The results of these two surgery studies suggest that there may be an underlying psychobiological basis for SI-defined Type A behavior, because increased cardiovascular responses[3] are observed under conditions where conscious mediation is minimized. That is, the impatience, hostility, and speech patterns exhibited by Type A individuals may, in part, *reflect* an underlying sympathetic nervous system responsivity (see Figure 1). Although this view is divergent from the conception that Type A appraisals or behaviors *produce* elevated sympathetic responses, the idea is nevertheless testable. Manipulations (e.g., pharmacologic) which act to decrease sympathetic responsivity should decrease intensity of Type A behavior as well.

Accordingly, we conducted a correlational analysis comparing behavioral and psychophysiological characteristics of coronary patients who, as part of their usual treatment, were either medicated or not medicated with the beta-adrenergic blocking drug propranolol (Krantz, Durel et al., 1982c). The beta-adrenergic blocking drugs act to selectively block a subset of sympathetic nervous system receptors that are located primarily in the heart and in smooth muscle of the blood vessels and lungs (Weiner, 1980).[4] Briefly, there appear to be two kinds of

---

[3] The cardiac surgery literature suggests that hypertension during or after coronary bypass surgery is probably caused by increased sympathetic nervous system activity (e.g., Estefanous & Tarazi, 1980).

[4] Comprehensive discussion of the physiology and pharmacology of the adrenergic system is beyond the scope of this chapter and can be found in Middlemiss et al. (1981), Obrist (1981), Patel and Turner (1981), and Weiner (1980).

Table 2 Comparisons of propranolol and no propranolol groups on measures of Type A behavior and components

	No propranolol group	Propranolol group	P
Interview Type A (4–point rating)	3.1	2.8	.05
Interview "style" components (5–point ratings)			
Loud/explosive speech	4.1	3.7	.01
Rapid/accelerated	4.3	3.8	.03
Response latency	4.5	4.1	.09
Potential for hostility	4.1	3.7	.02
Verbal competitiveness	4.1	3.8	NS
Interview "content" factors (5–point ratings)			
Pressured drive (mean of 5 items)	14.8	14.6	NS
Anger (mean of 4 items)	11.2	11.6	NS
Competitiveness (mean of 1 item)	3.2	3.3	NS
JAS Type A scale	6.5	4.3	NS

Note: Adapted from Krantz et al., 1982c.

beta receptors. The beta-1 cardiovascular response is increased force and rate of heart muscle contraction, and the beta-2 response is dilation of skeletal muscle blood vessels. There are also metabolic effects of beta-blocking drugs.

In our study, patients were given a Type A interview while heart rate and blood pressure were monitored, and results (see Table 1) indicated that patients taking propranolol (a beta-1 and beta-2 blocker) were significantly lower in intensity of Type A behavior compared to patients not taking propranolol. No such effects were found among patients medicated or not medicated with diuretics, nitrates, or central nervous system active drugs, suggesting an association specific to propranolol in this sample. The components of Type A that were lower in propranolol-treated patients included speech stylistics such as loud/explosive, rapid/accelerated, and potential-for-hostility. Content of responses to the SI and scores on the JAS did not differ between the groups. As one might expect, consistent with the physiologic effects of beta-blocking drugs, propranolol-treated patients also showed lesser cardiovascular responses to the interview.

A caution is in order in interpreting these results: These data are correlational and we cannot infer from this study alone that propranolol caused a lowering of Type A behavior. However, the data are at least suggestive because the effects were still present after controlling for possibly confounding factors associated with prescription of this medication, and also after considering the effects of other prescribed drugs.

Further corroboration for the hypothesis that sympathetic reactivity forms a substrate for Type A derives from a recent experiment (Schmieder, Friedrich, Neus, Rüddel, & Von Eiff, 1983) that pharmacologically blocked beta-adrenergic activity in seven patients by administering atenolol. Atenolol is another beta-blocking agent (beta-1 only) that, importantly, penetrates poorly into the brain (see below). A control group of nine patients received a diuretic. Results indicated the group receiving the beta-blocker atenolol, but not the controls, showed a decrease in intensity of SI-rated Type A behavior after receiving medication over a 4-6 week period. By attenuation of sympathetic responsivity with atenolol, behavioral manifestations of Type A appeared also to be dampened. These experimental findings provide further support for our suggestion that sympathetic nervous system reactivity forms a physiological substrate for Type A behavior.

BEHAVIORAL EFFECTS OF BETA-BLOCKERS: PERIPHERAL VIEWS OF EMOTION REVISITED

An understanding of the mechanisms responsible for the effects of beta-blockers on Type A must take into account what is known about the psychological effects of these drugs. Therefore, further speculation about mechanisms underlying Type A behavior and possible applications to anger control is justified here.

Since the introduction of beta-adrenoreceptor antagonists and their wide use for cardiovascular disorders, there have been reports of a variety of both desirable and untoward psychological effects. Foremost among these are beneficial effects in reducing anxiety. This observation has been made in a variety of acute stress situations, such as performing before an audience or race car driving, as well as in patients exhibiting chronic anxiety characterized by bodily symptoms. (See reviews by Frischman, Razin, Swencionis, & Sonnenblick, 1981; Middlemiss, Buxton, & Greenwood, 1981; Tyrer, 1976; Patel & Turner, 1981).

However, the precise mechanisms by which these anxiety-reducing effects occur are not entirely clear. Although all the commonly used beta-blockers penetrate into the central nervous system (CNS) to some extent, they vary widely in this characteristic with those that are very soluble in lipids (e.g., propranolol) crossing the blood-brain barrier readily, others (e.g., metoprolol) somewhat less so, and still others (e.g., atenolol), with low lipid solubility, penetrating into the brain very poorly (Patel & Turner, 1981) (see Table 3).

Nevertheless, it is important to note that penetration of beta-blocking drugs into the CNS is not sufficient to prove the drugs have a central action. In fact, it is thought by most reviewers (Middlemiss et al., 1981; Tyrer, 1976; Weiner, 1980) that the peripheral action of beta-blockers is sufficient to explain their anxiety-reducing (or anxiolytic) effects. This mechanism may involve the previously described role of processing of information concerning peripheral sympathetic responses in the subjective experience of emotion. As we have noted, peripheralist views of emotion suggest that the experience of anxiety is an end result of a sequence of events, beginning with sympathetic stimulation that gives rise to arousal manifestations such as palpitations and tremor. The perception, cognitive interpretation, and/or automatic processing of these responses acts to reinforce the psychic elements of anxiety. Based on this interpretation, beta-adrenergic blockade inhibits peripheral physiologic responses, interrupting the somatic-psychic interaction and thus reducing anxiety (Middlemiss et al., 1981; Tyrer, 1976).

This peripheral feedback explanation for the anxiolytic effects of beta-blockers receives support from several sources of data. First, there is evidence

Table 3 Ratios between plasma and brain tissue concentration of some β-adrenoceptor blocking drugs

Study	Drug	Brain/plasma ratio
Neil-Dwyer et al. (1981) (Neurosurgical patients)	Propranolol 160 mg daily	26
	Oxprenolol 160 mg daily	50
	Metoprolol 200 mg daily	12
	Atenolol 100 mg daily	0.2
Day et al. (1977) (Rats)	Propranolol	8.36
	Oxprenolol	3.26
	Practolol	0.18
	Atenolol	0.054

that beta-blockers such as atenolol, which do not readily penetrate into the CNS, may be as effective in reducing anxiety as propranolol, which does readily enter the brain (Middlemiss et al., 1981; Weiner, 1980). Secondly, beta-blockers are most effective for patients who exhibit anxiety particularly characterized by *somatic* or bodily symptoms (e.g., palpitations, tremor), rather than those who characterize their distress or anxiety in terms of purely cognitive or *psychic* terms (e.g., fearful ideation) (Tyrer, 1976). However, it should be noted that the degree to which peripheral versus central mechanisms are involved in the anxiolytic and other psychological effects of beta-blockers is an important concern, and we will discuss possible central actions of beta-blockers in a later section of this chapter.

A Somatopsychic Model of Type A Behavior

How might the aforementioned discussion of beta-blockers and anxiety be relevant to understanding mechanisms underlying Type A behavior? At first thought it may appear *irrelevant* because research (Chesney, Black, Chadwick, & Rosenman, 1981) indicates that SI-defined Type A behavior is virtually unrelated to various psychometric measures of anxiety and distress. However, the descriptive and empirical features of Type A (e.g., anger, hostility, irritability, vigorous mannerisms, etc.) do represent forms of emotional behavior apart from anxiety (cf. Chesney et al., 1981; Matthews et al., 1982).

Thus, if we view SI-defined Type A behavior in a larger context as emotional behavior, the pharmacologic data of Krantz et al. (1982c) and Schmieder et al. (1983) allow us to borrow from peripheral models of emotion and to conceptualize Type A as an interaction of cognitive/information-processing and physiological elements. Speech stylistics (e.g., loud/explosive and rapid/accelerated speech) which were sensitive to beta-blocking medication in the aforementioned studies might reflect underlying physiological processes. "Content" aspects of the SI and scores on the JAS, not related to beta-adrenergic blockade, might be more heavily linked to cognitive-perceptual or psychological factors. These cognitive and physiological components could interact to produce the expression of Type A behavior via a mechanism involving feedback from peripheral sympathetic responses (see Figure 3). Thus, the processing of information concerning cardiovascular or other peripheral responses would reinforce energetic Type A stylistics that contribute to assessments in the SI. By selectively attenuating these peripheral sympathetic responses, beta-blockers may reduce intensity of Type A. Indeed, the recent results (Schmieder et al., 1983) suggesting that Type A behavior may be reduced by atenolol—a beta-blocker with very poor CNS penetration—are particularly supportive of a peripheral feedback mechanism for Type A behavior. (Note the arrow labeled "somatopsychic effects" in Figure 1).

Stated in somewhat different language, this model would suggest that SI-defined Type A behavior (at least among cardiac patients) is the outcome of the interaction of both physiological and cognitive/information-processing factors. These factors include (1) an underlying sympathetic reactivity which may be constitutional (e.g., early conditioning or genetic)[5] in origin, and either (2a) the individual's reactions to peripheral sympathtic responses, which may be associated with his/her psychological set (e.g., psychological traits, interoceptive mechanisms), and/or (2b) the individual's cognitive reactions to a particular situational setting (see Krantz & Durel, 1983, for details for this model).

This view suggests that sympathetic reactivity alone is not sufficient to predict or explain the behavioral characteristics of Type A as measured in the SI. Somatopsychic mechanisms such as perception, evaluation, or automatic information processing of physiologic reactivity must also be considered. This explanation is also consistent with several puzzling or inconsistent lines of data which

[5] Although published studies have not indicated that Type A has a strong genetic component, it is possible that excessive or repetitive elicitation of sympathetic responses over the course of the life span may both enhance the expression of Type A and predispose to coronary disease as well. However, recent unpublished data have revealed significant heritability for certain components of SI-defined Type A behavior (Matthews, personal communication).

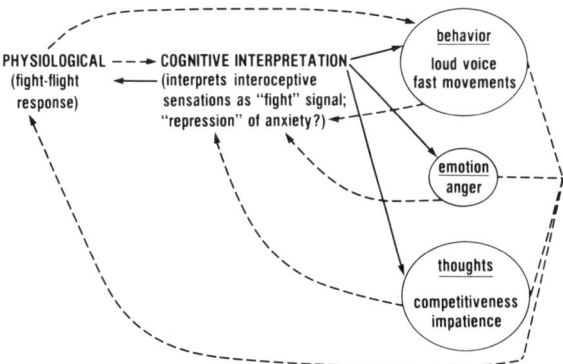

Figure 3 A possible somatopsychic model of Type A behavior illustrating bi-directional relationships between cognitive, physiological, and behavioral manifestations. (From Krantz & Durel, 1983). Reprinted with permission.

have recently emerged in the psychophysiological literature. First, there appear to be a variety of predictors of cardiovascular reactivity to stress, some of which are apprently independent of Type A (e.g., family history of hypertension; cf. Glass et al., under review; and Obrist, 1981). Secondly, there is considerable heterogeneity among Type A individuals in their extent of physiologic reactivity (cf. Dembroski et al., 1979; Glass & Contrada, 1984). Each of these findings would be consistent with the hypothesis that cardiovascular reactivity alone is not a sufficient criterion for predicting which individuals are classified as Type A or Type B in the SI. Instead, the individual's reactions to, or appraisals of, bodily responses must also be factored into the equation.

CENTRAL VERSUS PERIPHERAL ACTIONS OF BETA-BLOCKERS: ISSUES AND CAUTIONS

Before proceeding further in our discussion of the psychological effects of beta-blocking drugs, we must stop to consider that all the commonly-used beta-blockers (particularly propranolol) do penetrate into the brain and cerebrospinal fluid to some extent, although individual drugs vary widely in this characteristic. Several studies of human neurological patients and of animals have compared brain/plasma ratios of these drugs (see Table 3). It appears that their degree of CNS penetration can be explained largely on the basis of their lipid solubility, although other factors (e.g., amount of free drug in plasma, degree of ionization) also are determinants (Middlemiss et al., 1981; Patel & Turner, 1981). In addition to anxiety-reduction and apparent effects in decreasing Type A behavior, other psychological and behavioral effects of beta-blockers have been observed. These include fatigue, depression, sleep disturbance, and, infrequently, disturbed performance on some psychomotor and psychosensory tests (cf. Patel & Turner, 1981).

To make matters more complex, each of these effects may differ in the extent to which central versus peripheral sites of action are involved, and CNS activity—if it occurs—might itself result from a variety of mechanisms (Noyes, 1982). For example, CNS activity might take the form of a direct blocking of beta-adrenergic receptors which have been shown to exist in the CNS. On the other hand, central activity might be an indirect or learned result of peripheral blockade inhibiting feedback from the periphery, as discussed extensively in previous sections of this chapter.

Given that these issues presently remain unresolved, studies that systematically compare the effects of beta-blockers differing in extent of CNS-penetrability can yield potentially important information about the *relative* importance of central versus peripheral mechanisms. Accordingly, our present research involves a comparison of the behavioral effects of CNS penetrating (propranolol) and relatively non-CNS penetrating beta-blockers (atenolol and nadolol). We are assessing Type A behavior, administering measures of hostility and anger, and attempting to develop a typology to identify individuals who respond to autonomic cues with anger. Our research is also examining simple and complex psychomotor performance, and autonomic reactivity as well as other reported side-effects. Nevertheless, given the complexities and uncertainties of these questions, a central action for the effects of beta-blockers on emotion must be considered a potent alternative to the peripheral view described in this chapter.

FURTHER EVIDENCE FOR EFFECTS OF ADRENERGIC BLOCKERS ON ANGER AND AGGRESSION

Most research on pharmacologic treatment of aggressive disturbances has focused almost exclusively on central neurological mechanisms, particularly the role of central catecholamines in provoked aggression, and possible applications of anti-psychotics and benzodiazepines for aggressive disturbances. Discussion of central-neural mechanisms of anger and aggression is beyond the scope of this chapter, and comprehensive reviews of this area can be found elsewhere (Baldessarini, 1980; Eichelman, 1973; 1977). Similarly, we will not consider ethical and social issues in the treatment of anger and aggression. Suffice it to say that central noradrenergic activity is implicated in instances of rage and aggression, and that different types of aggressive behaviors (e.g., spontaneous vs. stress-induced) may be related to different neurotransmitters and/or different patterns of neurochemical activity (cf. Eichelman, 1973; 1977). Although the antipsychotic drugs are used primarily for their central effects, they also affect peripheral responses, but these are usually considered side-effects. As we have noted, the reverse is true of CNS-penetrating beta-blockers.

We have presented preliminary evidence that aspects of Type A behavior components described as "stylistic," rather than cognitive or attitudinal, may be decreased by beta-blockers, including atenolol which penetrates poorly into the CNS. This tentatively suggests that beta-blockers might be useful for the management of anger and hostility among individuals with chronic anger problems; individuals who characteristically respond to physiologically-arousing circumstances with anger might benefit from beta-blockers.

Other data from several research domains suggest possible effects of beta-blockers on anger and aggression, although mechanisms for these effects remain unresolved. These include: (1) clinical reports of pharmacologic treatment of neurologic patients with rage disorders; (2) some limited animal studies modeling "emotional" behavior; and (3) some laboratory psychopharmacologic research on human emotion.

First, several recent case studies report the effective use of propranolol in controlling explosive rage outbursts among patients with organic brain dysfunction (Elliot, 1977; Schreier, 1979; Williams, Mehl, Yudofsky, Adams, & Roseman, 1982). In the Williams et al. (1982) study, patients had prior unsuccessful medication treatment with stimulants, antipsychotics, or anti-convulsant drugs, and prior unsuccessful psychotherapeutic treatment. Results indicated that more than 75% of the sample showed marked decrease in rage outbursts and aggressive behavior when given a regimen of moderate-to-high doses of propranolol. Although a central action of propranolol is particularly compelling among these patients, the authors suggest that peripheral blockade of adrenergically-mediated physical sensations may also be plausibly involved in the therapeutic effects of this drug.

Secondly, there is also limited animal evidence which suggests that aggressive behaviors might be decreased by administration of beta-blockers. For example, Jaekel (1981) reported that rhesus monkeys given beta-blockers became less aggressive, less anxious, and showed increased positive social contacts.

Thirdly, a recent human laboratory study (Erdman & van Lindern, 1980) provides some equivocal evidence for the effects of adrenergic drugs on anger, but also reveals the complex relationships among situational factors, peripheral autonomic responses, and emotional responses of anger and anxiety. To examine the effects of beta-adrenergic stimulation and blockade on emotional reactions, Erdman and van Lindern (1980) administered either the beta-blocker oxprenolol, a placebo, or the beta-agonist orciprenaline (metaproterenol) in one of two situations designed to induce either anger-like or no emotional reactions (neutral control). Drug administration, given orally, was disguised so that changes in bodily activity would be more likely to be attributed to the situation than to the drug.

As expected, the anger manipulation increased ratings of anger among subjects given a placebo. However, the effects of the beta-blocker and beta-agonist were somewhat unexpected. While the beta-blocker slightly lessened anger self-ratings of provoked subjects compared to those of subjects receiving placebo, the effects of orciprenaline were, unexpectedly, similar in direction and almost of the same magnitude. However, orciprenaline also had the effect of increasing anxiety ratings of provoked subjects, whereas oxprenolol did not.

Physiologically, significant increases in systolic and diastolic blood pressure occurred in the anger situation. Beta-blockade resulted in significant decreases in heart rate (HR) and systolic blood pressure (SBP) but no change in diastolic blood pressure (DBP) over placebo. The beta-agonist resulted in significant HR and SBP increases but a *decreased* change in DBP. Thus, it appears that orciprenaline resulted in a more epinephrine-like than norepinephrine-like cardiovascular response pattern—one more typical of anxiety than anger (Ax, 1953; Schachter, 1957). This physiologic change may then have been interpreted by subjects as anxiety, rather than as anger.

Although the authors do not do so, this line of reasoning might be followed to account for the less than significant prevention of anger in the oxprenolol condition. To the extent that this drug did not prevent changes that might be associated with anger (e.g., increased DBP) it would not be expected to prevent the experience of anger. Although HR and SBP were significantly lower than in the neutral and anger conditions, such was not the case for DBP. DBP for oxprenolol subjects remained virtually identical to that in the anger condition. Of course, this explanation presumes an ability of subjects to differentiate these response patterns.

CONCLUDING COMMENTS

These data suggest that in a study with a strong situational manipulation of anger, a β_1 and β_2 adrenergic blocker such as oxprenolol—which would increase or leave unchanged DBP response—administered in relatively low doses may have limited effect in inhibiting resultant anger. However, given our earlier data on Type A, we might suggest that it would be fruitful to further examine the effects of beta-blockers among individuals with chronic anger problems. Such individuals may be cognitively predisposed to interpret or label peripheral sympathetic responses as anger. Recently, investigators (Schwartz et al., 1978; Tyrer, 1976) have explored the notion that it may be possible to characterize anxiety according to a "somatic" versus "psychic" typology. A similar typology for cognitive versus somatically triggered anger may also be possible. Indeed, the research on the pervasiveness of physiological symptoms associated with naturally-occurring anger suggests that this may be the case (Davitz, 1969).

Clearly, the role of peripheral sympathetic responses in anger remains a subset of larger unresolved theoretical issues concerning emotion. Research comparing various beta-blockers allows us to explore longstanding issues regarding central versus peripheral determinants of emotional behavior. However, the beta-blockers are among the most widely prescribed drugs in the United States (U.S.F.D.A., 1982). Systematic research on their *psychological* as well as physiologic effects and side effects is not only important for their mental health consequences but is also feasible ethically and practically, given their wide-ranging indications in clinical populations.

SUMMARY

This chapter reviews evidence suggesting that visceral sympathetic nervous system reactions can summate with other aspects of the emotional experience of anger, and thereby contribute to the intensity of anger and aggression. Such evidence supports the assumption that anger is the interactive outcome of physiological arousal and anger-related information processing. It is proposed here that beta-adrenergic blocking drugs, which selectively reduce peripheral sympathetic responses, might reduce anger among individuals predisposed to respond to autonomic changes in terms of anger. Preliminary data from the literatures on Type A behavior, rage disorders, and the psychophysiology of emotion are reviewed.

REFERENCES

Averill, J. R. *Anger and aggression: An essay on emotion.* New York: Springer-Verlag, 1982.

Ax, A. F. Physiological differentiation of emotional states. *Psychosomatic Medicine,* 1953, *15,* 433-442.

Brand, R. J., Rosenman, R. H., Jenkins, C. D., Sholtz, R. I., & Zyzanski, S. J. *Comparison of coronary heart disease prediction in the Western Collaborative Group Study using the Structured Interview and the Jenkins Activity Survey assessment of the coronary-prone Type A behavior pattern.* Paper presented at the Annual Conference on Cardiovascular Disease Epidemiology, American Heart Association, Orlando, Florida, March, 1978.

Cannon, W. B. *Bodily changes in pain, hunger, fear, and rage* (2nd ed.). New York: Appleton, 1929.

Chesney, M. A., Black, G. W., Chadwick, J. H., & Rosenman, R. H. Psychological correlates of the Type A behavior pattern. *Journal of Behavioral Medicine,* 1981, *4,* 217-230.

Chesney, M. A., & Rosenman, R. H. Specificity in stress models: Examples drawn from Type A behavior. In C. L. Cooper (Ed.), *Stress Research.* London: Wiley, 1983.

Davitz, J. R. *The language of emotion.* New York: Academic, 1969.

Day, M. D., Hemsworth, B. A., & Street, J. A. The central uptake of β-adrenoceptor antagonists. *Journal of Pharmacy and Pharmacology,* 1977, *29,* 52P.

Dembroski, T. M. Reliability and validity of methods used to assess coronary-prone behavior. In T. M. Dembroski, S. M. Weiss, J. L. Shields, S. G. Haynes, & M. Feinleib (Eds.), *Coronary-prone behavior.* New York: Springer-Verlag, 1978.

Dembroski, T. M., MacDougall, J. M., Herd, J. A., & Shields, J. L. Effects of level of challenge on pressor and heart rate responses in Type A and B subjects. *Journal of Applied Social Psychology,* 1979, *9,* 208-228.

Dembroski, T. M., MacDougall, J. M., Shields, J. L., Petitto, J., & Lushene, R. Components of the Type A coronary-prone behavior pattern and cardiovascular responses to psychomotor performance challenge. *Journal of Behavioral Medicine,* 1978, *1,* 159-176.

Eichelman, B. The catecholamines and aggressive behavior. *Neuroscience Research,* 1973, *5,* 109-129.

Eichelman, B. Pharmacological treatment of aggressive disturbances. In J. D. Barchas, P. A. Berger, R. D. Ciaranello, G. R. Elliott (Eds.), *Psychopharmacology: From theory to practice.* New York: Oxford University Press, 1977.

Eliot, F. Propranolol for the control of the belligerent behavior following acute brain damage. *Annals of Neurology,* 1977, *1,* 489-491.

Estefanous, F. G., & Tarazi, R. G. Systemic arterial hypertension associated with cardiac surgery. *American Journal of Cardiology,* 1980, *46,* 685-694.

Frishman, W. H., Razin, A., Swencionis, C., & Sonnenblick, E. H. Beta-adrenoceptor blockade in anxiety states: A new approach to therapy? *Cardiovascular Reviews and Reports,* 1981, *2,* 447-459.

Gates, G. S. An observational study of anger. *Journal of Experimental Psychology,* 1926, *9,* 235-331.

Geen, R. G., Rakosky, J. J., & Pigg, R. Awareness of arousal and its relation to aggression. *British Journal of Social and Clinical Psychology,* 1972, *11,* 115-121.

Glass, D. C. *Behavior patterns, stress, and coronary disease.* Hillsdale, N.J.: Erlbaum, 1977.

Glass, D. C. & Contrada, R. J. Type A behavior and catecholamines: A critical review. In C. R. Lake & M. Ziegler (Eds.), *Norepinephrine: Clinical aspects.* Baltimore: Williams & Wilkins, 1984.

Glass, D. C., Lake, C. R., Contrada, R. J., Kehoe, K., & Erlanger, L. R. Stability of individual differences in physiological responses to stress. *Health Psychology,* 1983, *2*(4), 317-341.

Jaekel, J. Influence of selected β-blockers on social interaction of rhesus monkeys. Paper presented at the symposium on Psychophysiological risk factors of cardiovascular diseases: Psychosocial stress, personality, and occupational specificity. Karlovy Vary, CSSR, 1981.

James, W. What is an emotion? *Mind,* 1884, *9,* 188-205.

Jenkins, C. D. A comparative review of the interview and questionnaire methods in the assessment of the coronary-prone behavior pattern. In T. M. Dembroski, S. M. Weiss, J. L. Shields, S. G. Haynes, & M. Feinleib (Eds.), *Coronary-prone behavior.* New York: Springer-Verlag, 1978.

Jenkins, C. D., Zyzanski, S. J., & Rosenman, R. H. Progress toward validation of a computer scored test for the Type A coronary prone behavior pattern. *Psychosomatic Medicine,* 1971, *33,* 193-202.

Kahn, J. P., Kornfeld, D. S., Frank, K. A., Heller, S. S., & Hoar, P. F. Type A behavior and blood pressure during coronary artery bypass surgery. *Psychosomatic Medicine,* 1980, *42,* 407-414.

Konecni, V. J. Annoyance, type, and duration of postannoyance activity, and aggression. *Journal of Experimental Psychology: General,* 1975a, *104,* 75-102.

Konecni, V. J. The mediation of aggressive behavior: Arousal level versus anger and cognitive labeling. *Journal of Personality and Social Psychology,* 1975b, *32,* 706-712.

Krantz, D. S., Arabian, J. M., Davis, J. E., & Parker, J. S. Type A behavior and coronary artery bypass surgery: Intraoperative blood pressure and perioperative complications. *Psychosomatic Medicine,* 1982, *44,* 273-284.

Krantz, D. S. & Durel, L. A. Psychobiological substrates of the Type A behavior pattern. *Health Psychology,* 1983, *2,* 393-411.

Krantz, D. S., Durel, L. A., Davia, J. E., Shaffer, R. T., Arabian, J. M., Dembroski, T. M., & MacDougall, J. M. Propranolol medication among coronary patients: Relationship to Type A behavior and cardiovascular response. *Journal of Human Stress,* 1982, *8*(3), 4-12.

Krantz, D. S., Glass, D. C., Schaeffer, M. A., & Davia, J. E. Behavior patterns and coronary disease: A critical evaluation. In J. T. Cacippo & R. E. Petty (Eds.), *Perspectives on cardiovascular psychophysiology.* New York: Guilford, 1982.

Lange, C. G. *Om sindsbevaegelser.* Kjobenhavn, 1885.

Leventhal, H. Toward a comprehensive theory of emotion. In L. Berkowitz (Ed.), *Advances in Experimental Social Psychology.* New York: Academic, 1980.

Matthews, K. A. Psychological perspectives on Type A behavior pattern. *Psychological Bulletin,* 1982, *91,* 293-323.

Matthews, K. A., Krantz, D. S., Dembroski, T. M., MacDougall, T. M. Unique and common variance in Structured Interview and Jenkins Activity Survey assessments of the Type A behavior pattern. *Journal of Personality and Social Psychology,* 1982, *42,* 303-313.

Middlemiss, D. N., Buxton, D. A., & Greenwood, D. T. Beta-adrenoreceptor antagonists in psychiatry and neurology. *Pharmacology and Therapeutics,* 1981, *12,* 419-437.

Obrist, P. A. *Cardiovascular psychophysiology: A perspective.* New York: Plenum, 1981.
Patel, L., & Turner, P. Central actions of beta-adrenoreceptor blocking drugs in man. *Medicinal Research Reveiews,* 1981, *1,* 387-410.
Rosenman, R. H. The interview method of assessment of the coronary-prone behavior pattern. In T. M. Dembroski, S. M. Weiss, J. L. Shields, S. G. Haynes, & M. Feinleib (Eds.), *Coronary-prone behavior.* New York: Springer-Verlag, 1978.
Schachter, S., & Singer, J. E. Cognitive, social, and physiological determinants of emotional state. *Psychological Review,* 1962, *69,* 379-399.
Schachter, J. Pain, fear, and anger in hypertensives and normotensives. *Psychosomatic Medicine,* 1957, *19,* 17-29.
Scherwitz, L., Barton, K., & Leventhal, H. Type A assessment and interaction in the behavior pattern interview. *Psychosomatic Medicine,* 1977, *39,* 229-240.
Schmieder, R., Friedrich, G., Neus, H., Rüddel, H., & Von Eiff, A. W. Effect of β-blockers on Type A coronary-prone behavior. *Psychosomatic Medicine,* 1983, *45,* 417-423.
Schreier, H. Use of propranolol in the treatment of postencephalitic psychosis. *American Journal of Psychiatry,* 1979, *136,* 840-841.
Schucker, B., & Jacobs, D. R. Assessment of behavioral risk for coronary disease by voice characteristics. *Psychosomatic Medicine,* 1977, *39,* 219-228.
Schwartz, G. E., Davidson, R. G., & Goleman, D. J. Patterning of cognitive and somatic processes in the self-regulation of anxiety: Effects of meditation versus exercise. *Psychosomatic Medicine,* 1978, *40,* 321-328.
Tyrer, P. J. *The role of bodily feelings in anxiety.* London: Oxford University Press, 1976.
U.S. Food and Drug Administration. *Drug utilization in the U.S. 1981: Third annual review.* Washington, D.C.: National Center for Drugs and Biologics, 1982.
Weiner, N. Drugs that inhibit adrenergic nerves and block adrenergic receptors. In A. G. Gilman, L. S. Goodman, & A. Gilman (Eds.), *Goodman and Gilman's the pharmacological basis of therapeutics* (6th ed.). New York: MacMillan, 1980.
Williams, D. T., Mehl, R., Yudofsky, S., Adams, D., & Roseman, B. The effect of propranolol on uncontrolled rage outbursts in children and adolescents with organic brain dysfunction. *Journal of the American Academy of Child Psychiatry,* 1982, *21,* 129-135.
Zillmann, D. Excitation transfer in communication-mediated aggressive behavior. *Journal of Experimental Social Psychology,* 1971, *7,* 419-434.
Zillman, D., Johnson, R. C., & Day, K. D. Attribution of apparent arousal and proficiency of recovery from sympathetic activation affecting excitation transfer to aggressive behavior. *Journal of Experimental Social Psychology,* 1974, *10,* 503-515.

15

Anger and Hostility: Future Implications for Behavioral Medicine

Margaret A. Chesney
SRI International

Anger and hostility have been considered to be causal factors in a number of serious health problems, including coronary heart disease—the leading cause of death among adults in the United States and other western countries. Detrimental effects of anger, hostility, and aggression that were discussed in the preceding chapters in this volume, may include relationships with hypertension, cancer, and psychophysiologic disorders, in addition to interpersonal discord, conflict, and violence.

In spite of the serious consequences of excessive anger, hostility, and aggression, these constructs have received relatively little attention from behavioral scientists until recently. The strong evidence that hostility and anger expression are causally related to coronary heart disease promotes these variables to target behaviors, which require attention to issues of their assessment and treatment or intervention.

Elevating these behaviors to target status constitutes a mandate for the behavioral research community in behavioral medicine. Considering the potential impact of anger and hostility on public health, this research agenda represents a challenge that is more than academic. This chapter will discuss some issues that need to be addressed by behavioral science in terms of assessment of and intervention for anger, and suggests avenues for exploration of the many questions raised by these issues.

ANGER: DEFINING THE TARGET BEHAVIOR

Anger now assumes a position similar to that assigned in the past to anxiety. Like anxiety, anger has been identified as a causal factor in behavioral, as well as psychophysiological, disorders. Moreover, as with anxiety, anger can be a consequence of, or reaction to, illness (Burish & Bradley, 1983). However, unlike anxiety, an accepted operational definition distinguishing anger from hostility, aggression and other related emotional states (e.g., irritation) does not yet exist.

A consensus among leading researchers in the field is not far off, as indicated by those chapters in the first section of this volume. This is likely to describe hostility as an enduring disposition or attitude, anger as an emotional reaction or state, and aggression as a behavior or action. Furthermore, the consensus will probably describe these factors as being interrelated, while varying in intensity frequency, duration, and mode of expression.

The development of questionnaires to assess anger, hostility and aggression has received renewed interest and will undoubtedly result in relevant scales that are reliable and valid in terms of their agreement with existing measures. When selecting or considering assessment strategies, the purpose of the assessment is of central importance. For the investigation of relationships between hostility or anger and health status, paper and pencil self-report questionnaires may be adequate. This belief is supported by the causal relationships discussed by Rosenman, Julius, Williams and their colleagues in chapters in this volume. However, the assessment of anger, as well as hostility and aggression, must go beyond paper and pencil self-report questionnaires, such as those proposed by Spielberger et al. and by Seigel in Chap. 3. For the study of pathogenetic mechanisms and the design and assessment of interventions, for example, such measurements will fall short of the mark. More comprehensive assessment strategies, such as those discussed in the next section, need to be developed and validated in order to meet the needs and demands of research on anger mechanisms and treatment.

BEHAVIORAL ASSESSMENT OF ANGER

Valid measurement of anger is predicated on an understanding of the anger construct and a conceptualization of the process underlying anger arousal and related behaviors. Anger arousal, as conceptualized by Novaco (1979; Chap. 11) and Konecni (1975a) is determined by cognitive expectations and appraisals of environmental events. Events alone do not directly lead to anger arousal and the emotional experience of anger, but are mediated by cognitive processes. As Berkowitz has noted (1983), Leventhal's (1980) perceptual motor theory of emotion offers an appealing analysis of the cognitive pathway to the emotional experience of anger. According to Leventhal, a subject perceives the occurrence of an event, interprets it, and responds with an involuntary expressive motor reaction that is outside focal awareness. This motor reaction is spontaneous, often involving facial expression that can range from momentary narrowing of the eyes to a distinct frown. The reaction is fed back into the central nervous system and plays a primary role in generating the emotional feeling of anger. Once aroused, anger influences future cognitive expectations and appraisals. According to Leventhal, this influence would be exerted by schematic or emotional memories that "act as selective devices, focusing attention on particular stimulus features (of environmental events) and generating anticipations about later experience." Arousal of angry emotions is a major precipitator of aggressive behavior (Rule & Nesdale, 1976), and, while anger is not necessary for occurrence of aggression, anger and aggression interact with one another such that the level of anger influences the level of aggression, and vice versa (Konecni, 1975b). Aggressive behavior, as documented by the work of Bandura (1983) and of Patterson, Reid and their associates (discussed in this volume), not only reflects the level of anger, but is also influenced by the environment's response (e.g., support for reinforcement, punishment or sanctions) to the aggression.

This complex conceptual model is presented in Figure 1. In addition, an

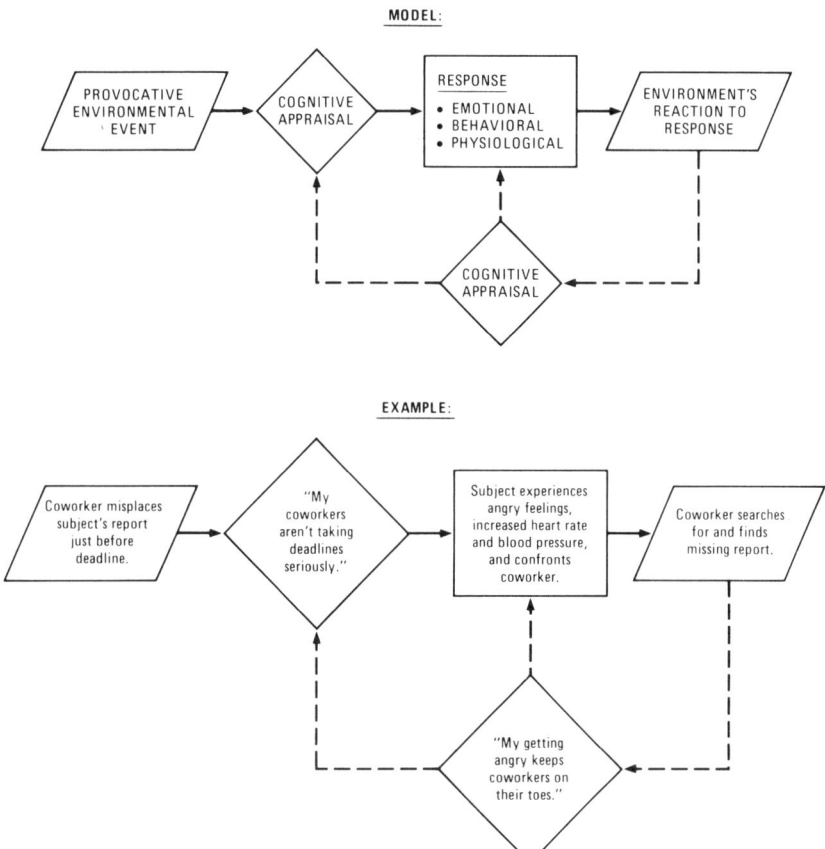

Figure 1 Conceptual model and specific example of anger arousal.

example illustrating the dynamic interdependencies between environmental events among the elements of the model is presented. In this example, the coworker misplaces the subject's report just before a deadline and the subject perceives this event to mean that the coworker is not taking the deadline seriously. The result of this perception or cognitive appraisal in turn leads to the target subject feeling angry, experiencing increased heart rate and blood pressure, and confronting the coworker. The coworker responds to the confrontation by searching for and ultimately finding the misplaced report. The subject is relieved that the report is found so quickly and sees the value of his anger expression. This not only provides positive feedback for, or reinforces, his anger response but also reinforces his cognitive expectancy and appraisal that coworkers are careless and need to be monitored. This, in turn, increases the likelihood that similar environmental events in the future will also lead to anger arousal.

Research investigations of the interactive processes and psychosocial or physiological mechanisms represented in this model require measures that capture more of the dynamics that determine anger arousal than those afforded by brief self-report questionnaires.

Alternative measures, most of which have not been previously applied to anger assessment, might include direct observation, the use of analogue or simulated situations, assessment of articulated thoughts, and ambulatory monitoring of cardiovascular arousal and other variables. Future research in anger assessment should consider using these measures, either separately or in combination, in order to obtain a more accurate portrait of anger arousal.

Direct Observation: Capturing the Naturally Occurring Event and Response

One approach to the assessment of anger is to directly monitor a subject's behavior in the natural environment. This approach is exemplified by the microsocial analysis described by Patterson in this volume. Environmental events that provoke anger, behavioral responses to those events, and the environment's reaction to the behavior are observed and noted in sequence. Such monitoring, while providing rich detail in terms of processes and chains of events, is not without difficulties. Among these is the potential that the observer's presence may influence the behavior of the subject. Videotaping behavior can reduce the risk of this contamination but is only feasible when observations are made in restricted settings; otherwise, the subject is likely to move in and out of the observational setting during the assessment period. Direct observation in the natural environment may be accurate, but is costly in terms of the personnel and time required for data collection, and presents major challenges from the perspective of data reduction and analysis. The fact that the environment is not altered constitutes an advantage of this method; however, the situations of data collection may vary considerably across observational sessions. Thus, a large number of data samples are required to obtain a valid and reliable behavioral assessment of behavioral patterns. These problems have inhibited the widespread use of this procedure, although the insights it can foster reserve a place for direct observation in behavioral assessment, particularly in the early stages of concept formulations.

Analogues: Present the Event in Simulation

As an alternative to direct observation, behavioral scientists interested in assessing actual behavior responses to certain environmental events have developed a useful strategy. Standard analogue situations designed to simulate the natural environment are presented to subjects who are instructed to respond as they typically would to similar circumstances in the natural environment (Nay, 1977).

The method of presenting these stimuli can vary considerably. The least costly and most readily administered analogue is a variant of the paper and pencil questionnaire. The subject reads through an analogue situation and is instructed to respond to such a situation by providing a written response or by endorsing one of a range of presented alternatives. Other analogues include audiotape or videotape-recorded stimuli where subjects' verbal responses are recorded for subsequent analysis. A further step toward naturalistic assessment is the laboratory analogue in which the subject is brought into a situation designed to provide certain elements of anger provocation, while responses to the situation are monitored and evaluated. Such a procedure was followed in the assessment of assertive behavior in the research reported by Manuck in Chap. 10. In many respects the Structured Interview, used to classify individuals according to the Type A behavior pattern (Rosenman, 1978), is a well-known example of analogue assessment. This interview is a standard interpersonal interactive situation in which the interviewer presents the subject with subtle challenges and provocations and evaluates the subject's response. The behavioral analogue nature of this assessment procedure has been cited as the primary reason for its superiority over pencil and paper questionnaire scales in predicting coronary heart disease (Chesney, Eagleston, & Rosenman, 1981).

Assessing Cognitive Appraisal

A pivotal feature in the conceptual model proposed by Novaco (1979) and Konecni (1975a) described previously is the subject's cognitive expectation and appraisal of environmental events. Despite the preeminence given to cognitive appraisal in conceptualizations of anger arousal, little if any attention is given to assessment of cognitions, making this an area where further attention is warranted. One recently developed approach to assessing cognitive appraisal is a paradigm known as "Articulated Thoughts During Simulated Situations" (Davison, Robins, & Johnson, 1983). Subjects are told to imagine that an audiotaped recording of an analogue or simulated situation presented on the tape is actually occurring, to attend to the thoughts and feelings that the situation evokes, and to say these thoughts aloud after the situation is presented. These verbalizations are recorded on audiotape for analysis.

This approach provides a record of ongoing thoughts or cognitions, including appraisals and expectations, and allows an examination of variables that influence cognitive appraisal. In a study of cognitive appraisals of stressful situations, for example, subjects were found to articulate more hostile or aggressive cognitions to situations involving personally salient uncontrollable stress than to a less personally relevant situation (Lerman & Davison, Note 1). As this example suggests, the "articulated thoughts" paradigm may be an approach to the assessment of cognitive appraisal in anger arousal. In particular, this paradigm appears to be effective in the study of the cognitive appraisals of environmental events—cognitive factors that determine anger responses. Further research to develop this and similar cognitive assessment strategies should be followed by data collection or anger cognitions underlying anger arousal and its behavioral correlates. Together, they will serve to document and track the influence of cognitive appraisal and expectations in the conceptualization of anger and hostility.

Assessing Anger Response: Emotional, Behavioral, and Physiological Components

The central feature in anger assessment is the subject's angry response with its emotional, behavioral, and physiological components. Understanding the physiological mechanisms underlying these responses will ultimately require integrated assessments of the components as they occur in response to perceived provocation. For example, the research linking beta-adrenergic arousal and anger emotions reviewed by Durel and Krantz in Chap. 14 suggests that under some circumstances physiological arousal occurs first, and subjects subsequently label this arousal as anger. Sorting out this chain of events will require assessing both emotional responses and physiological arousal.

It will also be important to assess the behavioral component of the anger response. Definitions of anger recognize the importance of distinguishing between the emotional component and the behavioral component of anger responses. For example, the scales developed by Spielberger and his associates, described in Chapter 1, reflect this distinction. The State Anger Scale measures the emotional experience of anger while the Anger Expression Scale assesses the subject's typical behavior in terms of the extent to which the anger is typically expressed ("anger-out") or suppressed ("anger-in").

Comprehensive assessment of the emotional, behavioral, and physiological components of anger responses as they occur in time is essential to the study of anger in behavioral medicine—from research addressing questions of pathophysiologic mechanisms, to patient evaluation and assessment of treatment outcome. Casual or resting measures of physiological parameters will not meet the needs of these applications nor will paper and pencil questionnaires, as they are typically administered. There is a great need for dynamic monitoring of the responses. One approach to a more comprehensive assessment that not only would provide these integrated measurements, but could also be used in conjunction with direct observation of responses in the natural setting or to analogue simulation situations, is an extension of ambulatory physiological assessment. Specifically, physiological responses could be measured automatically using such devices as Holter and ambulatory blood pressure monitors. In conjunction with the regular physiological recordings, subjects could report on their behavior and on their current emotional state, such as the extent to which they are experiencing feelings of anger. A diary or an automatically activated audiotape recorder worn by the subject could record this self-report. In fact, to the extent that the subject's anger expression had verbal features, this expression would become part of the audiotaped record that could be analyzed later. Such a procedure was used by Whitehead, Blackwell, DeSilva, and Robinson (1977) in a study of 29 hypertensive patients. In this study, the patients took their own blood pressures four times daily and rated their feelings of anxiety and anger on simple scales. Interestingly, anxiety was found to be more highly correlated with increased blood pressure than was anger.

The technology for more automated integrated assessments is now available (Chesney, 1984) and is directly applicable to behavioral evaluation of anger responses. Moreover, this strategy could be combined with direct observation in the environment, the study of responses to analogue simulated strategies, and the "articulated thoughts" procedures described above. Thus, while observers monitor environmental events or present analogue situations, subjects wearing an ambulatory device could verbalize cognitive appraisals of the environmental events, reports on their mood in response to these situations, and appraisals of their reactions. The monitor, in addition to recording these self-reported thoughts and moods, would record physiological parameters. Reactions by the environment to the subject's responses would also be observed or, as in the case of an analogue situation, these reactions could even be manipulated by the observer. Thus, by behavioral assessment, the complex model of anger arousal would be translated from a conceptual framework to a measurable chronology of events.

INTERVENTION

Treatment of inappropriate, excessive or habitual states of anger, hostility, and aggression has lagged far behind the recognition of their detrimental effects. The conceptual model presented previously reflects research conducted to date, and it suggests issues that need to be addressed in therapeutic approaches. As Novaco discussed in his chapter in this volume, a change in this situation, perhaps spurred by the evidence of the etiological role of anger in such serious, life-threatening diseases as coronary heart disease, is underway.

Barriers to Treatment

From a social learning perspective, anger, hostility, and aggression can be conceptualized as acquired styles of coping with or responding to environmental demands. A full discussion of the social learning orientation is not possible here, but stated simply it assumes that the anger and accompanying behavior are "reinforced." This constitutes a major potential obstacle for intervention efforts.

In their introduction to one of the few clinical studies of intervention for anger, Moon and Eisler (1983) wrote that anger is an "aversive state" with "social sanctions." Depending on the individual, however, anger may be perceived as a state of power and strength that society *reinforces* rather than punishes. This reinforcement can take many forms, the most common being that subjects tend to maintain or repeat those anger responses to which they perceive the environment reacting in a desired direction. For example, subjects who express anger by complaining will then be likely to complain in the future, if they perceive that their environment reacted to remedy their situation as a result of their complaint.

Averill (1982) presents data in support of the functional effectiveness of anger in a survey of community residents and students. Subjects evaluated the consequences of angry episodes, both situations in which they were the aggressor and those in which they were the targets. As would be expected, subjects rating their angry behavior in terms of its consequences perceived their anger as being beneficial three times as often as being harmful. However, subjects who evaluated episodes in which they were the target also tended to perceive the aggressor's anger against them as being more often beneficial than harmful (ratio 2.5:1). These target subjects rated 76 percent of the episodes as resulting in their coming to "realize their own faults" because of the other person's anger. Averill concluded from his survey that, in everyday experience, anger is sufficiently reinforced to maintain its high rate of occurrence.

For successful treatment, the importance of actual or perceived reinforcement of angry behaviors resides in the perception of many individuals that their angry, hostile or aggressive responses are adaptive, or even necessary, for achieving personal goals. This barrier is likely to be even more pervasive than suggested by Novaco's discussion in this volume of certain individual and societal groups. In some cases, for example, the angry behavior is an effective strategy to secure a desired environmental reaction. In other cases, the angry behavior probably leads to a desirable short-term reaction but an undesrable long-term effect. In either case, alternative behaviors to anger, hostility, and aggression will be considered by the individuals in terms of their perceived ability to elicit desirable results. This issue is an important aspect of what Bandura (1977) has termed "self-efficacy"—a set of expectations about potential treatment outcomes (including the individuals' expectations regarding their ability to modify target behaviors) that determine whether treatment is sought or initiated, how much effort individuals will expend toward treatment, and how long this effort will be sustained. Unless these issues are carefully examined prior to intervention, the subject's motivation for behavior change could be inadequate to sustain interest in intervention.

Need for Clarification of Treatment Objectives

Among anger treatment studies (cf. Moon & Eisler, 1983), the emphasis is on reducing the emotional and physiological components of anger arousal by teaching subjects alternative ways of handling their anger. One such alternative is to express negative emotions in a constructive, assertive manner. This treatment objective reflects what Averill (1983) referred to as "traditional moral teaching." For example, just as it may be undesirable to express anger inappropriately, it is also undesirable to suppress anger or be "unassertive" under certain circumstances. The concept of assertiveness or of expression of anger as being more beneficial than anger suppression was given support by research indicating that hypertensive individuals are often characterized by low levels of assertiveness (see the review by Manuck in Chapter 8). Furthermore, ameliorating effects of anger expression, "catharsis," or assertiveness have been inferred from the often cited research by Hokanson (Hokanson & Burgess, 1962a; Hokanson & Shetler, 1961), which indicates that expression of aggression by college students toward a fellow student reduced elevations of systolic blood pressure and heart rate produced by presenting a frustrating situation. However, in a subsequent study (Hokanson & Burgess, 1962b), the influence of the status of the frustrator was examined. While the previously observed effects were replicated with a low status frustrator (i.e., the experimenter introduced as a student), the expression of aggression toward a high status frustrator (i.e., the same investigator introduced as a faculty member) did not *reduce* frustration-produced physiologic changes but instead led to *increases* in systolic blood pressure. Considering the model proposed here, it is possible that the subjects perceived negative environmental reactions as likely to result from their anger expression, and this concern may have overridden the blood pressure reduction typically observed when anger is expressed.

A series of reports by Harburg and associates (Harburg, Erfurt, Hauenstein et al., 1973; Gentry, Harburg, & Hauenstein, 1973) indicated that low levels of anger expression in response to specific anger-provoking situations may be a behavioral contributor to elevated blood pressure and, thus, to essential hypertension. In subsequent analyses of this data set, Gentry and his associates (Gentry, Chesney, Gary, et al., 1982) extended this finding beyond the specific situations studied by Harburg by confirming an association between habitual low levels of anger expression and elevated blood pressure. In his chapter in this volume, Gentry discusses these and more recent results showing that black Americans who are high in hostility and tend to keep anger suppressed have excessive blood pressure elevations.

Taken together, these findings firmly support the concept of training subjects in anger expression to avoid the negative effects of anger arousal.

There is a third treatment alternative, first described by Harburg and his associates (Harburg, Blakelock, & Roeper, 1979), "reflective coping," which involves the subject's cognitive appraisals of environmental events. As shown in Figure 1 and discussed above, cognitive appraisal mediates the effect that environmental events have on emotions and behavior. Thus, if a subject modified cognitive appraisals that would typically lead to the experience of anger and its behavioral and physiological correlates, then the otherwise resulting anger is prevented.

In the research by Harburg et al., (1979), this style of coping was associated with lower blood pressures than either the anger-in or anger-out alternatives. Responses that characterized reflective coping upon anger-provocation included trying to reason with provocateurs at the time, as well as talking with them after they "cooled down." Harburg examined the frequency with which coping styles are used by various subjects and found that reflective coping was more often reported by women than by men and by those in middle classes more often than those in the lower classes.

In Harburg's view, reflective coping involves an inhibition of impulsive reactions, appraisal of situations as less anger-provoking, and internal processing of coping alternatives to achieve beneficial and avoid harmful outcomes. Thus reflective coping, in addition to its association with lower physiological arousal, would be less likely to lead to interpersonal conflict than either anger-in or anger-out. It should therefore be a candidate for serious consideration as a treatment objective in anger intervention.

Phases of Anger Management

The model presented earlier (see Figure 1), when viewed at an individual level, suggests that strategies in anger management, of which some are included in the treatment approaches discussed in the treatment section of this volume, may be arranged in a sequence of phases or stages. A prerequisite for treatment, as noted above, would be to evaluate motivation for change and, in particular, the extent to which anger is perceived as functionally effective or responsible for achieving personal goals, objectives and desired societal responses.

Following this satisfactory resolution of issues of motivation, the first phase of treatment in anger management involves teaching subjects to modify their cognitive appraisals of environmental events in order to prevent anger provocation. Novaco, who includes cognitive reappraisal in his treatment protocol (Novaco, 1979), works to help subjects to keep situations in perspective, to "consider the source," and to focus on the task of resolving potential conflicts rather than responding to the event as a personal affront or ego threat. According to Novaco, "The fundamental idea is to promote flexibility in the cognitive structuring of a situation that previously has elicited anger" (Novaco, 1979, p. 269).

The specific strategies employed in this cognitive restructuring are similar to the "articulated thoughts" assessment described earlier. In this application, subjects are given specific examples of thoughts to articulate when appraising situations. Indeed, subjects are encouraged to "think aloud" (Camp, 1977) as they confront anger-provoking situations. With practice, new appraisals replace the previously anger-arousing ones, and even in response to previously provoking situations anger is prevented.

The second phase of treatment involves modifying the behavioral and physiological correlates of the emotional anger response. Specific training and systematic practice in social skills, such as assertiveness (Frederiksen & Eisler, 1977; Frederikson, Jenkins, Foy, & Erston, 1976), and problem solving (D'Zurilla & Goldfield, 1971), as well as instruction in impulse control and strategies of arousal reduction using relaxation techniques (Hart, 1984) or pharmacological intervention (see Durel and Krantz, Chap. 14) come into play in the phase. Its objective is to provide individuals with a repertoire of alternatives to typical anger responses of inappropriate anger expression, suppression of anger, and physiological arousal. However, as discussed by Hecker and Lunde in their chapter in this volume, not all individuals who are candidates for anger or hostility intervention will benefit equally from training in each of these strategies.

For example, coronary-prone Type A individuals, while often characterized by an elevated potential for hostility and anger, are not lacking in assertive behavior (Rosenman, 1978). On the other hand, Type As have been shown to be low in impulse control (Chesney, Black, Chadwick, & Rosenman, 1981) and to show elevated cardiovascular arousal to perceived stressors (see Houston, 1983, or Dembroski, MacDougall, Herd, & Shields, 1983, for reviews). This enhanced responsivity is particularly true of Type As who are high in hostility (Dembroski, MacDougall, Herd, & Shields, 1979). Type As who are interested in anger intervention might benefit from training in self-monitoring of anger reactions and techniques for impulse control, such as self-control techniques that create a pause between initial arousal of anger impulses and action. Conversely, as discussed above, some hypertensive individuals experience high levels of anger but may lack assertiveness skills. These subjects might benefit more from assertion training than other anger management skills, such as strategies to enhance impulse control.

The third phase of treatment involves the reaction of the environment to anger responses. Most approaches to anger intervention discuss some or all of the foregoing phases but typically do not include this third phase, which is likely to be of major importance in maintaining treatment gains—a problematic issue in behavior change. The power exerted by the social environment in maintaining or modifying behavior is reflected in programs designed to induce behavior change solely through manipulation of the environment's responses to undesirable (aggressive) and desirable behaviors. This approach is an essential element in the programs developed by Patterson and Reid for the modification of childhood aggression (Patterson & Reid, 1973; Patterson, 1976) and is incorporated in their treatment of child-abusing parents discussed by Reid and Kavanagh in this volume.

The individual's conscious monitoring of the environment's reactions to anger responses may provide an alternative avenue to directly manipulating social reactions. By attending to positive social feedback as well as modifying cognitive appraisals of ambiguous or negative social reactions, maintenance of new anger coping strategies can be enhanced. As a prerequisite for treatment, it was noted that perceptions of the effects of, and particularly the social reinforcements for, anger behavior would need to be examined, because these provide a feedback that supports the individual's maladaptive approach to handling anger. These perceptions can be modified in the same manner as the appraisals of anger-provoking environmental events discussed in the first phase of treatment. However, at this third phase of treatment, the focus of cognitive reappraisal should be upon the positive effects of new strategies for preventing or handling anger. For example, managers who previously enjoyed the intense, quick response of their staff to anger outbursts might, after reducing the frequency of anger outbursts, observe a reduction in the frequency of the staff's intense, quick responses and conclude that their effectiveness as managers was diminishing. If this perception is not evaluated and challenged, it is likely that the new anger management strategies will not be maintained and that the anger outbursts will return. Conversely, the manager could be guided in comparing the long-term, as well as the short-term, effects of the contrasting previous and the new styles of handling anger. While the short-term effects of the anger outbursts may have been attention and compliance, the long-term effects may have been a reduction in morale and productivity coupled with high turnover. On the other hand, the short-term effects of the new approach may be negligible, while the long-term effects may be to increase morale, productivity, and commitment.

Newly acquired anger management strategies will not always lead to reactions that can be so readily translated into positive outcomes for individuals. In some cases, previous anger responses may have been more effective than new behaviors in eliciting certain environmental reactions that may be valued by the individual. This problem returns "full circle" to the initial issue of existing reinforcement conditions and motivation of change raised earlier and brings the individual and the therapist to issues of values. Perhaps the mounting evidence that incriminates anger in the development of cardiovascular and other diseases discussed in the second section of this volume will provide a persuasive argument for the efficacy of prevention of anger arousal and adoption of anger management strategies that increases personal effectiveness.

Efforts to intervene in anger arousal or hostility at any of the phases discussed above will be more effective when tailored to the specific characteristics of individuals seeking treatment. Initially, these characteristics will be represented by categories such as those proposed by Megargee and by Hecker and Lunde in their chapters in this volume. In the future, with further advances in anger assessment, it might be possible to replace such typologies with an evaluation of needs and a selection of treatment alternatives on an individual basis. Compared to the group-based approaches that reflect the current state-of-the-art in anger and hostility interventions, individualized programs will permit concentration of treatment efforts on those specific components of anger arousal and hostility that have adverse effects on health and well-being.

CONCLUSION

Until recently, when the detrimental effects of anger and hostility on health became more apparent, anger had received little attention in the behavioral and medical science communities. The chapters in this volume provide a persuasive testimony that this situation is changing. Efforts to define and assess anger, document its adverse health correlates, and design effective treatment strategies are well under way. Despite the progress already made, certain assessment and treatment issues will need to be addressed by behavioral scientists if they are to meet the challenge presented by the research evidence linking anger and hostility to disease incidence and severity. These issues include the necessity to go beyond self-report paper and pencil questionnaires to more comprehensive behavioral assessment of anger. Future measurement batteries will likely include observation of behavior in the natural or simulated environment, assessment of cognitive behavior, and ambulatory monitoring of physiological arousal

The demand to reduce health risk through anger interventions will not wait for new behavioral assessment batteries or basic research on the pathophysiologic mechanisms that underlie the association between anger and its negative health consequences. Indeed, it may be beneficial to move ahead with treatment studies. When viewed as basic research, clinical studies yield valuable information related to definition, assessment, and mechanisms. There are certain issues that will need to be addressed as these studies advance, including barriers to treatment, clarification of treatment objectives, and tailoring of treatment approaches to individuals.

Finally, as interventions to prevent anger arousal and modify anger responses are designed and implemented, it is essential that behavioral and medical scientists are alert to important ethical issues. Among these is the need to convey that anger is only one of a number of factors that contribute to adverse health consequences, and that treatment should not concentrate solely on anger to the exclusion of other risk factors. Another ethical issue involves the appropriateness of anger. There are situations, such as the social injustice of apartheid, in which anger responses are not only justified but are appropriate. These situations can often be identified by weighing the risks to health and welfare from the situation per se versus the risks associated with anger arousal. When these issues arise, rather than to focus on modifying a subject's responses, the ethical choice would be to make the situation the target of intervention. It is fortunate that these situations are rare; however, their potential presence requires vigilance.

In the majority of cases, personal effectiveness and health enhancement will benefit from efforts of anger and hostility prevention and treatment. The success of these intervention efforts will, in turn, depend upon advances in research on the assessment of anger, hostility and aggression, and on further explication of the processes by which these factors exert their adverse health and behavioral consequences.

REFERENCES

Averill, J. R. *Anger and aggression: An essay on emotion.* New York: Springer-Verlag, 1982.
Averill, J. R. Studies on anger and aggression: Implications for theories of emotion. *American Psychologist,* 1983, *38,* 1145–1160.
Bandura, A. Self-efficacy: Towards a unifying theory of behavioral change. *Psychological Review,* 1977, *84,* 191–215.
Bandura, A. Psychological mechanisms of aggression. In R. G. Geen & E. I. Donnerstein (Eds.), *Aggression: Theoretical and methodological issues.* New York: Academic, 1983.
Berkowitz, L. Aversively stimulated aggression: Some parallels and differences in research with animals and humans. *American Psychologist,* 1983, *38,* 1135–1144.
Burish, T. G., & Bradley, L. A. Coping with chronic disease. In T. G. Burish & L. A. Bradley (Eds.), *Coping with chronic disease: Research and applications.* New York: Academic, 1983.
Camp, B. W. Verbal mediation in young aggressive boys. *Journal of Abnormal Psychology,* 1977, *86,* 145–153.
Chesney, M. A. Non-invasive ambulatory blood pressure monitoring. In J. A. Herd, A. M.

Gotto, P. G. Kaufmann, & S. M. Weiss. *Cardiovascular instrumentation: Proceedings of the working conference on applicability of new technology to behavioral research.* U.S. Department of Health and Human Services: Public Health Service. NIH Publication No. 84-1654, March 1984, 79-84.

Chesney, M. A., Black, G. W., Chadwick, J. H., & Rosenman, R. H. Psychological correlates of the Type A behavior pattern. *Journal of Behavioral Medicine,* 1981, *4,* 217-229.

Chesney, M. A., Eagleston, J. E., & Rosenman, R. H. The Type A structured interview: A behavioral assessment in the rough. *Journal of Behavioral Assessment,* 1980, *2,* 255-272.

Davison, G. C., Robins, C., & Johnson, M. Articulated thoughts during simulated situations: A paradigm for studying cognition in emotion and behavior. *Cognitive Therapy and Research,* 1983, *17,* 17-39.

Dembroski, T. M., MacDougall, J. M., Herd, J. A., & Shields, J. L. Effect of level of challenge of pressor and heart rate responses in Type A and Type B subjects. *Journal of Applied Social Psychology,* 1979, *9,* 209-228.

Dembroski, T. M., MacDougall, J. M., Herd, J. A., & Shields, J. L. Perspectives on coronary-prone behavior. In D. S. Kranta, A. Baum, & J. E. Singer (Eds.), *Cardiovascular disorders and behavior.* Hillsdale, N.J.: Erlbaum, 1983.

D'Zurilla, T. J., & Goldfried, M. R. Problem solving and behavioral modification. *Journal of Abnormal Psychology,* 1971, *78,* 107-126.

Frederiksen, L. W., & Eisler, R. M. The control of explosive behavior: A skill development approach. In D. Upper (Ed.), *Perspectives in behavior therapy.* Kalamazoo, Mich.: Behaviordelia, 1977.

Frederiksen, L. W., Jenkins, J. O., Fow, D. W., & Eisler, R. M. Social skills training in the modificaiton of abusive outbursts in adults. *Journal of Applied Behavior Analysis,* 1976, *9,* 117-125.

Gentry, W. D., Chesney, A. P., Gary, H. E., Hall, R. P., & Harburg, E. Habitual anger-coping styles: I. Effect on mean blood pressure and risk for essential hypertension. *Psychosomatic Medicine,* 1982, *44,* 195-202.

Gentry, W. D., Harburg, E., & Hauenstein, L. Effects of anger expression/inhibition and guilt on elevated diastolic blood pressure in high/low stress and black/white females. *Proceedings of the American Psychological Association,* 1973, 115-116.

Harburg, E., Blakelock, E. H., & Roeper, R. J. Resentful and reflective coping with arbitrary authority and blood pressure: Detroit. *Psychosomatic Medicine,* 1977, *41,* 189-202.

Harburg, E., Erfurt, J. C., Hauenstein, L. S., Chape, C., Schull, W. J., & Schork, M. A. Socioecological stress, suppressed hostility, skin color, and black-white male blood pressure: Detroit. *Psychosomatic Medicine,* 1973, *35,* 276-296.

Hart, K. E. Anxiety management training and anger control for Type A individuals. *Journal of Behavior Therapy and Experimental Psychiatry,* 1984, *15,* 1-7.

Hokanson, J. E., & Burgess, M. The effects of three types of aggression on vascular process. *Journal of Abnormal and Social Psychology,* 1962a, *64,* 446-449.

Hokanson, J. E., Burgess, M. The effects of status, type of frustration and aggression on vascular processes. *Journal of Abnormal and Social Psychology,* 1962b, *65,* 232-237.

Hokanson, J. E., & Sheter, S. The effect of overt aggression on physiological arousal. *Journal of Abnormal and Social Psychology,* 1961, *63,* 446-448.

Houston, B. K. Psychophysiological responsivity and the Type A Behavior Pattern. *Journal of Research in Personality,* 1983, *17,* 22-39.

Konecni, A. J. Annoyance, type and duration of post-annoyance activity and aggression: The "cathartic effect." *Journal of Experimental Psychology,* 1975a, *104,* 76-102.

Konecni, V. J. The mediation of aggressive behavior: Arousal level versus anger and cognitive labeling. *Journal of Personality and Social Psychology,* 1975b, *32,* 706-712.

Leventhal, H. Toward a comprehensive theory of emotion. In L. Berkowitz (Ed.), *Advances in experimental social psychology,* (Vol. 13). New York: Academic, 1980.

Moon, J. R., & Eisler, R. M. Anger control: An experimental comparison of three behavioral treatments. *Behavior Therapy,* 1983, *14,* 493-505.

Nay, W. R. Analogue measures. In A. R. Ciminero, K. S. Calhoun, & H. E. Adams (Eds.), *Handbook of behavioral assessment.* New York: Wiley, 1977.

Novaco, R. W. The cognitive regulation of anger and stress. In P. C. Kendall, & S. D. Hollon (Eds.), *Cognitive-behavioral interventions: Theory, research, procedures.* New York: Academic, 1979.

Patterson, G. R. The aggressive child: Victim and architect of a coercive system. In E. J. Mash,

L. A. Hamerlynck, & L. C. Handy (Eds.), *Behavior modification and families*. New York: Brunner/Mazel, 1976.

Patterson, G. R., & Reid, J. B. Intervention for families of aggressive boys: A replication study. *Behaviour Research and Therapy*, 1973, *11*, 383-394.

Rosenman, R. H. The interview method of assessment of the coronary-prone behavior pattern. In R. M. Dembroski, S. M. Weiss, J. L. Shields, S. G. Haynes, & M. Feinleib (Ed.), *Coronary-prone behavior*. New York: Springer-Verlag, 1978.

Rule, B., & Newdale, A. Emotional arousal and aggressive behavior. *Psychological Bulletin*, 1976, *83*, 851-863.

Whitehead, W. E., Blackwell, B., De Silva, H., & Robinson, A. Anxiety and anger in hypertension. *Journal of Psychosomatic Research*, 1977, *21*, 383-389.

REFERENCE NOTE

Lerman, C. E., & Davison, G. C. *Salience of environmental stress on the evocation of Type A articulated thoughts.* Unpublished manuscript, University of Southern California, 1984.

Index

Abusive families, 250-251
   parent-child conflict, 247-248
   research on, 250-251
Abusive parent, 242
Action-emotion complex, 205
Aggression, 7, 33-36, 173, 208-209
   and anger, differences in definition, 31
   animal model, 112, 190
   antagonistic appraisal, 212
   assessment issues in, 278
   cardiovascular disease and, 52-54
   and coronary heart disease, 5, 31, 115
   cultural factors of, 112-114
   extrapunitive/intropunitive factors of, 32-34
   extrinsic motivation for, 42-45
   frustration and, 37
   habit strength, 34, 42-45
   hostile, 11, 97
   inhibitions against, 34, 45-48
   instrumental, 11, 97, 112
   intrinsic motivation of, 34, 36-42
   as personality trait, 5, 180, 205
   pharmacological treatment of, 265-267, 271-272
   physiological arousal and, 260
   research on, 206-207
   as response competition, 52
   sex differences, 114, 215
   situational factors, 34, 49-52
   social dominance and, 190
   Type A, 38
   typology, 32-33
Aggressive children, 215
AHA syndrome 7-8
Anger, 173, 206, 208, 210, 277-278
   adaptive functions and, 203
   as affective stress reaction, 213
   appraisal of, 211-212, 281
   -arousal model, 210, 212, 279
   autonomic reactions, 261
   cardiovascular effects of, 23, 104-107, 116-117, 127, 131, 160, 281-282, 287
   cognitive factors of, 261, 281
   as coping style, 145, 210, 288
   as defense mechanism, 142
   escalation of, 87
   expectations, 211-212
   expression of (anger-in, anger-out), 11, 13-18, 66, 131, 139, 141, 209, 284
   minorities, effects on, 140-145, 209, 284
   person-environment transactions, 222
   reinforcing properties of, 283
   self-efficacy and, 284
   trait/state, 9-10, 13, 15
   ventilation hypothesis 39, 203
Anger assessment, 6-10, 140, 142, 221-222, 287-288
   analogue situations of, 280-281
   anger expression (AX) scale, 4, 10-13
   development of, 14-23
   anger inventory, 8
   anger self-report scale, 8, 14
   Beck depression inventory, 8, 207
   behavioral evaluation of, 272, 282
   Buss-Durkey hostility inventory and, 8, 9, 14, 64-65, 131
   Harburg assessment procedure, 13, 64-65, 70-72, 131
   MMPI hostility scale, 23, 53-54, 62, 108-109, 207
   multidimensional anger inventory, 9, 63-64, 78-82
   Novaco inventory, 64-65, 70-72
   development of, 64-76
   projective techniques of, 8
   reaction inventory, 8
   social interaction, 86, 88-92
   state-trait scale, 6, 9-10, 15, 23, 157, 175, 182
   videotaping, 280
Anger treatment, 41-42, 45, 48, 51, 117-119, 145, 203-204, 234-238, 284
   anger management training of, 64, 244-249, 285-287
   assertiveness training, 118, 142, 158, 218-219, 283
   classical conditioning in, 215
   cognitive-behavioral and, 211-213, 218-219, 238-239, 281
   difficulties with, 204-208, 283-284
   ethical issues in, 288
   exercise in, 118
   familial approaches to, 95, 243-254

Anger treatment (*Cont.*):
  humor in, 40, 119
  operant conditioning for, 215-217
  pharmacologic approaches to, 118
  reflective coping and, 285
  social skills training for, 215
Animosity, 13, 41-42
Anxiety, 31, 282
  assessment of, 15, 23, 131, 157
  blood pressure correlates and, 103
Assertiveness, 106, 166
  training for, 167, 284
Atherosclerosis:
  animal model of, 188-190, 192-194
  cardiac responsivity and, 194
  chronic hate and, 62-63
  estradiol, 115, 183
  psychosocial factors of, 191-192
  testosterone and, 183
  Type-A, 59, 188, 195

Beta-blockers, 128-130, 267
  animal studies with, 271
  anxiety reduction and, 267-268
  blood pressure reduction with, 270-272
  side effects of, 151, 270
  treatment effects of, 271-272
  Type A treatment and, 265-267
Black Americans:
  anger expression in, 140-143
  blood pressure in, 12-13, 284-285
  hypertension risk of, 143-144
  research issues on, 144-145
Blood pressure, 131, 150
  anger and, 12, 60, 103, 139-140, 282, 284
  assertiveness and, 151
  AX scale and, 23-25
  cardiac output in, 128
  coronary patients, 265
  failing heart, 132
  sex differences in, 25-26
  stress, effects on, 134
  (*See also* Hypertension)

Cardiac responsivity, 105, 153-157, 161, 166
  behaviorally induced model of, 157
  engagement/involvement and, 158, 161-162
  genetic basis of, 158
  heart rate, 194

hypertension and, 154
  individual differences in, 149, 153, 156
  microsocial analysis of, 254
  normalization of, 133
  Type A-B differences in, 133-134, 263-264
Catecholamines, 106, 132, 152-153, 183, 193
  aggression and, 271
  sex differences and, 115-116
  Type A-B differences in, 263
  (*See also* Epinephrine; Norepinephrine)
Central nervous system, 128, 156, 267-268, 278
  pharmacological penetration of, 117, 270
Child abuse, 113, 217-219, 249-250, 286
  anger in, 252
  coercive family chain, 88-90
  discipline in, 45, 87, 243-244, 248-249, 252
  family interaction patterns and, 86
  incidence of, 241-242
  parental anger in, 87, 92-95, 244, 252
  prevention of, 242
  protective agencies for, 253
  treatment of, 219, 244-249, 251
Coping styles, 12, 109, 158, 205, 210, 218, 283-285
Coronary heart disease, 195
  anger and, 23, 107-111, 277, 287
  dietary factors in, 195
  morbidity and, 177-179
  Type-A, 5, 150, 187
  (*See also* Type A Behavior Pattern; Western Collaborative Group Study)
Cynicism scale, 181
  disease, 183
  hostility scale, relation to, 180

Delayed Stress Syndrome, 204, 220
  Vietnam veterans and, 204
Discipline, 245

Emotion:
  beta-blockers, role in, 259
  bio-informational process model of, 83
  pituitary adrenal, effects on, 105
  theories of, 259-260

INDEX

Exercise:
 cardiac output, relation to, 128
 treatment for anger, 118
Epinephrine, 104-105, 182
 anger and, 260
 excessive secretion of, 117
 (*See also* Norepinephrine)
Escalation hypothesis, 87
Extrinsic instigation, 34, 42-49

Family:
 entrapment hypothesis, 96
 health risks associated with, 114, 154-155, 161
 interaction coding system of, 89
 management skills in, 95
 negative affect and, 93-95
 process code of, 85
Framingham study, 62, 135
Frustration, 37, 41-42
 autonomic response to, 157
 blood pressure and, 60, 284
 proneness to, 157
 Type A-B differences in, 38

Habit strength, 34, 45
 acquisition of, 43
 decreasing, 44
Heart rate:
 anger expression, effects on, 105
 catecholamine effects on, 153
 pharmacological treatment for, 272
Hemodynamic patterns, 127-128, 130, 162
 assessment of, 130
 phases of hypertension and, 155
Hostility, 7, 173, 227-228, 277
 coronary artery disease and, 6, 174-179
 disposition of, 277
 health correlates of, 175-181, 184
 pathophysiology and, 111, 113, 181-184
 racial factors in, 143
 treatment of, 117-119, 228, 234-239
 typology of, 229
  overcontrolled, stable, 231-232, 237
  overcontrolled, unstable, 32, 232, 237-238
  suppressed, normal, 233-234, 238
  suppressed psychotic, 234, 238
  undercontrolled, deliberate, 33, 230-231, 236-237
  undercontrolled, impulsive, 33, 230, 235-236

Hostility assessment, 109
 Cattell 16PF Questionnaire, 180
 hostility (HO) scale, 53-54, 62, 108-109, 174, 176, 177-180, 184
 MMPI o-h (overcontrolled hostility), 33
 sex differences in, 175
 trait anger scale, 175, 180
Hypertension:
 anger in, 5, 10, 23-28, 60-61, 63, 103-105, 131, 139-145, 151, 162, 213, 284
 assertiveness and, 150-151, 162-167
 assessment of, 130-132
 autonomic mechanisms of, 151-153
 borderline, 104, 110, 127-130, 134-135, 152
 cardiac reactivity in, 104, 132-133
 established, 128, 132
 etiology of, 107, 127-130, 132-135, 139-149, 150, 155-156
 familial predisposition toward, 154-155, 159-160
 hostility and, 63, 233
 neurogenic factors in, 132
 personality characteristics of, 106, 150
 psychosocial factors in, 153
 psychosomatic factors in, 127
 racial factors in, 139-145
 renin and, 104, 107, 131
 treatment of, 116-117, 129

Immune function, 183
Irritable motor behaviors, 84, 92
Israeli Ischemic Heart Disease Study, 60

Managers, 287
 diseases of, 40
Maternal behaviors, 91
Microsocial analysis:
 anger assessment, role in, 88, 280
 cardiovascular response in, 254
 child abuse assessment in, 254
 family interactions in, 88-92
Multidimensional Anger Inventory (MIA):
 factor analysis of, 67, 74
 reliability of, 70-71, 75-76
 validation of, 64-72
Myocardial hypertrophy, 133

Negative affect, 93-96
 health consequences and, 97

Neuroendocrine response pattern:
   fight/flight, 104–105, 181–182
   cognitive appraisal (vigilance), 104–105, 181–182
Neurohormonal responses, 104–105
   cortisol and, 105, 110
Norepinephrine, 105, 130, 132
   aggression, 110
   dopamine and, 116
   neuroleptic drugs, effects of, 116
   (*See also* Epinephrine)
Normotensive patterns, 154

Parent training, 29, 253
   research on, 249–251
   techniques of, 245–248
Passion, 209
Person-situation interactions, 50–51
Poorly socialized child, 84
Problem solving behavior, 213, 247
Propranolol in Type-A treatment, 128, 130, 266–267
   (*See also* Beta-blockers)
Post-combat stress reactions, 220
   (*See also* Delayed stress reaction)
Punishment, 248
   fear of, 46
   time-out, 45, 248, 252

Rage, 59
   elevated blood pressure and, 139
Rape as a conditioned response, 113
Reaction inventory, 8
Renin:
   aldosterone release, 107
   borderline hypertensives and, 130, 152
   sodium renin profiles and, 104
Risk factors for coronary heart disease, 59, 187

Social competence:
   assertiveness and, 163, 166
   assessment of, 163–167
   health correlates and, 162–165
   Type-A behavior and, 164
Social environment:
   anger arousal and, 279
   disruption of, 189
   effects on health, 83, 86
   exchange of, 166
   feedback in, 286
   programming, 85
   status in, 207

Spouse abuse, 220
State-trait anxiety inventory, 157
Stress:
   cardiac responsivity to, 155–156, 193, 270
   child abuse and, 213, 254
   engagement/involvement, 159
   long-term effects of, 213
   treatment of, 213, 219–220, 238–239
   Type-A, 263
Suppressed anger, 7, 153, 162–163
   in black Americans, 12, 141–144
   coronary artery disease and, 214
Sympathetic responsivity, 265–266
   excessive, 61

Testosterone, 182
   aggression and, 114
   puberty and, 115
Type-A assessment:
   structured interview, 62, 108, 162, 174–175, 261–262, 281
   Jenkins activity survey of, 261–262
Type-A behavior pattern, 5, 6, 59, 61, 96, 150, 159, 164, 187–188, 197, 268–270, 281
   anger, relation to, 41, 108, 205, 214, 230, 269
   child abuse and, 243–244, 254
   components of, 61–62, 107–111, 180, 260–261
   engagement/involvement, 159
   health correlates of, 108, 110, 160–161, 174, 182, 187, 262–263, 281
   hyperactivity (or impulsivity) and, 117, 230, 286
   physiology, 262–265, 268, 270
   responsivity of, 109–111, 134, 160–161, 262–265
   treatment for, 265–268, 270, 286

Violence, 32–33
   corporate, 207
   criminal, 33
   domestic, 209
   treatment of, 46

Western Collaborative Group Study (WCGS), 5, 6, 61–62, 108, 180
Western Electric Study:
   of coronary heart disease, 179
   of hostility measures, 108, 176–177